Kidney Disease in the Elderly

Holly Kramer • Edgar V. Lerma • Holly Koncicki

Editors

Kidney Disease in the Elderly

A Case-Based Guide

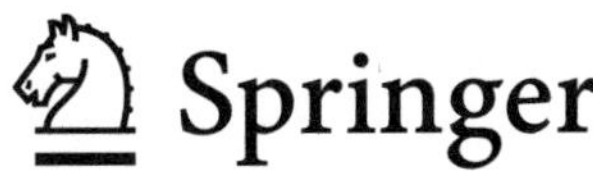 Springer

Editors
Holly Kramer
Dept of Public Health Sciences & Med
Loyola University Chicago
Maywood, IL, USA

Edgar V. Lerma
Advocate Christ Medical Center
University of Illinois at Chicago
Oak Lawn, IL, USA

Holly Koncicki
Nephrology
Mount Sinai Hospital
New York, NY, USA

ISBN 978-3-031-68462-3   ISBN 978-3-031-68460-9   (eBook)
https://doi.org/10.1007/978-3-031-68460-9

This Springer imprint is published by the registered company Springer Nature Switzerland AG
The registered company address is: Gewerbestrasse 11, 6330 Cham, Switzerland

If disposing of this product, please recycle the paper.

To all my mentors and friends at the University of Santo Tomas, Faculty of Medicine and Surgery and the University of Santo Tomas, College of Science, in Manila, Philippines, and Northwestern University Feinberg School of Medicine in Chicago, IL, who have, in one way or another, influenced and guided me to become the physician that I am.

To all the medical students, interns, and residents at Advocate Christ Medical Center, whom I have taught or learned from, particularly those who eventually decided to pursue Nephrology as a career.

To my parents and my brothers, without whose unwavering love and support through the ups and downs, I would not have persevered and reached my goals in life.

And most especially to my two lovely and precious daughters Anastasia Zofia and Isabella Ann, whose smiles and laughter constantly provide me unparalleled joy and happiness, and my very loving and understanding wife Michelle, who has always been supportive of my endeavors both personally and professionally, and who sacrificed a lot of time and exhibited unwavering patience as I devoted significant amount of time and effort to this project. Truly, they provide me with motivation and inspiration.

—Edgar V. Lerma, MD

To my mother Carol

—Holly Kramer

To my mom and dad, whose encouragement, love, and sacrifice provided me with the opportunity to pursue my dream of becoming a physician.
To my patients and their families, who inspire me through their strength and perseverance and are the motivation behind this work.
To my mentors and colleagues at Mount Sinai and Northwell Health, who have been an integral part of my professional career.

Patients' Foreword

I am an 18-year kidney transplant recipient and a former hemodialysis patient. I spent close to 2 years on in-center hemodialysis and received my transplant in 2006. I am the Past President of the American Association of Kidney Patients (AAKP) and serve on numerous advisory boards and committees. I am a Lecturer at Bowie State University (BSU) and a founding member of BSU's College of Business Advisory Council. Additionally, I am a Board Member of the Personalized Medicine Coalition, advocating for adopting personalized medicine to benefit patients and health systems.

More recently, I have held significant roles, including membership in the National Diabetes and Digestive and Kidney Diseases (NIDDK) Advisory Council, Co-Chair of the NIDDK Strategic Plan Stakeholder Engagement Subgroup, and participation in the Steering Committee for NIDDK's Kidney Precision Medicine Project (KPMP) and the Scientific Registry of Transplant Recipients (SRTR) Visiting Committee. I have also contributed to six Centers for Medicare and Medicaid Services (CMS) Technical Expert Panels (TEPs).

By many standards, I enjoy a good quality of life. I want to share the rest of my story. My history with chronic kidney disease dates back to 1996, when I was denied life insurance. Perplexed and surprised, I visited my primary care physician (PCP) for an explanation. After a review of my labs and a urine analysis, he explained that the reason for the life insurance company's rejection of insuring me was due to protein in my urine. Unfortunately, there was never any discussion about me potentially having chronic kidney disease.

I continued taking prescribed high blood pressure medication but began to slowly experience problems such as not sleeping well, nocturia, lightheadedness, and worse off all in 2004, constantly regurgitating. As I later discovered, the blood pressure medication was ineffective. To be clear, I remained under the care of my PCP from 1996 to 2004. *I was never referred to a nephrologist!*

My older brother, John, had issues with his prostate and suggested that I see a urologist because an enlarged prostate could cause constant urination. His suggestion made sense because no one in my family of seven experienced chronic kidney disease. I visited a urologist on a Tuesday. He asked if I was seeing a PCP, and I replied of course. Less than a week later, he called me with a sense of great urgency and told me to go to the emergency room immediately. This sudden urgency underscored the seriousness of my condition.

My visit to the emergency room was life-altering—my blood pressure was 215/95 mmHg, and my creatinine was 13.5 mg/dL, which confirmed the diagnosis made by my urologist. From that point, time passed very quickly. I remember it as if it happened yesterday. A representative from my PCP's practice met me at the hospital and began to query me about the care I received from their practice. I sensed he was more interested in defending the PCPs than my health.

I met with a nephrologist for the first time, and Dr. Razi is still my nephrologist. He asked what I knew about dialysis. In short, I was familiar with the word but did not know what was involved in being on dialysis. Of course, I asked him if he could give me medication so I could get back to my life—my kids, my wife, and running my business. Being able to pursue my personal goals and aspirations were at stake.

I had a procedure to give me a central venous catheter (CVC). I was concerned about having a CVC. After a week in the hospital, where I received my initial dialysis session, I was referred to a DaVita dialysis facility near my house. Thus, began my education in the world of chronic kidney disease. I remember my initial visit to the facility. I was curious to see how my body would respond after four dialysis hours.

I began doing research and concluded that a transplant was my best option, but I would have to make that happen. In reviewing the transplant list and being shocked at the abysmal transplant data for African Americans in the Washington, DC, metro area, I knew that I had to be engaged in getting a kidney. I viewed the transplant system as inefficient, particularly for African Americans (regulations in 2014 made the system more favorable to African Americans).

While on dialysis, I was active with the Baltimore Washington Corridor Chamber of Commerce (BWCC). While serving on the BWCC BOD, I attended a fundraiser where a fellow BOD member approached me to talk about my health situation. She knew I needed a kidney from an article written about me in a local newspaper. The gist of the article was how much I continued to do in the community despite being on dialysis. She offered to donate a kidney to me. I asked if she was serious but remained cautiously optimistic. Her offer was great, but the match between us was to be determined.

Success, she was a very good match! I was humbled that a woman in her mid-fifties would offer me the gift of life. I also learned that race was not a determining factor. I was 55 years old, getting a new lease on life. The transplant was a success. I woke up in the recovery room thinking I was drugged because I felt so well. I learned the kidney worked immediately. Toxins began draining from my body so much so it felt as if someone removed a 50-lb weight from my back.

I recovered very quickly. I had no comorbidities and was in great shape. During the next few months as I walked and healed, I began reflecting on my journey and knew I had to do something to help others avoid what I experienced. I was fortunate because I have good health and a supportive network that exposed me to potential donors.

Why did my PCP not refer me to a nephrologist? Why was home dialysis not offered as an option? Why was there no focus on slowing the progression to dialysis? I addressed these questions by becoming a champion of patient engagement. I remain engaged in educating patients and healthcare professionals that the status quo is unacceptable.

While I enjoy a good quality of life, I am keenly aware of the need to engage with the nephrology community and the many healthcare professionals. The care I need as a person in my seventies is important to my well-being. I am excited about the future of kidney care. Innovations, the implementation of the Kidney Care Choices Model, and increased focus on slowing the progression to dialysis are encouraging trends.

Because of my experiences and the experiences of so many other older adults, this book is important. This book teaches clinicians about multiple aspects of the patient experience such as diagnosis, treatment, and management. Understanding the nuances of kidney disease in older adults can improve care and heighten quality. While numerous advances have been made in the diagnosis and treatment of kidney disease, these discoveries will not improve patients' lives unless clinicians use them. It is my hope that clinicians will read the chapters of this book and think about their own patients and reflect on how any new knowledge can help them deliver better care. I don't want anyone to experience the difficulties I did. If we all work together through education, practice, and advocacy, we can improve the lives of individuals living with kidney diseases and prevent a large proportion of kidney failure. I congratulate the authors who submitted the chapters and editors for their hard work. And congratulations to you the reader. Thank you for taking the time to further your education so you can constantly strive to be better.

Richard A. Knight

Preface

In 1972, Richard Nixon signed the Social Security Amendment Act which made persons with kidney failure eligible for Medicare coverage and created the U.S. End-Stage Renal Disease (ESRD) Program. At the time of its creation, this ESRD Program served approximately 10,000 individuals in the United States, who required dialysis. Fifty years later, the number of individuals requiring dialysis in the United States is 60-fold higher and the cost of treating kidney failure now exceeds 140 billion US dollars annually. The highest growth in kidney failure incidence and dialysis initiation is among adults aged 75 years and older, both within the United States and in other industrialized countries. This growth in dialysis initiation among older adults reflects the changing demographics in high- and middle-income countries. Approximately 10% of the global population is aged 65 years and older, and by 2050, this proportion will likely approach 20%. By 2030, 20% of the United States population will be aged 65 years and older and 12% will be over the age of 75 years. Changing population demographics is gradually altering the landscape of healthcare and its delivery, especially in the field of nephrology. Given the dynamics of demography, the introduction of this textbook is extremely timely.

This textbook entitled, *Kidney Disease in the Elderly*, is a case-based guide to the clinical care for older patients with or at risk for kidney diseases. Each chapter starts with a clinical scenario and the chapter then delves into information that provides education on patient evaluation, treatment, and the reasons for the clinical decisions. The first chapter provides an overview of the older patient with kidney disease. As a person ages, organ functions decline and this leads to the gradual onset of symptoms such as shortness of breath, memory loss, and lower physical functioning. With kidney diseases, symptoms may be absent or subtle. In this first chapter, the authors point out age group differences in natriuretic hormones and diurnal variations in urine output. The authors also discuss the controversies in CKD diagnosis and staging due to lack of incorporation of age in the current CKD staging system. The second chapter extends the discussion of how aging affects renal physiology by pointing out the distributions of CKD prevalence across age groups, country, and region. CKD prevalence among older adults is high but varies widely, even within the European continent. Despite the high prevalence of CKD, the incidence of kidney failure is overall low because death is three times more likely among adults aged 75–84 years and 25-fold more likely among adults aged 85 years and older. This chapter discusses conservative kidney management, and this topic is further addressed in Chaps. 15 and 17.

Chapter 3 provides the biological explanation for nephron loss with aging. The authors provide an overview of nephron senescence and help the reader discern normal kidney aging from chronic disease processes. Readers will also learn how serum biomarkers of senescence may be used to gauge aging and how cellular stressors can induce senescence. Aging can be accelerated and possibly slowed, and this chapter provides the reasons for this phenomenon at the cellular level. Aging is also associated with changes in brain function, which can lead to mental health disorders and vice versa. Chapters 4 and 5 address mental and cognitive health in the older adult with kidney diseases. Chapter 4 guides the reader on the diagnosis and treatment of depression and how to select the optimal antidepressant. Anxiety is also discussed along with common patient symptoms that frequently accompany anxiety such as insomnia and sexual dysfunction. Issues of brain health in the older adult are further outlined in Chap. 5 using the geriatric 5Ms model. The 5Ms model helps the clinician frame the potential mental and cognitive issues an older patient may face by using existing tools such as the Mini-Mental Status Examination, the Mini-Cog™, or the Montreal Cognitive Assessment. Cognitive decline is a common factor in the older adult with CKD yet frequently not diagnosed, discussed, or treated. This chapter provides the tools a clinician can use at the bedside to assess cognition in an older patient with CKD.

Just as the kidneys age, so does the bladder. Chapter 6 discusses urinary symptoms in the older adult with CKD and why that matters. The case discussion describes an older male with urinary incontinence, and the reader is then guided on how the urinary issue affects CKD management. Chapter 7 addresses hypertension in the older patient with CKD and provides case scenarios. The clinical benefits and risks of blood pressure reduction and treatment goals in older adults are discussed along with a presentation of existing evidence. While hypertension guidelines recommend blood pressure goals <130/80 mmHg in most older adults to prevent cardiovascular disease, this blood pressure goal may be problematic in certain individuals. This chapter discusses the pitfalls in blood pressure lowering in older adults. Another common condition that affects approximately one-third of adults over the age of 65 years is diabetes mellitus. Chapter 8 provides a case vignette of an older patient with both diabetes mellitus and CKD. This chapter describes the natural history of CKD development and its progression in a patient with diabetes mellitus and how disease progression can be modified by other factors, including advancing age. Whether a patient with CKD and diabetes mellitus should undergo kidney biopsy and the safety and benefits of treatment are also discussed.

Polycystic kidney disease accounts for 5–10% of kidney failure, and due to the development of cysts with aging and the heterogeneity of cystic kidney diseases, diagnosis can be challenging in older adults. Chapter 9 outlines the diagnostic approach and treatment decisions for cystic kidney diseases in the older adult. This interactive chapter provides case presentations, computed tomography images of cystic kidney disease cases, and a discussion of the pathogenesis and genetic mutations associated with cystic kidney diseases. In the older adult, the extrarenal manifestations can be as important or even more important than the kidney disease itself. The chapter discusses these extrarenal manifestations and how the clinician should approach them. Glomerular diseases can also be extremely challenging to manage in the older patient due to concerns of infections and other adverse effects of immunosuppressants. Chapter 10 provides strong guidance on the diagnosis and treatment of glomerular diseases. The chapter first focuses on diseases associated with nephrotic syndrome and then moves on to discuss diseases associated with a nephritic presentation. The authors provide a summary of previous studies that examined clinical outcomes for treated elderly patients with ANCA-associated vasculitis. Readers will gain understanding of when treatments for glomerular diseases may have more harm than benefits and vice versa.

Fractures affect almost 20% of older patients with non-dialysis dependent CKD and 50% of patients receiving dialysis. Bone health remains a critical factor for fracture risk and is especially important in patients with CKD. Chapter 11 is written by endocrinologists and focuses on bone and mineral metabolism in the older adult with CKD. While acknowledging that bone biopsies may not be readily available to most practicing nephrologists, the authors provide guidance on the practical diagnosis and management of impaired bone health such as osteoporosis and osteomalacia. Readers are guided on whom and when to treat.

Hyponatremia is commonly encountered in both the outpatient and inpatient setting when caring for older adults with CKD. Chapter 12 outlines the age-related physiologic changes that impair water excretion due to reduced ability to dilute the urine. The authors walk the reader through a case presentation and discuss the multitude of factors that can cause inappropriate antidiuretic hormone levels. Safe treatment of low serum sodium levels in older adults is also discussed. This chapter also includes a table that provides urine concentration and dilution in the older adult and their implications for sodium disorders. Chapter 13 addresses acute kidney injury (AKI) in older adults. As noted in Chap. 3, nephron senescence occurs with aging which makes advanced age a major risk factor for AKI due to reduced reserve. This chapter outlines the molecular, cellular, and structural changes associated with aging that may contribute to kidney injury. The chapter also provides information on the diagnostic and therapeutic issues for AKI in the older adult. Chapter 14 covers pharmacotherapeutic considerations in the older adult with CKD and includes tables of common medications with altered pharmacokinetics in older adults. As a person ages, the absorption, distribution, and metabolism of many drugs changes and understanding these issues can strengthen prescribing practices and mitigate adverse effects.

The last three chapters discuss dialysis, nutrition, and kidney supportive care in the older adult with CKD. Mortality remains high for the older adult facing kidney failure, and determining the best mode of care for the patient can be extremely challenging for the patient, caregivers, and clinicians. These three chapters provide an overview of the options for patients with kidney failure, including in-center dialysis, home dialysis, and conservative management. Regardless of the choice, strong nutritional support is required, and Chap. 16 discusses how and why nutritional support can augment care and improve the quality of life for a patient. The chapter on supportive care provides an overview of the role of multidisciplinary care, including palliative care for the management of the older patient with advanced kidney disease.

We congratulate you because you are obviously motivated to continue your education. In the last 10 years, the knowledge and advancement in kidney care have never been greater. The 17 chapters in this textbook provide the reader with the education they will need to heighten the quality of care delivered for the older adult with CKD. We were fortunate to have fantastic thought leaders in nephrology and endocrinology to contribute to this textbook. These authors are responsible for advancing the clinical and diagnostic care of older adults with CKD and we are grateful for their contributions. We hope this textbook leads not only to better care but will also inspire research that can improve the care for patients with kidney diseases.

Maywood, IL, USA   Holly Kramer
Oak Lawn, IL, USA   Edgar V. Lerma
New York, NY, USA   Holly Koncicki

Contents

Chapter 1
The Elderly Patient with Kidney Disease: Overview and Evaluation

Dawn Wolfgram and Christina Mariyam Joy

Case

A 78-year-old woman is referred to nephrology clinic due to routine labs indicating an eGFR of 57 mL/min. She has a medical history of migraines, osteoporosis, and gastroesophageal reflux disease for which she takes sumatriptan as needed, a daily vitamin D and calcium tablet, and omeprazole that she buys over-the-counter. She was recently diagnosed with high blood pressure and was started on losartan 50 mg daily. She was confused by this recent diagnosis of hypertension because she did not think her blood pressure had been elevated. However, her physician explained that her goal blood pressure should be lower. She is worried about having kidney disease as a friend of hers was on dialysis and recently died. She says she tries to be healthy and exercises by walking daily. Her blood pressure at the visit is 120/60 with a pulse of 70, and her BMI is 22. Her main question is how this kidney disease will affect her life.

D. Wolfgram (✉) · C. Mariyam Joy
Zablocki VA Medical Center, Milwaukee, WI, USA

Department of Medicine, Medical College of Wisconsin, Milwaukee, WI, USA
e-mail: dwolfgram@mcw.edu

© The Author(s), under exclusive license to Springer Nature Switzerland AG 2024
H. Kramer et al. (eds.), *Kidney Disease in the Elderly*,
https://doi.org/10.1007/978-3-031-68460-9_1

Structural Changes in the Kidney with Aging

Macrostructural Changes

A common part of the evaluation for a change in estimated glomerular filtration rate (eGFR) is completion of a kidney ultrasound (US), which can detail several macro-anatomy changes that occur with aging. A kidney US provides information on kidney size, cortical thickness, echogenicity, and presence of lesions or cysts to screen for potential malignancies that are higher risk in older adults. Aging-associated changes can occur that affect these parameters, so interpretation of findings should be done in the context of age. Macroscopically, the kidney increases in mass to about 400 g until about the fourth decade of life when decline in kidney mass typically begins. Most of the decline in kidney volume with aging is within the cortex, while medullary volume increases slightly to compensate for total volume until age 50–60 years. After age 60 years, kidney volume declines overall, and this decline becomes more dramatic beginning after age 70 years [1–3]. See Fig. 1.1, for changes in kidney volume by age [4]. Although kidney length by ultrasound is only a crude measure of one dimension of overall size, it can be helpful in determining if the kidneys are appropriate in size. Although kidney length does decrease with age, the change is small, and body height is a more important contributor to kidney length, thus there is no useful age-adjusted kidney length [5]. However, a kidney length that is less than 9 cm in an average-height individual is suggestive of pathology, even in an older person.

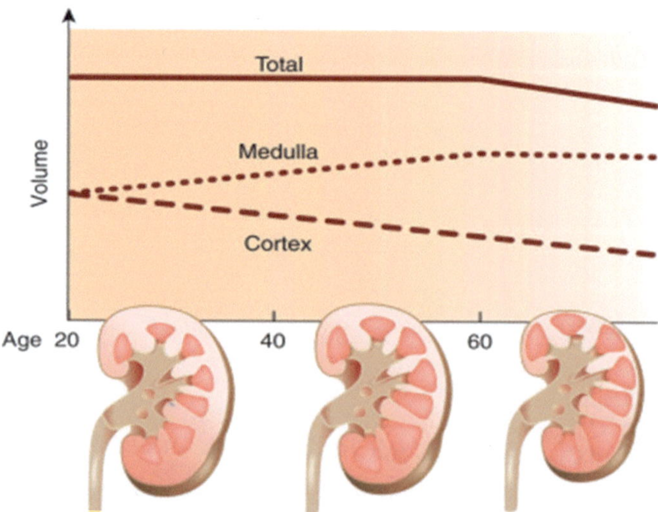

Fig. 1.1 The changes in cortical, medullary, and total volumes of the kidney with aging. (Used with permission from reference [4])

Another parameter obtained from the kidney ultrasound includes the number of kidney cysts. Cysts are a common finding, and the presence of cysts, the size, and the number of cysts do increase with aging. The older age group is more likely to have cysts, and their cysts are more numerous and wider in diameter, particularly in the cortex and in men [6, 7]. In fact, the upper limit for normal number of cysts between both kidneys may be as high at 10 for a male over the age of 60 years, although having only 1–3 is more common [6]. However, this is only for simple cysts. Cysts that are complex, with septations, vascularity, solid components, or calcifications, may be premalignant or malignant and require further evaluation.

Finally, if using duplex ultrasound to also evaluate the renal arteries, the incidence of renal artery narrowing is higher in older adults due to arthrosclerosis. In one study, the prevalence of renal artery narrowing was 25% in potential kidney donors over the age of 60 years [8]. Indications of significant stenosis that may lead to hypoperfusion include size differential between the kidneys with the smaller kidney having the narrowed or stenotic artery, a peak systolic velocity > 200 cm/sec, or a trans-lesion pressure gradient from 10 to 15 mmHg [9]. In addition, difficult-to-control hypertension may be due to renal artery stenosis and would be accompanied by a high renin level. In women, the presence of fibromuscular dysplasia should also be considered when finding narrowed renal arteries.

Microstructural Changes

In addition to imaging, there are several histologic changes that occur. The most common histologic change with aging includes nephrosclerosis with nephron loss and compensatory nephron hypertrophy. These changes can have effects on glomerular filtration rate, which will be discussed later in this chapter.

Nephrosclerosis with normal aging includes glomerulosclerosis that is focal and global, as opposed to the pathological glomerular feature of focal and segmental glomerulosclerosis. Focal and global glomerulosclerosis is often referred to as obsolescent, which indicates shrunken and retracted glomerular capillary tuft and fibrous matrix replacing Bowman's space. In a study of over 1000 biopsies completed on donated kidneys at the time of transplantation, the number of samples with more than 25% global glomerulosclerosis increased from 1% in donors aged 40–49 to 4.3% and 9.1% in those aged 60–69 and 70–79, respectively. Having any global glomerulosclerosis was noted in 82% of samples from those aged 70–79 years compared to slightly less than half of those aged 40–49 [10]. This and other studies led to the development of an age-appropriate reference for the number of globally sclerotic glomeruli in a kidney biopsy based on number of glomeruli in the section. A representative section of 9–16 glomeruli is shown in Figure 1.2 [11]. When including at least two features of nephrosclerosis (glomerulosclerosis, tubular atrophy, interstitial fibrosis, and arteriosclerosis), the prevalence of sclerotic glomeruli increases from 16% in those aged 30–39 to 58% and 73% in those aged 60–69 and 70–79, respectively [10]. Nephrosclerosis with aging is linked with arteriosclerosis

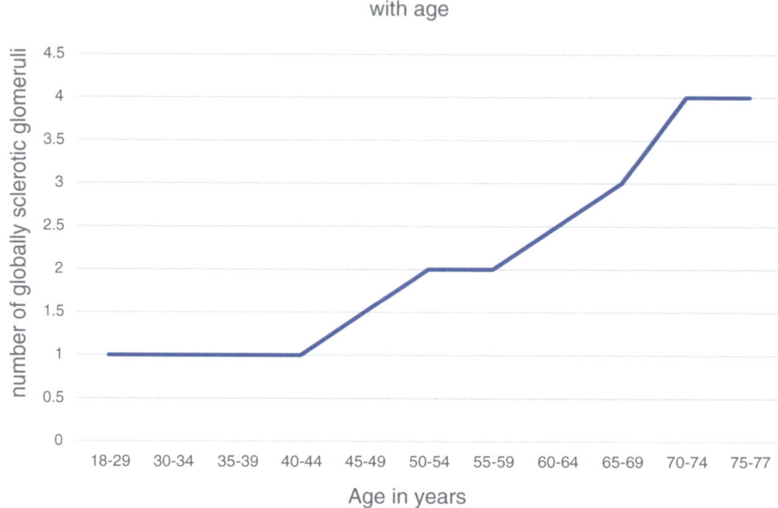

Fig. 1.2 The upper limit of normal for number of globally sclerotic glomeruli based on age and a section containing 9–16 glomeruli. (Data from reference [11])

as it leads to ischemic injury that over time causes glomerulosclerosis and tubular atrophy. The interstitial fibrosis then occurs in places of tubular atrophy and shrunken glomeruli. Although the loss of nephrons typically leads to compensatory nephron hypertrophy in kidney diseases, loss of nephrons with aging is usually not accompanied by substantial hypertrophy. The presence of glomerular hypertrophy is much more pronounced when seen with nephron loss due to diabetes, obesity, or other comorbidities compared to hypertrophy that occurs with normal aging [1, 12].

Physiological Changes

The macro- and microanatomical changes we discussed above are also accompanied by a reduction in glomerular filtration rate (GFR) that occurs starting after age 40 years. The decline in GFR with aging varies among individuals, and the decline is steeper in men compared to women. Most studies have demonstrated a decline of 6–8 mL/min/decade [13, 14]. Although comorbidities play a role in GFR decline, even normotensive individuals and those without cardiovascular disease show a reduction in GFR with advancing age. [15] Changes in glomerular arterial pressure due to changes in renin–angiotensin levels and responsiveness and reduction in nitric oxide levels with age can have a significant impact on GFR. Given the important role of age in the normal range of values for GFR, age-specific thresholds for defining chronic kidney disease have been suggested but never incorporated into guidelines. The rationale and guidance on the use of age-adjusted eGFR thresholds are described later in this chapter.

Table 1.1 Example of differences in urine volume and concentration in young vs elderly. Used with permission from reference [17]

	Young		Elderly	
	Day	Night	Day	Night
Plasma AVP (pg/mL)	1.1	2.0	1.9	1.3
Plasma ANH (pg/mL)	19	17	40	55
Urine osmolality (mosm/kg)	700	830	510	450
Urine volume (mL/h)	75	35	50	70
Urine volume for 8 h sleep		280		560

When discussing physiological changes in kidney function, the tubular concentrating changes should be considered. While tubular concentrating changes with age do not influence GFR, they can have an impact on patient symptoms. In normal aging, the kidneys' ability to maximally concentrate the urine declines due to a decline in maximal urine osmolarity. This decline in urine concentrating ability is due to resistance of the distal tubules to antidiuretic hormone (ADH) and changes in the diurnal release of antidiuretic hormone (ADH) [16]. In addition, aging is accompanied by an increase in atrial natriuretic hormone levels and a decrease in renin and aldosterone levels, and these changes lead to an increase in sodium wasting [16]. The decrease in urine concentrating ability combined with higher sodium excretion results in a higher urine production overall or polyuria and a shift toward greater urine production at night or nocturia. See Table 1.1 for a comparison of typical parameters in urine volume and concentration levels that lead to the common age-related symptoms of polyuria and nocturia [17].

Estimating Kidney Function

Assessment of Glomerular Filtration Rate

Glomerular filtration rate remains the best overall index to assess kidney function in health as well as in disease states. In addition, GFR estimation helps determine drug dosing, especially among the elderly, minimizing side effects. Currently, available GFR calculators utilize endogenous biomarkers such as creatinine and cystatin-C. However, it is important to note that there are no "ideal molecules" that are 100% filtered without being secreted or reabsorbed by the kidney tubules. Creatinine is a waste product of muscle metabolism. It is freely filtered by the glomerulus, secreted by the tubules, and also has limited extra-renal elimination from the gastrointestinal tract. Creatinine is the most used molecule for kidney function estimates, as it is inexpensive, widely accepted, and universally available. Creatinine levels often vary with muscle mass, exogenous creatine/protein intake, as well as certain drugs, like cimetidine and triamterene, that can decrease tubular secretion. Cystatin-C is a ubiquitous molecule present in all nucleated cells, freely filtered by the kidney, metabolized by the tubules, and its metabolites subjected to extra-renal elimination. Cystatin-C is not present in the urine. Its levels are affected by obesity, inflammatory states, thyroid diseases, smoking, steroid use, etc.

The current gold standard for GFR calculation is the 24 h Inulin clearance, but this measurement is often tenuous to perform, difficult to access, and costly. Alternatively, Iothalamate and Iohexol clearance can be used as alternatives to Inulin clearance. The Cockcroft and Gault (1976) [18] equation was the first equation used to estimate creatinine clearance and is still utilized for drug dosing. Creatinine clearance combines glomerular filtration rate and tubular secretion of creatinine. Therefore, when GFR declines, tubular secretion of creatinine becomes substantially higher, and, therefore, at very low GFR, creatinine clearance overestimates kidney function.

The Modification of Diet in Renal Disease (MDRD) GFR estimating equation by Levey et al. [19] was validated in 1999, and later redeveloped in 2002 to its current form today and remains widely utilized. As the MDRD equation was developed among individuals with chronic kidney disease (CKD), its major limitation is the underestimation of GFR when >60 mL/min/1.73 m^2. To rectify this bias, the CKD-EPI (Chronic Kidney Disease Epidemiology Collaboration) group developed a new equation in 2009 to accurately estimate GFR (eGFR) across the spectrum of CKD stages [20]. There are multiple variations to the CKD-EPI equation, using creatinine, cystatin-C, as well as a combination of both. It is important to note that the combined equations using cystatin-C and creatinine are better estimates of glomerular function than either of these markers used alone [21]. In light of recent outcry to reassess predictive algorithms pointing out that race is a social, not a biological construct, KDIGO and CKD-EPI combined task force validated two new creatinine, cystatin-C-based equations in 2021, that do not include race to determine eGFR [22]. Non-race based estimations of GFR are particularly important among people of African–American race/ethnicity, in whom the equation falsely estimates a higher GFR, which was previously delaying earlier diagnosis and management.

Interpretation of eGFR should be done carefully with advancing age. Most laboratories report eGFR based on creatinine. However, it is important to know which of the prediction equations was utilized by the lab in the estimation of kidney function. It is well-recognized that MDRD equations underestimate eGFR, especially at higher degrees of renal function. Therefore CKD-EPI-based equations often provide a better estimate. In addition, a combined creatinine–cystatin-C-based formula may also be better among older adults who may have muscle decline with aging the elderly where there are alterations to muscle mass with age.

Assessment of Albuminuria

The presence of albumin in the urine is often considered an early marker of kidney damage. Increased urine albumin excretion portends a higher likelihood of kidney disease progression and cardiovascular events regardless of the presence of diabetes

Prognosis of CKD by GFR and albuminuria categories: KDIGO 2012			Persistent albuminuria categories Description and range		
			A1	**A2**	**A3**
			Normal to mildly increased	Moderately increased	Severely increased
			< 30 mg/g < 3 mg/mmol	30–300 mg/g 3–30 mg/mmol	> 300 mg/g > 30 mg/mmol
GFR categories (ml/min/1.73 m²) Description and range	**G1**	Normal or high	≥ 90			
	G2	Mildly decreased	60–89			
	G3a	Mildly to moderately decreased	45–59			
	G3b	Moderately to severely decreased	30–44			
	G4	Severely decreased	15–29			
	G5	Kidney failure	< 15			

Green: low risk (if no other markers of kidney disease, no CKD); Yellow: moderately increased risk; Orange: high risk; Red: very high risk.

Fig. 1.3 Prognosis of CKD by GFR and albuminuria categories

mellitus. Although the exact mechanism is unclear—albuminuria is hypothesized as a sign of endothelial dysfunction or chronic inflammation [23, 24]. The gold standard test for assessment of urine albumin excretion is a 24-h urine collection, but this is often difficult to perform as a routine screening test. Hence a spot urine albumin-to-creatinine ratio (UACR) may be calculated instead as an initial screening test, followed by a 24 h urine albumin for confirmation. It is important to understand that UACR assumes a steady state and a daily creatinine excretion of 1 g/day. Older adults with lower muscle mass may have daily creatinine excretion less than 1 g/day; hence UACR may overestimate actual urine albumin excretion. There are also benign entities like orthostatic and exercise-induced proteinuria, which can present with diurnal variations in albumin excretion and timed urine collections may be needed to accurately assess the urine albumin excretion. UACR may be then used to follow over time. Urine protein measurements are not routinely recommended due to high sample-to-sample variability in the quantity and composition of the proteins measured. KDIGO 2012 recognizes that UACR above 30 mg/g (or 0.03 g/g) portends a high risk of CKD progression.

The purpose of obtaining eGFR and UACR is for risk stratification as well as prognostication of patients. Fig. 1.3 shows the KDIGO 2012 prognostic classification in patients with CKD [25].

Age Thresholds for eGFR

The concept of an age-adjusted eGFR threshold has been gaining momentum recently. An eGFR of <60 mL/min/1.73 m^2 has been recognized as an important risk factor for increased morbidity and mortality among adults with CKD, based on CKD-EPI consortium epidemiological studies and adopted by KDIGO guidelines. Most controversies focus on using 60 mL/min/1.73 m^2 as GFR cutoff, especially among those categorized as CKD G3aA1 and 65 years and older. There are other epidemiology studies that show that the mortality risk among the elderly does not substantially increase until eGFR is below 45 mL/min/1.73 m^2. In addition, the risk of progression to ESKD for a given eGFR value is lower in the elderly compared to younger counterparts. Individuals over the age of 70 years with eGFR 45–60 mL/min/1.73m^2 and normal-to-mild albuminuria (< 30 mg/g) have a similar risk to those with eGFR of 60–89 mL/min/1.73m^2 [26, 27]. The lower risk of progression to ESKD may be due to the competing risk of death. With greater incidence of death compared to ESKD in older age groups when eGFR is above 15 mL/min/1.73M^2 (see schematic in Fig. 1.4) [26]. CKD may also progress slower in older adults.

Use of age-adjusted thresholds does have a small risk of identifying older patients with CKD later in life, but it may also identify CKD earlier among younger adults. Further use of age-adjusted thresholds can reduce the anxiety of being labeled with "kidney disease" when there is little evidence to suggest a strong negative health impact. In addition, it also decreases the cost of diagnostic and therapeutic interventions, costs of life insurance premiums, etc. It is also noted that patients with known CKD are often limited from receiving life-saving medical interventions like cardiac catheterizations, contrast-based imaging, or even cancer therapies. Hence, an age adjustment could help minimize creatinine-based medical

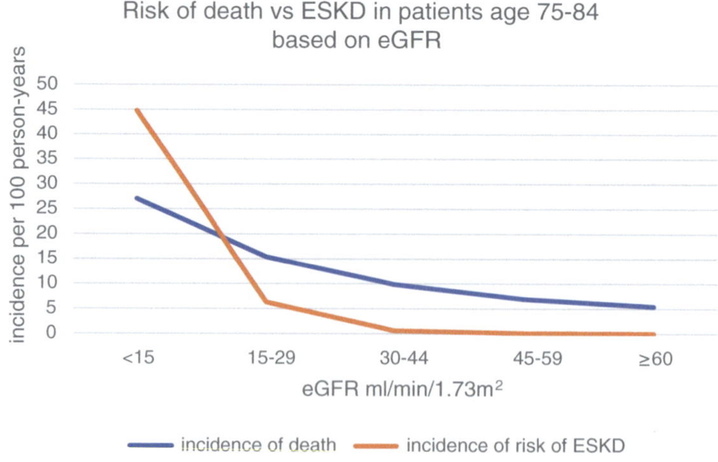

Fig. 1.4 The risk of death is higher than the risk of ESKD for eGFR levels >15 mL/min/1.73m^2 in older age groups. (Data from reference [25])

bias. However, it is important to note that clinically significant proteinuria is always pathological, no matter what the kidney function. Delanaye et al. have proposed the following adapted thresholds for CKD: 75 mL/min per 1.73 m^2 for ages below 40 years, 60 mL/min per 1.73 m^2 for ages between 40 and 65 years, and 45 mL/min per 1.73 m^2 for ages above 65 years [28]. Age-adjusted thresholds for eGFR seem like a reasonable option, but it is not widely adopted into current practice guidelines. Although more data is emerging, studies are often limited by smaller sample sizes. The studies often use creatinine as a measure of estimating kidney function, but this might be inaccurate among older adults with a declining muscle mass. KDIGO currently recommends the use of cystatin-C to verify lower GFR in the elderly. More importantly, the current staging system is simplistic and can be universally adopted without creating confusion and complications among its users.

A Summary of Approach to Kidney Disease Among Elderly

Approach to specific kidney diseases will be discussed in detail in subsequent chapters. Included here is an initial investigative approach when evaluating an elderly individual for kidney disease and some important considerations on management.

History and Physical: The first step in any diagnostic algorithm includes obtaining a detailed medical history, a physical examination, as well a review of current and past medications. It is worth mentioning that many elderly patients take over-the-counter medications including non-steroidal anti-inflammatory agents (NSAIDs), herbal supplements, and proton pump inhibitors; such medications are often not included in the list of active medications; but their use can lead to decline in kidney function. Also, if evaluating a recent change in eGFR, the use of renin–angiotensin–aldosterone systems blockers should be assessed to determine recent dose adjustments. Other medications to note include diuretics since elderly patients are more sensitive to changes in volume status affecting kidney perfusion due to decrease in kidney autoregulation [29]. Use of anticholinergics for treatment of polyuria or nocturia can lead to urinary retention. This is especially true among men with prostatic hypertrophy. Other medications that can have anti-cholinergic effects include antihistamines, tricyclic antidepressants, and sleep aids.

To complete the history, discuss in detail any current ongoing symptoms, with specific emphasis on urogenital system. A head-to-toe review of symptoms, including recent weight changes, night sweats or fevers, bony pain, and rash, should be obtained. Past medical history, including information on gestation and birth, including birthweight, gestational age at birth, higher-order pregnancies, and childhood illnesses are needed to determine the risk of decreased nephron mass. History of prolonged illnesses with known kidney involvement, even if the kidney function normalized, as previous AKI is a predecessor of CKD. History of all chronic ailments, along with occupational as well as environmental exposures, can also be important. For example, a person who immigrated from the Balkans is at risk for CKD as well as urothelial malignancies and should be screened appropriately. Similarly, individuals with prior heavy metals/agricultural chemicals are also prone to CKD. Previous whole-body irradiation or myeloablative therapy for stem cell transplantation and previous or ongoing chemo or immunotherapy also give up vital clues to the nature of underlying kidney disease. A positive family history is also very helpful.

A thorough physical exam should follow next. Evaluation of blood pressure and establishing age-adjusted BP goals is also an important part of the initial visit. This is discussed in detail later in the book.

Investigations: Reviewing previous laboratory data is paramount while investigating kidney diseases. A basic laboratory workup can include but not be limited to a complete blood count, basic metabolic panel (or renal function panel, including albumin, phosphorus, and a calculated anion gap), and serum cystatin-C whenever readily available, etc. A combined Creatinine–cystatin-C eGFR should be calculated based on CKD-EPI formulas using online tools. The presence of anemia with elevated calcium levels and elevated creatinine should warrant evaluation for paraproteinemia, especially among the elderly, as reduced GFR is often the first indicator for this entity.

The role of urinalysis in the diagnosis of kidney disease is often underappreciated. Check for evidence of hematuria, proteinuria, isosthenuria, presence of casts, inflammatory cells, crystals, etc. It is also important to quantify proteinuria—a spot urine protein to creatinine or spot urine albumin-to-creatinine ratio can be used. A negative dipstick for albumin but a positive quantifiable protein can suggest non-albumin proteinuria like Bence–Jones proteinuria, which should warrant additional testing. Isolated persistent hematuria should warrant imaging as well as referral to urology. Kidney ultrasonography can be requested to check for kidney sizes, echogenicity, presence of cysts, masses, stones, or hydronephrosis. If any one or more of the initial tests are suggestive of a possible pathology, additional workup is warranted.

Case Continued

History: During her visit, you ask about any other medical history, which she denies. She only takes the medications listed and no other supplements; specifically, she does not take any NSAIDs. She has been on her medications for years, except for the losartan that was started 3 months ago. She takes her current medications consistently. She denies any dysuria, gross hematuria, incontinence, or hesitancy but does not occasionally need to void overnight. She has had some trouble with mild dizziness when getting up after lying that usually resolves after 30 s or if she gets up slowly. She has not had any falls. She says she was a healthy child and was born at term. She has not had any hospitalizations and was never told she had a kidney injury.

Physical: Her sitting BP was 120/60 with pulse of 70 and standing was 100/55 with a pulse of 88. She is 5′4″ and weight 129 pounds. She has a normal cardiovascular and pulmonary exam. Her abdomen is soft and nontender. She has no peripheral edema and no skin rashes.

Evaluation: You review her labs and note that a prior lab from 1 year ago shows an eGFR of 69 mL/min. The rest of her electrolytes are normal. You have her complete a urinalysis and urine albumin-to-creatine rations. There is no hematuria on urinalysis, and her albumin-to-creatinine ratio is within normal at 15 mg/g. You also check a cystatin-C with eGFR panel that results in an eGFR of 64 mL/min. You proceed with a kidney ultrasound that demonstrates the right kidney with length of 9.5 cm and left kidney with length of 9.8 cm. The report indicated that there is mild decrease in cortical thickness and two simple cysts on the right kidney and three simple cysts on the left kidney.

You explain that the changes noted in her eGFR likely represent natural decline in kidney function with a component of reduced intraglomerular arterial pressure after starting the losartan to achieve the lower blood pressure goal. Given her age, she likely has some arteriosclerosis that impairs kidney autoregulation. The lack of protein in the urine and normal age changes on the kidney ultrasound indicate that there is no pathology. Since she did have orthostatic hypotension and had issues with some dizziness upon standing you reduced her dose of losartan and explained that her blood pressure target can be slightly liberalized to under 140/90 mmHg. You reassure her that her kidney function is appropriate for her age, and that it should not lead to any worsening in her overall health.

References

1. Denic A, Glassock RJ, Rule AD. Structural and functional changes with the aging kidney. Adv Chronic Kidney Dis. 2016;23(1):19–28. https://doi.org/10.1053/j.ackd.2015.08.004.
2. Emamian SA, Nielsen MB, Pedersen JF, Ytte L. Kidney dimensions at sonography: correlation with age, sex, and habitus in 665 adult volunteers. AJR Am J Roentgenol. 1993;160(1):83–6. https://doi.org/10.2214/ajr.160.1.8416654.
3. Piras D, Masala M, Delitala A, et al. Kidney size in relation to ageing, gender, renal function, birthweight and chronic kidney disease risk factors in a general population. Nephrol Dial Transplant. 2020;35(4):640–7. https://doi.org/10.1093/ndt/gfy270.
4. O'Neill WC. Structure, not just function. Kidney Int. 2014;85(3):503–5. https://doi.org/10.1038/ki.2013.426.
5. Akpinar IN, Altun E, Avcu S, Tuney D, Ekinci G, Biren T. Sonographic measurement of kidney size in geriatric patients. J Clin Ultrasound. 2003;31(6):315–8. https://doi.org/10.1002/jcu.10178.
6. Rule AD, Sasiwimonphan K, Lieske JC, Keddis MT, Torres VE, Vrtiska TJ. Characteristics of renal cystic and solid lesions based on contrast-enhanced computed tomography of potential kidney donors. Am J Kidney Dis. 2012;59(5):611–8. https://doi.org/10.1053/j.ajkd.2011.12.022.
7. Laucks SP Jr, McLachlan MS. Aging and simple cysts of the kidney. Br J Radiol. 1981;54(637):12–4. https://doi.org/10.1259/0007-1285-54-637-12.

8. Lorenz EC, Vrtiska TJ, Lieske JC, et al. Prevalence of renal artery and kidney abnormalities by computed tomography among healthy adults. Clin J Am Soc Nephrol. 2010;5(3):431–8. https://doi.org/10.2215/CJN.07641009.

9. Drieghe B, Madaric J, Sarno G, et al. Assessment of renal artery stenosis: side-by-side comparison of angiography and duplex ultrasound with pressure gradient measurements. Eur Heart J. 2008;29(4):517–24. https://doi.org/10.1093/eurheartj/ehm631.

10. Rule AD, Amer H, Cornell LD, et al. The association between age and nephrosclerosis on renal biopsy among healthy adults. Ann Intern Med. 2010;152(9):561–7. https://doi.org/1 0.7326/0003-4819-152-9-201005040-00006.

11. Kremers WK, Denic A, Lieske JC, et al. Distinguishing age-related from disease-related glomerulosclerosis on kidney biopsy: the aging kidney anatomy study. Nephrol Dial Transplant. 2015;30(12):2034–9. https://doi.org/10.1093/ndt/gfv072.

12. Denic A, Alexander MP, Kaushik V, et al. Detection and clinical patterns of nephron hypertrophy and Nephrosclerosis among apparently healthy adults. Am J Kidney Dis. 2016;68(1):58–67. https://doi.org/10.1053/j.ajkd.2015.12.029.

13. Weinstein JR, Anderson S. The aging kidney: physiological changes. Adv Chronic Kidney Dis. 2010;17(4):302–7. https://doi.org/10.1053/j.ackd.2010.05.002.

14. Lindeman RD, Tobin J, Shock NW. Longitudinal studies on the rate of decline in renal function with age. J Am Geriatr Soc. 1985;33(4):278–85. https://doi.org/10.1111/j.1532-5415.1985. tb07117.x.

15. Hollenberg NK, Rivera A, Meinking T, et al. Age, renal perfusion and function in Island-dwelling indigenous Kuna Amerinds of Panama. Nephron. 1999;82(2):131–8. https://doi. org/10.1159/000045389.

16. Cugini P, Lucia P, Di Palma L, et al. Effect of aging on circadian rhythm of atrial natriuretic peptide, plasma renin activity, and plasma aldosterone. J Gerontol. 1992;47(6):B214–9. https:// doi.org/10.1093/geronj/47.6.b214.

17. Miller M. Fluid balance disorders in the elderly. In: ASN geriatrics task force. ASN geriatrics nephrology online curriculum. American Society of Nephrology; 2009. https://www.asn-online.org/education/distancelearning/curricula/geriatrics/. Accessed 5 Aug 2022.

18. Cockcroft DW, Gault MH. Prediction of creatinine clearance from serum creatinine. Nephron. 1976;16(1):31–41. https://doi.org/10.1159/000180580.

19. Levey AS, Bosch JP, Lewis JB, Greene T, Rogers N, Roth D. A more accurate method to estimate glomerular filtration rate from serum creatinine: a new prediction equation. Modification of diet in renal disease study group. Ann Intern Med. 1999;130(6):461–70. https://doi.org/1 0.7326/0003-4819-130-6-199903160-00002.

20. Levey AS, Stevens LA, Schmid CH, et al. A new equation to estimate glomerular filtration rate. Ann Intern Med. 2009;150(9):604–12. https://doi.org/10.7326/0003-4819-150-9 -200905050-00006.

21. Inker LA, Schmid CH, Tighiouart H, et al. Estimating glomerular filtration rate from serum creatinine and cystatin C. N Engl J Med. 2012;367(1):20–9. https://doi.org/10.1056/ NEJMoa1114248.

22. Delgado C, Baweja M, Crews DC, et al. A unifying approach for GFR estimation: recommendations of the NKF-ASN task force on reassessing the inclusion of race in diagnosing kidney disease. Am J Kidney Dis. 2022;79(2):268–288 e1. https://doi.org/10.1053/j.ajkd.2021.08.003.

23. Weir MR. Microalbuminuria and cardiovascular disease. Clin J Am Soc Nephrol. 2007;2(3):581–90. https://doi.org/10.2215/CJN.03190906.

24. Stehouwer CD, Smulders YM. Microalbuminuria and risk for cardiovascular disease: analysis of potential mechanisms. J Am Soc Nephrol. 2006;17(8):2106–11. https://doi.org/10.1681/ ASN.2005121288.

25. Kidney Disease: Improving Global Outcomes (KDIGO) CKD Work Group. KDIGO. Clinical practice guideline for the evaluation and management of chronic kidney disease. Kidney Int Suppl. 2012;3(2013):1–150.

26. O'Hare AM, Choi AI, Bertenthal D, et al. Age affects outcomes in chronic kidney disease. J Am Soc Nephrol. 2007;18(10):2758–65. https://doi.org/10.1681/ASN.2007040422.
27. Liu P, Quinn RR, Lam NN, et al. Accounting for age in the definition of chronic kidney disease. JAMA Intern Med. 2021;181(10):1359–66. https://doi.org/10.1001/jamainternmed.2021.4813.
28. Delanaye P, Jager KJ, Bokenkamp A, et al. CKD: a call for an age-adapted definition. J Am Soc Nephrol. 2019;30(10):1785–805. https://doi.org/10.1681/ASN.2019030238.
29. Abuelo JG. Normotensive ischemic acute renal failure. N Engl J Med. 2007;357(8):797–805. https://doi.org/10.1056/NEJMra064398.

Chapter 2
Epidemiology of Kidney Disease in the Elderly

Gregorio T. Obrador

Introduction

Chronic kidney disease (CKD) and acute kidney injury (AKI) are increasingly common in the elderly population. Several factors contribute to the rising incidence and prevalence of CKD, most notably an age-related glomerular filtration rate (GFR) loss and the comorbid conditions that often accompany aging. Glomerular diseases are also common in the elderly and pose significant diagnostic and therapeutic challenges. This chapter reviews the controversies surrounding the definition of and the epidemiology of CKD, AKI, and glomerular diseases in the elderly population.

Chronic Kidney Disease

The Kidney Disease: Improving Global Outcomes (KDIGO) has defined CKD as the presence of more than 3 months of markers of kidney damage or an estimated glomerular filtration rate (eGFR) of less than 60 ml/min per 1.73 m^2 that has health implications. KDIGO has also classified CKD into five stages based on eGFR (G1 to G5) and three levels based on albuminuria (A1 to A3) (Fig. 2.1) [1].

Leaving aside the issue of the accuracy and precision of current equations to estimate GFR, there has been significant controversy regarding the KDIGO definition of CKD, particularly when applied to older adults [2–5]. Since GFR declines with normal aging and there is an absolute threshold of an eGFR <60 mL/min per

G. T. Obrador (✉)
Epidemiology, Biostatistics, and Public Health, Universidad Panamericana School of Medicine, Mexico City, CDMX, Mexico
e-mail: gobrador@up.edu.mx

H. Kramer et al. (eds.), *Kidney Disease in the Elderly*,
https://doi.org/10.1007/978-3-031-68460-9_2

Prognosis of CKD by GFR and Albuminuria Categories: KDIGO 2012

				Persistent albuminuria categories Description and range		
				A1 Normal to mildly increased <30 mg/g <3 mg/mmol	**A2** Moderately increased 30-300 mg/g 3-30 mg/mmol	**A3** Severely increased >300 mg/g >30 mg/mmol
GFR categories (ml/min/ 1.73 m²) Description and range	G1	Normal or high	≥90	Green	Yellow	Orange
	G2	Mildly decreased	60-89	Green	Yellow	Orange
	G3a	Mildly to moderately decreased	45-59	Yellow	Orange	Red
	G3b	Moderately to severely decreased	30-44	Orange	Red	Red
	G4	Severely decreased	15-29	Red	Red	Red
	G5	Kidney failure	<15	Red	Red	Red

Green: low risk (if no other markers of kidney disease, no CKD); Yellow: moderately increased risk; Orange: high risk; Red, very high risk.

Fig. 2.1 Prognosis of CKD by GFR and albuminuria category. Green, low risk (if no other markers of kidney disease, no CKD); Yellow, moderately increased risk; Orange, high risk; Red, very high risk. CKD, chronic kidney disease; GFR, glomerular filtration rate; KDIGO, Kidney Disease: Improving Global Outcomes. (With permission from [1])

1.73 m² for defining CKD, an increasing proportion of older people are diagnosed with CKD. Indeed, approximately half of the adults older than 70 years supposedly have "CKD," as determined by a measured or estimated GFR ≤ of 60 mL/min per 1.73 m² [6]. Some argue that many elderly individuals with a stable eGFR between 45 and 59 mL/min per 1.73 m² and without abnormal albuminuria are erroneously labeled as having CKD [7]. Others propose that identifying older individuals with an eGFR <60 ml/min per 1.73 m² is justified because they are more susceptible to toxic accumulation of medications cleared by the kidney and develop metabolic or endocrine complications associated with CKD. They also have an increased risk of all-cause and cardiovascular mortality, kidney failure, AKI, and CKD progression [1]. As the debate continues, some authors have suggested amending the current CKD definition to include age-specific thresholds for GFR [8, 9].

Despite the above caveats, several studies that used the current KDIGO definition have reported that the prevalence of CKD increases with age. In a meta-analysis of observational studies, estimating CKD prevalence in general populations, univariate meta-regressions confirmed that CKD prevalence increases with age (Fig. 2.2). Studies of this meta-analysis that evaluated CKD stages 1–5 found the following mean prevalence (95% CI) for people in their 30s, 40s, 50s, 60s, and 70s: 13.7% (10.8–16.6%), 12.0% (9.9–14.1%), 16.0% (13.5–18.4%), 27.6% (26.7–28.5%), and 34.3% (31.9–36.7%). Likewise, studies that evaluated CKD stages 3–5 found the following mean prevalence for the same age groups (95% CI): 8.9% (4.7–13.1%), 8.7% (6.9–10.5%), 12.2% (9.8–14.5%), 11.3% (8.1–14.5%), and 27.9% (16.4–39.3%) [10].

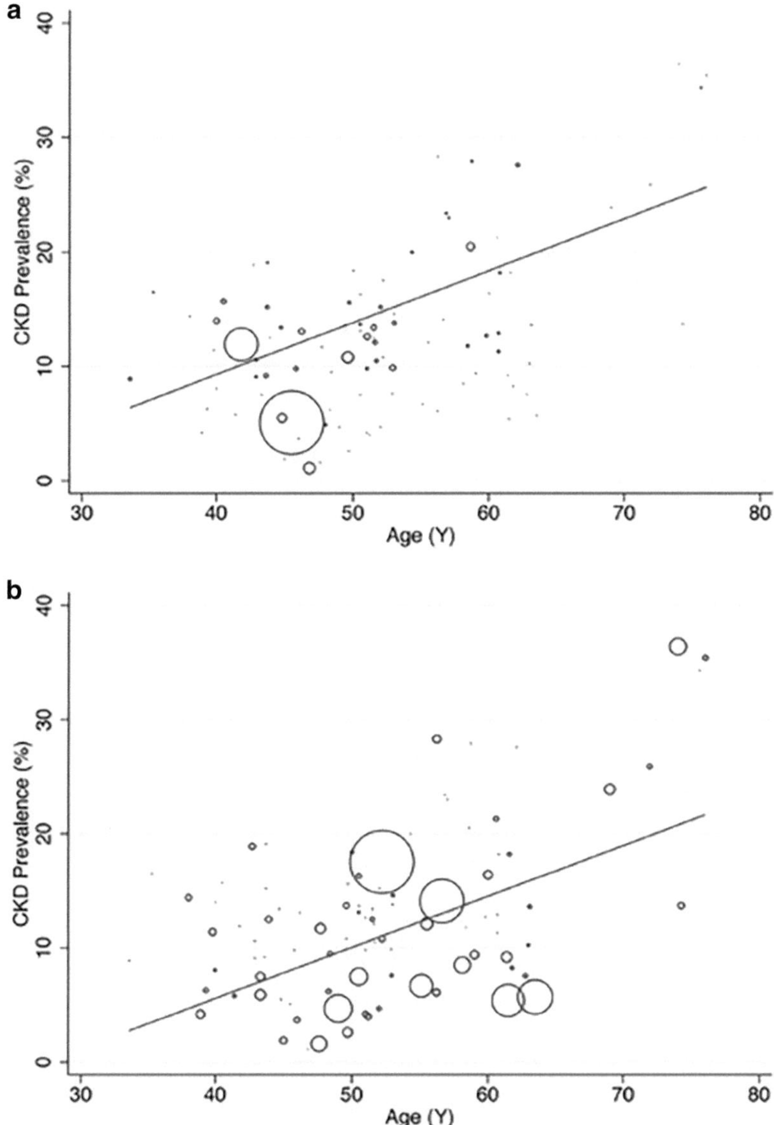

Fig. 2.2 Meta-regression of CKD prevalence and mean sample population age (**a**) Studies report-ing stages 1–5 (**b**) Studies reporting stages 3–5. Each circle represents a study prevalence estimate, with the size denoting the estimate's precision. (*With permission from* [10])

CKD prevalence among older adults varies by country and region. In a system-atic analysis of worldwide-based population data, the prevalence of CKD (Stages 1–5 and 3–5) increased with age and was higher in women than in men in both high-income and low-and middle-income countries. Age-specific prevalence of CKD was higher in low-and middle-income countries, except in those aged ≥70 years, whose prevalence was higher in high-income countries for both men and women (Fig. 2.3) [11]. Also, based on data from 19 general-population studies from 13 European countries, the age-and sex-adjusted CKD stages 1–5 prevalence among adults aged 65–74 years varied from 14.3% in Central Norway, 16.7% in North Netherlands, 19.5% in Northeast Italy, 29.2% in Spain, 34.5% in Ireland, and 41.3% in Northeast Germany. Differences in the prevalence of diabetes, hypertension, and obesity did not fully explain this regional variation in CKD prevalence [12].

In the United States, the National Health and Nutrition Examination Survey (NHANES) 2017–2020 reported that the crude prevalence of CKD stages 1–4 in adults aged 70 years or older, 60–69, 40–59, and 18–39 years was 43%, 20%,11%, and 6%, respectively. It should be noted, however, that these estimates were based on a single measurement of albuminuria or serum creatinine, and thus, they can overestimate CKD prevalence [13].

Regarding trends over time, the United States Renal Data System (USRDS) compared the prevalence of CKD, defined as eGFR <60 ml/min per 1.73 m^2 or urinary albumin to creatinine ratio ≥ 30 mg/g, between the NHANES 2003–2006 and the NHANES 2015–2018. CKD prevalence changed slightly from 8.6% to 8.8% among adults under age 65 and decreased from 43.2% to 36.8% among individuals ≥65 between the two periods. The reduction in CKD in the older group was driven mainly by fewer people with low eGFR rather than a reduction in the prevalence of albuminuria. Although the eGFR decline among older individuals has slowed over time, the percentage of individuals over age 65 with diabetes and cardiovascular disease has increased simultaneously, highlighting the importance of addressing these risk factors to reduce the prevalence of CKD effectively [14].

Impaired kidney function has been associated with adverse outcomes. The Screening for CKD among Older People across Europe (SCOPE) study involved a cohort of 2464 patients from seven European countries. Through cross-sectional analyses and comprehensive geriatric evaluations, it showed the negative impact of advanced CKD on nutritional status, sarcopenia, falls mental health, quality of life, physical function, and multimorbidity [15].

| Age, years | High-income countries | | | | Low- and middle-income countries | | | |
| | CKD stages 1–5 | | CKD stages 3–5 | | CKD stages 1–5 | | CKD stages 3–5 | |
	Men	Women	Men	Women	Men	Women	Men	Women
Prevalence % (95% CI)								
20–29	3.7 (2.7–5.1)	5.3 (3.8–6.3)	0.7 (0.3–1.4)	0.9 (0.4–1.6)	7.3 (6.4–9.0)	6.6 (6.2–7.3)	3.0 (1.7–5.4)	2.0 (1.4–3.3)
30–39	5.0 (4.0–6.0)	5.9 (4.4–6.9)	1.3 (0.7–2.1)	1.6 (0.9–2.6)	8.1 (6.8–10.3)	9.0 (8.6–9.7)	3.1 (1.9–5.0)	3.1 (2.1–5.1)
40–49	6.8 (5.5–8.2)	7.7 (5.9–9.0)	2.1 (1.4–3.1)	3.2 (2.0–4.8)	10.2 (9.0–12.6)	11.5 (11.0–12.7)	3.0 (1.8–6.2)	4.0 (2.5–7.7)
50–59	10.2 (8.6–12.2)	11.1 (8.6–13.8)	4.6 (3.2–6.7)	7.4 (5.2–10.2)	12.0 (10.4–15.1)	15.7 (14.7–17.8)	4.9 (3.5–8.1)	6.7 (4.5–11.7)
60–69	16.0 (13.6–18.1)	15.6 (12.6–18.9)	9.4 (7.8–11.6)	12.2 (9.6–15.8)	16.3 (14.7–20.0)	21.3 (19.6–24.9)	9.7 (6.1–15.6)	13.1 (9.5–19.7)
≥70	28.1 (23.4–33.0)	28.9 (22.7–34.3)	22.7 (20.0–26.4)	28.5 (26.1–31.5)	20.6 (19.4–24.1)	28.4 (26.3–32.7)	11.8 (9.0–17.6)	17.3 (12.6–27.2)
Total	10.1 (8.8–11.1)	12.1 (9.9–13.7)	5.4 (4.6–6.5)	8.6 (6.9–10.7)	10.2 (9.1–12.4)	12.1 (11.6–13.3)	4.3 (2.9–7.1)	5.3 (3.8–8.2)
Age-standardized	8.6 (7.3–9.8)	9.6 (7.7–11.1)	4.3 (3.5–5.2)	5.7 (4.4–7.6)	10.6 (9.4–13.1)	12.5 (11.8–14.0)	4.6 (3.1–7.7)	5.6 (3.9–9.2)
Absolute numbers in thousands (95% CI)								
20–29	3453 (2485–4718)	4647 (3307–5500)	694 (288–1275)	800 (307–1570)	37,121 (32,209–45,651)	32,054 (30,213–35,932)	14,998 (8471–27,644)	9863 (6,746–16,328)
30–39	4699 (3802–5684)	5298 (4000–6235)	1221 (659–1957)	1440 (712–2514)	33,274 (27,740–42,285)	35,920 (34,256–38,727)	12,499 (7803–20,591)	12,365 (8185–20,402)
40–49	6326 (5158–7691)	7120 (5519–8306)	2004 (1290–2934)	2,990 (1731–4700)	35,322 (31,190–43,673)	39,012 (37,165–43,201)	10,253 (6328–21,335)	13,495 (8579–26,111)
50–59	8531 (7149–10,157)	9752 (7541–12,136)	3874 (2625–5549)	6485 (4218–9418)	29,618 (25,640–37,287)	38,337 (35,959–43,651)	12,167 (8612–19,988)	16,355 (10,900–28,611)
60–69	9579 (8155–10,849)	10,425 (8411–12,690)	5608 (4694–6963)	8291 (6329–11,264)	22,434 (20,338–27,637)	31,136 (28,731–36,396)	13,420 (8430–21,497)	19,232 (13,883–28,848)
≥70	15,099 (13,066–18,416)	24,426 (19,150–29,003)	12,690 (11,136–14,745)	24,065 (21,769–27,161)	19,606 (18,459–22,925)	33,637 (31,150–38,706)	11,176 (8541–16,673)	20,509 (14,912–32,240)
Total	48,285 (42,349–53,284)	61,669 (50,394–69,929)	26,091 (22,014–31,078)	44,071 (35,296–54,831)	177,375 (159,157–215,924)	210,096 (200,787–231,704)	74,513 (50,324–123,460)	91,719 (66,697–143,121)

Abbreviations: CI, confidence interval; CKD, chronic kidney disease.

Fig. 2.3 Age-specific and age-standardized prevalence estimates and absolute numbers of men and women with chronic kidney disease in high-income and low-and middle-income countries. (*With permission from* [11])

The age-related increase in CKD prevalence does not necessarily translate into higher demand for kidney failure treatment in older adults. In a population-based cohort study of nearly four million people in the province of Alberta, Canada, 30,801 adults had stage 4 CKD (eGFR between 15 and 30 ml/min/1.73 m^2), with a mean (SD) age of 76.8 (13.3) years. Although the yearly incidence rate of stage 4 CKD increased sharply with age, death was three times more likely to occur than kidney failure, and death was six times more likely than kidney failure among those aged 75–84 years, and 25 times more likely among those aged 85 years or older [16].

Kidney Replacement Therapy

The incidence and prevalence of treated end-stage kidney disease (ESKD) in older adults is higher than in younger people. In the USRDS 2021 Annual Data Report, the adjusted incidence of ESKD in 2019 among individuals aged 18–44 and 45–64 years was 123 and 622 cases per million population (pmp), respectively, whereas among individuals aged 65–74 and ≥ 75 years it was 1307 and 1587 pmp. However, between 2009 and 2019, the adjusted ESKD incidence declined by 13.1% in individuals aged 65–74 and by more than 17.5% in those aged ≥75 years. Likewise, the adjusted prevalence of ESKD in 2019 among individuals aged 18–44 and 45–64 years was 930 and 4169 cases per million population (pmp), respectively, whereas, in individuals aged 65–74 and ≥ 75 years, it was 7419 and 7473 pmp. In the latter two age groups, compared to 2009, there has been an increase in ESKD prevalence of 11.9% and 15.6%, respectively [14].

Regarding KRT modalities, among incident US patients in 2019, as age increased, the percentage of patients initiating in-center hemodialysis (HD) increased, and the percentage of patients initiating peritoneal dialysis (PD) or receiving a preemptive kidney transplant decreased. A similar pattern was seen among prevalent US patients. For example, the percentage of ESKD patients aged 65–74 years receiving in-center HD, home HD, PD, or with a functioning kidney transplant was 64.6, 1.3, 7.3, and 26.8%, respectively, whereas, among ESKD patients ≥75 years, the percentage was 79.1, 1.0, 7.0, and 12.9% [14].

While the overall 5-year survival for ESKD patients on hemodialysis and peritoneal dialysis in 2015 was 42% and 48%, respectively, it is significantly shorter in the elderly. Indeed, in 2019, the expected remaining years of life of prevalent dialysis patients aged 70–74 and 75–79 were approximately 4.2 and 3.6 years, respectively, compared to 14 and 10.7 years, for the 2018 general US population. Likewise, the expected remaining years of life of prevalent dialysis patients aged 80–84 and 85+ were approximately 3.0 and 2.5 years, respectively, compared to 7.8 and 4.0 years for the general US population. The mortality rates were more than two and three times higher for dialysis patients aged 66–74 years than those with heart failure and cancer [14].

In the European Renal Association (ERA) Registry 2019 Annual Report, the percentage of incident and prevalent patients on KRT aged ≥65 years was 54% and

45%, respectively, and their median age was 67.9 and 60.5 years. On December 31, 2019, the unadjusted incidence of KRT ranged from around 1 per 170,000 persons aged 0–19 years to about 1 per 1900 persons aged ≥75 years. In the same year, the unadjusted prevalence of KRT ranged from around 1 per 19,000 persons aged 0–19 years to 1 per 300 persons aged ≥75 years. The 5-year patient survival of dialysis patients ranged from 90% in patients aged 0–19 years to 25% in patients aged ≥75 [17].

Withdrawal of dialysis, which means discontinuing maintenance dialysis, is frequent, especially in the elderly. In the United States in 2015, dialysis withdrawal occurred in 23% of hemodialysis and peritoneal dialysis patients before death [18]. Compared to patients aged 20–44, dialysis withdrawal was nearly four times as common among those older than 85 and was the second most common cause of death in patients older than 80. Older age, female sex, comorbid conditions, and poor quality of life, among other factors, contribute to the risk of withdrawing from dialysis [18, 19]. Canada, the United Kingdom, and other European countries have also reported increasing rates of withdrawal from dialysis, and it is a leading cause of death, especially among the elderly [20].

Regarding kidney transplantation, in 2019 in the United States, 19% of kidney transplant recipients were aged 65–74 years, and 2.2% were aged ≥75. The percentage of US recipients aged ≥65 years has tripled since 1999, while the percentage of recipients aged <45 decreased by over 60%. As a result, transplant recipients in recent years have been older than in the past on average. Older recipients are less likely to receive a living-donor kidney, and their long-term mortality is higher than younger patients [14]. According to the ERA Registry, in 2019, 93% of patients aged ≥75 received deceased donor grafts, and the 5-year patient survival after the first kidney transplant ranged from 97% in patients aged 0–19 years to 66% in patients aged ≥75 [17].

Conservative Kidney Management

Conservative kidney management (CKM) is a holistic, patient-centered treatment option for individuals with stage 5 CKD that aims to improve quality of life through the provision of kidney supportive care without pursuing dialysis or transplantation. CKM involves (a) interventions to delay the progression of kidney disease and minimize the risk of adverse events and complications, (b) active symptom management, (c) advance care planning and shared decision-making, (d) psychological, spiritual, and family support, and (e) end-of-life care [21]. Observational evidence shows no apparent net survival or quality of life benefit of dialysis compared to CKM among the oldest individuals with major comorbid conditions [22–25]. CKM can be offered to patients who elect or are medically advised not to pursue KRT; also, as a choice-restricted option if KRT is not available.

Knowledge and utilization of CKM vary substantially. In a survey of 40 nationally representative French renal clinics, nephrologists reported CKM was widely available and easily discussed. However, CKM was an infrequent option for older patients, who said they needed to be made aware of this option. A person or team responsible for CKM and precise information was critical to CKM implementation [26]. In another survey of US nephrologists, only 37% reported routinely discussing CKM with their patients [27].

Regarding the availability of CKM, in a study conducted by the International Society of Nephrology of 150 countries comprising most of the world's population, 81% ($n = 124$) of the countries reported offering CKM. Although there was no association between country-income level and offering CKM, only 38% of countries said that CKM services were readily available. 46% and 36% of countries reported utilization of multidisciplinary teams and shared decision-making, and 26% reported offering CKM training to their healthcare professionals [28].

Despite the above caveats, registry data from Australia and Canada suggests that "untreated" kidney failure is becoming increasingly common in patients aged ≥75, but there are differences among countries. In a study of ESKD patients aged ≥85, 41% began dialysis in the United States, compared to only 7% in Canada and less than 5% in Australia and New Zealand [29–31]. However, it is essential to note that "untreated" kidney failure does not necessarily mean that patients received full CKM. Many gaps, including lack of uniform CKM terminology, methodological issues of studies evaluating outcomes, shortcomings of available prognostic tools, and lack of knowledge and availability of CKM services, limit current information about CKM use [21].

Acute Kidney Disease

Acute kidney disease is increasingly common in the elderly. Fees et al. reported a three-to eight-fold, progressive, age-dependent increase in the frequency of development of community-acquired acute kidney injury (AKI) in patients older than 60. The 2021 USRDS Annual Data Report showed that among individuals aged ≥66 years, the annual adjusted rate for first hospitalization with AKI increased 42% between 2009 and 2019, from 36.1 to 51.3 admissions per 1000 person-year. The adjusted hospitalization rate for AKI requiring dialysis was 2.3 admissions per 1000 person-year. Patients hospitalized with AKI were much more likely to be ≥75 years old than those 66–74 years old [14]. Several factors contribute to the increased risk, including (a) age-related structural and functional changes of the kidneys, (b) high frequency of comorbidities, (c) exposure to medications and interventions that may be potentially nephrotoxic or alter kidney function, and d) alterations in drug metabolism and clearance associated with aging [32].

Regarding causes, prerenal factors are the leading cause of AKI in the general geriatric population, and acute tubular necrosis is the most frequent form of intrinsic AKI. Acute interstitial nephritis due to medications and postrenal causes is also frequent in this population [33]. AKI is associated with a higher risk of mortality and development of CKD and dialysis dependency in the elderly. Data from the

USRDS indicate that the in-hospital mortality for patients older than 66 who had a first AKI hospitalization was 8.2% compared to 1.8% for non-AKI hospitalizations. Moreover, the cumulative probability of a recurrent AKI hospitalization within 1 year was 36%, and 30.8% developed CKD in the year following the AKI hospitalization. The risk of developing kidney failure after an AKI episode is substantially higher in patients with underlying CKD [14]. Lastly, mortality rates in elderly patients admitted to the intensive care unit are over 50%.

Glomerular Diseases

As the general population ages, the prevalence of glomerular diseases (GDs) in the elderly increases and faces significant diagnostic and therapeutic challenges. A shorter life expectancy, multiple comorbid conditions, potential complications of a kidney biopsy, and side effects of immunosuppressive medications contribute to the complexity of managing these patients. The epidemiology of GDs varies among countries due to differences in ethnic predisposition, approaches to indications of kidney biopsy, and methods used in epidemiological studies. Information usually derives from biopsy or glomerulonephritis (GN) registries and single-center data. In most countries, membranous nephropathy (MN) is the leading cause of primary GN and nephrotic syndrome in the elderly. Minimal change disease (MCD) and focal and segmental glomerulosclerosis are other frequent causes of nephrotic syndrome. Pauci-immune crescentic GN is also very common and reportedly the leading GN in the United States in this age group. IgA nephropathy and membranoproliferative GN are also frequent causes of nephritic syndrome. AKI often accompanies the nephrotic syndrome, particularly in patients with MN or MCD. Multiple myeloma and amyloidosis are common secondary causes of GN. Older patients generally respond well to treatment, but therapeutic decisions about immunosuppressants are difficult due to patient-related factors and limited clinical trial evidence of the risk-benefit of therapy in this patient population [34–37].

References

1. Kidney Disease: Improving Global Outcomes CKD Workgroup. KDIGO 2012 Clinical practice guideline for the evaluation and management of chronic kidney disease. Kidney Inter Suppl. 2013;3:1–150.
2. Delanaye P. Too much nephrology? The CKD epidemic is real and concerning. A CON view. Nephrol Dial Transplant. 2019;34(4):581–4.
3. Gansevoort RT. Too much nephrology? The CKD epidemic is real and concerning. A PRO view. Nephrol Dial Transplant. 2019;34(4):577–80.
4. Glassock RJ, Delanaye P, Rule AD. Should the definition of CKD be changed to include age-adapted GFR criteria? YES Kidney Int Suppl. 2020;97(1):34–7.

5. Levey AS, Inker LA, Coresh J. "should the definition of CKD be changed to include age-adapted GFR criteria?": con: the evaluation and management of CKD, not the definition, should be age-adapted. Kidney Int Suppl. 2020;97(1):37–40.
6. Ebert N, Jakob O, Gaedeke J, van der Giet M, Kuhlmann MK, Martus P, et al. Prevalence of reduced kidney function and albuminuria in older adults: the Berlin initiative study. Nephrol Dialy Trans. 2016;32(6):997–1005.
7. Denic A, Glassock R, Rule A. The kidney in Normal aging. Clin J Am Soc Nephrol. 2021;17:137.
8. Delanaye P, Jager KJ, Bokenkamp A, Christensson A, Dubourg L, Eriksen BO, et al. CKD: a call for an age-adapted definition. J Am Soc Nephrol. 2019;30(10):1785–805.
9. O'Hare AM, Rodriguez RA, Rule AD. Overdiagnosis of chronic kidney Disease in older adults-an inconvenient truth. JAMA Intern Med. 2021;181(10):1366–8.
10. Hill NR, Fatoba ST, Oke JL, Hirst JA, O'Callaghan CA, Lasserson DS, et al. Global prevalence of chronic kidney disease—a systematic review and meta-analysis. PLoS One. 2016;11(7):e0158765.
11. Mills KT, Xu Y, Zhang W, Bundy JD, Chen CS, Kelly TN, et al. A systematic analysis of worldwide population-based data on the global burden of chronic kidney disease in 2010. Kidney Int Suppl. 2015;88(5):950–7.
12. Bruck K, Stel VS, Gambaro G, Hallan S, Volzke H, Arnlov J, et al. CKD prevalence varies across the European general population. J Am Soc Nephrol. 2016;27(7):2135–47.
13. Centers for Disease Control and Prevention. Chronic Kidney Disease Surveillance System—United States. http://www.cdc.gov/ckd. Accessed 28 Dec 2023.
14. System USRD. 2021 USRDS annual data report: epidemiology of kidney disease in the United States. Bethesda, MD: National Institutes of Health, National Institute of Diabetes and Digestive and Kidney Diseases; 2021.
15. Corsonello A, Freiberger E, Lattanzio F. The screening for chronic kidney disease among older people across Europe (SCOPE) project: findings from cross-sectional analysis. BMC Geriatr. 2020;20(Suppl 1):316.
16. Ravani P, Quinn R, Fiocco M, Liu P, Al-Wahsh H, Lam N, et al. Association of age with Risk of kidney failure in adults with stage IV chronic kidney Disease in Canada. JAMA Netw Open. 2020;3(9):e2017150.
17. Boenink R, Astley ME, Huijben JA, Stel VS, Kerschbaum J, Ots-Rosenberg M, et al. The ERA registry annual report 2019: summary and age comparisons. Clin Kidney J. 2022;15(3):452–72.
18. United States Renal Data System. 2018 USRDS annual data report: epidemiology of kidney disease in the United States. Bethesda, MD: National Institutes of Health, National Institute of Diabetes and Digestive and Kidney Diseases; 2018.
19. Murphy E, Germain MJ, Cairns H, Higginson IJ, Murtagh FE. International variation in classification of dialysis withdrawal: a systematic review. Nephrol Dial Transplant. 2014;29(3):625–35.
20. Wetmore JB, Yan H, Hu Y, Gilbertson DT, Liu J. Factors associated with withdrawal from maintenance dialysis: a case-control analysis. Am J Kidney Dis. 2018;71(6):831–41.
21. Harris DCH, Davies SJ, Finkelstein FO, Jha V, Bello AK, Brown M, et al. Strategic plan for integrated care of patients with kidney failure. Kidney Int. 2020;98(5):S117–S34.
22. Brown MA, Collett GK, Josland EA, Foote C, Li Q, Brennan FP. CKD in elderly patients managed without dialysis: survival, symptoms, and quality of life. Clin J Am Soc Nephrol. 2015;10(2):260–8.
23. Chandna SM, Da Silva-Gane M, Marshall C, Warwicker P, Greenwood RN, Farrington K. Survival of elderly patients with stage 5 CKD: comparison of conservative management and renal replacement therapy. Nephrol Dial Transplant. 2011;26(5):1608–14.
24. Hussain JA, Mooney A, Russon L. Comparison of survival analysis and palliative care involvement in patients aged over 70 years choosing conservative management or renal replacement therapy in advanced chronic kidney disease. Palliat Med. 2013;27(9):829–39.

25. Murtagh FE, Marsh JE, Donohoe P, Ekbal NJ, Sheerin NS, Harris FE. Dialysis or not? A comparative survival study of patients over 75 years with chronic kidney disease stage 5. Nephrol Dial Transplant. 2007;22(7):1955–62.
26. Hamroun A, Speyer E, Ayav C, Combe C, Fouque D, Jacquelinet C, et al. Barriers to conservative care from patients' and nephrologists' perspectives: the CKD-REIN study. Nephrol Dial Transplant. 2022;37(12):2438–48.
27. Ladin K, Pandya R, Kannam A, Loke R, Oskoui T, Perrone RD, et al. Discussing conservative management with older patients with CKD: an interview study of nephrologists. Am J Kidney Dis. 2018;71(5):627–35.
28. Bello AK, Levin A, Lunney M, Osman MA, Ye F, Ashuntantang GE, et al. Status of care for end stage kidney disease in countries and regions worldwide: international cross sectional survey. BMJ. 2019;367:l5873.
29. Hemmelgarn BR, James MT, Manns BJ, O'Hare AM, Muntner P, Ravani P, et al. Rates of treated and untreated kidney failure in older vs younger adults. JAMA. 2012;307(23):2507–15.
30. Sparke C, Moon L, Green F, Mathew T, Cass A, Chadban S, et al. Estimating the total incidence of kidney failure in Australia including individuals who are not treated by dialysis or transplantation. Am J Kidney Dis. 2013;61(3):413–9.
31. Wong SP, Hebert PL, Laundry RJ, Hammond KW, Liu CF, Burrows NR, et al. Decisions about renal replacement therapy in patients with advanced kidney Disease in the US Department of veterans affairs, 2000-2011. Clin J Am Soc Nephrol. 2016;11(10):1825–33.
32. Coca SG. Acute kidney injury in elderly persons. Am J Kidney Dis. 2010;56(1):122–31.
33. Abdel-Kader K, Palevsky PM. Acute kidney injury in the elderly. Clin Geriatr Med. 2009;25(3):331–58.
34. Chen Y, Li P, Cui C, Yuan A, Zhang K, Yu C. Biopsy-proven kidney diseases in the elderly: clinical characteristics, renal histopathological spectrum and prognostic factors. J Int Med Res. 2016;44(5):1092–102.
35. Glassock RJ. An update on glomerular disease in the elderly. Clin Geriatr Med. 2013;29(3):579–91.
36. Molnar A, Thomas MJ, Fintha A, Kardos M, Dobi D, Tisler A, et al. Kidney biopsy-based epidemiologic analysis shows growing biopsy rate among the elderly. Sci Rep. 2021;11(1):24479.
37. Sumnu A, Gursu M, Ozturk S. Primary glomerular diseases in the elderly. World J Nephrol. 2015;4(2):263–70.

Chapter 3
Nephron Senescence and Mechanisms

Helen Healy, Andrew J. Kassianos, Monica S. Y. Ng, and Eoin D. O'Sullivan

Take Home Points
1. Senescence is a specific cellular process that is distinct from aging.
2. Senescent cells in the kidney may drive fibrosis and inflammation.
3. Removal of senescent cells shows promise as a therapeutic pathway in both acute and chronic kidney disease.

Helen Healy and Andrew J. Kassianos contributed equally with all other contributors.

H. Healy · A. J. Kassianos
Conjoint Internal Medicine Laboratory, Chemical Pathology, Pathology Queensland, Brisbane, QLD, Australia

Kidney Health Service, Royal Brisbane and Women's Hospital, Brisbane, QLD, Australia

Faculty of Medicine, University of Queensland, Brisbane, QLD, Australia

M. S. Y. Ng
Conjoint Internal Medicine Laboratory, Chemical Pathology, Pathology Queensland, Brisbane, QLD, Australia

Kidney Health Service, Royal Brisbane and Women's Hospital, Brisbane, QLD, Australia

Faculty of Medicine, University of Queensland, Brisbane, QLD, Australia

Institute of Molecular Biosciences, University of Queensland, Brisbane, QLD, Australia

Department of Nephrology, Princess Alexandra Hospital, Brisbane, QLD, Australia

E. D. O'Sullivan (✉)
Kidney Health Service, Royal Brisbane and Women's Hospital, Brisbane, QLD, Australia

Department of Renal Medicine, Royal Infirmary of Edinburgh, Edinburgh, UK

QIMR Berghofer Medical Research Institute, Brisbane, Australia

H. Kramer et al. (eds.), *Kidney Disease in the Elderly*,
https://doi.org/10.1007/978-3-031-68460-9_3

Introduction

Contemporary definitions of aging emphasize a time dependant progressive decline in normal organ functions and impairment of biological pathways that have been preserved across evolution for host survival [1]. This chapter explores the proposition that senescence in the kidney is more than just the chronological organ age but also encompasses the cellular phenotype that results after accumulating a range of cellular insults that result in undesirable effects on the kidney tissue and impaired function.

Aging is characterized by altered molecular pathways driven by both intracellular and extracellular factors. These pro-aging factors are summarized in Fig. 3.1, alongside an overview of the resulting changes to the kidney. Heterogeneity in organ aging and senescence exists within populations. Drivers of organ aging and cellular senescence, and their interactions, are dynamic and vary across an individual's lifespan. It leads to the preservation of kidney function into advanced age in some individuals, but not in others.

The term senescence derives from the Latin word "senex" meaning old and continues to be used in this sense in common language. It was originally used by biologists interchangeably with the term aging to describe the decline in organ function over time. This led to confusion in the early literature, with organismal aging and cellular senescence used indiscriminately before the biology of senescence was described. The need to delineate senescence from aging is succinctly summarized by George C. Williams in 1957: No one would consider a man in his thirties senile, yet, according to athletic records and life tables, senescence is rampant during this decade [2].

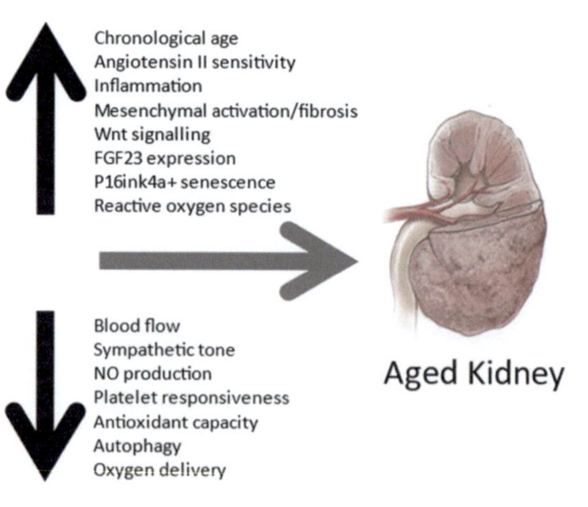

Fig. 3.1 Causes and consequences of kidney aging

Senescence has a different and precise meaning at the level of our cells. Leonard Hayflick published the seminal paper on senescence in 1961, describing the loss of cellular replicative features, i.e., changes are irreversible, based on his observations of long-term in vitro cell cultures. Cellular senescence is a state of permanent growth arrest and cessation of cell division [3]. The key biological feature of cellular senescence is the cell permanently exits cell cycling. It is accompanied by a distinct set of phenotypical alterations, metabolic reprogramming and altered secretomes, known as the senescence-associated secretory phenotype or SASP. Senescent cells accumulate following triggers from either inside the cell (e.g. telomere shortening) and/or outside the cell (e.g., post-injury in a range of diseases). Senescence is a non-negotiable biological process protecting survival of the organism. However, it may not be desirable at the level of specific tissue. While vital for embryogenesis or wound healing, for example, a senescent cell may be detrimental to health in other contexts, where the senescent cell triggers inflammation, accelerates the processes of aging and promotes tissue fibrosis.

To avoid ambiguity, this chapter will define aging as the loss of tissue and organ function over time [1]. In contrast, senescence is a loss of cell proliferation resulting in canonical changes in cell functioning.

Case Study 1

A 32-year-old man was referred with an asymptomatic 6-month decline of kidney function— eGFR from 75 to 55 mL/min/1.73m^2 with 1.5 g/d proteinuria. He reported an episode of acute kidney injury 3 years ago in the context of salmonella gastroenteritis and kidney function returned to baseline. His history was notable for lymphoblastic leukemia at 10 years, treated with an allogeneic hematopoietic stem cell transplant protocol that included total body irradiation and etoposide conditioning. He was taking ibuprofen 400 mg three times daily and ramipril 5 mg daily for hypertension.

Investigations were unremarkable, with normal-sized kidneys on ultrasound.

A kidney biopsy reported acute tubular injury and chronic changes of glomerulosclerosis in 40% of sampled glomeruli and interstitial fibrosis and tubular atrophy in 30–40% of the cortex. The decline in kidney function was attributed to non-steroid anti-inflammatory drug use and he experienced partial improvement in eGFR (to 62) 3 months after stopping ibuprofen. Further staining of biopsy tissue showed increased numbers of cortical senescent tubular and endothelial cells and dramatically increased senescence-associated beta-galactosidase (SA-β-gal) staining and p21/p16^{INK4a} immunofluorescence relative to age-matched control kidney. Case 1 demonstrates the aging-associated morphology of the kidney does not always reflect chronological age. In this case, the injury-associated aging and premature senescence were likely the outcome of the earlier kidney hit of total body irradiation and chemotherapy. His senescent cell burden is high which may lead to increased acute kidney injury risk and poorer post-injury recovery and progression to chronic kidney disease.

Aging and Senescence Reciprocity

The role of cellular senescence in the biology of aging in vivo is complex and continues to be debated in the presence of emerging literature. Many of the biomarkers of senescence (i.e., increased p16^{INK4a} expression, molecules of the SASP) are also found in aging tissue [4, 5]. The co-expression may, in part, be a consequence of stem cell senescence. As somatic cells reach the end of their replicative lifespan or are damaged and removed from tissue, they are replenished from a stem cell pool. A feature of aging is a reduced stem cell pool and tissue reconstitution is consequently compromised. Supporting this concept, depleting the SRY-box transcription factor 2 (Sox2$^+$) stem cell pool in mice promotes both cellular senescence and premature aging [6].

Senescence is increased in models of aging. For example, p16^{INK4a}, a cell cycle protein that slows progression from G1 to S phase of the cell cycle, is increased in the presence of stem cell senescence and tissue dysfunction in the brain, bone marrow, and pancreas [7–9]. p16^{INK4a} is increased in the BubR1 mutant mouse model in which skeletal muscle and adipose tissue develop premature aging-associated phenotypes. The changes can be mitigated by either genetic inactivation of p16^{INK4} or inducible elimination of p16^{INK4a}-expressing cells [10, 11]. Collectively, the data report that some tissue features of aging are driven by cell cycle arrest, a key characteristic of senescent cells.

In addition to p16^{INK4a} expression, circulating concentrations of SASP proteins have been identified as candidate biomarkers of age and exposure to medical risk in humans. A pre-specified panel of 7 SASP proteins (growth differentiation factor 15 (GDF15), tumor necrosis factor (TNF) receptor superfamily member 6 (FAS), osteopontin (OPN), TNF receptor 1 (TNFR1), ACTIVIN A, chemokine (C-C motif) ligand 3 (CCL3), and Interleukin-15) predict biologically significant age-related adverse events (higher frailty score, adverse post-operative outcomes) better than a single SASP protein or chronological age [12]. SASP proteins are an exciting area of biomarker and prognostic research.

Biology of Cellular Senescence: Mechanisms and Associated Pathways

Multiple cellular stressors induce senescence are summarized in Fig. 3.2. Different stressors trigger distinct pathways to senescence, but the majority culminate in induction of one or both of the cyclin-dependent kinase inhibitor checkpoint proteins, p16^{INK4a} and p53/p21cip1. Upregulated inhibitor checkpoint activity down-modulates downstream cyclin-dependant kinases 2, D, 4 and 6 [13, 14] and their regulation of the cell cycle, i.e., inhibits cell cycling. The cell cycle arrests at the G1/S checkpoint and the cell assumes the senescent phenotype. Typical senescent cells have a flat and large cellular morphology, intracellular vacuoles, positive

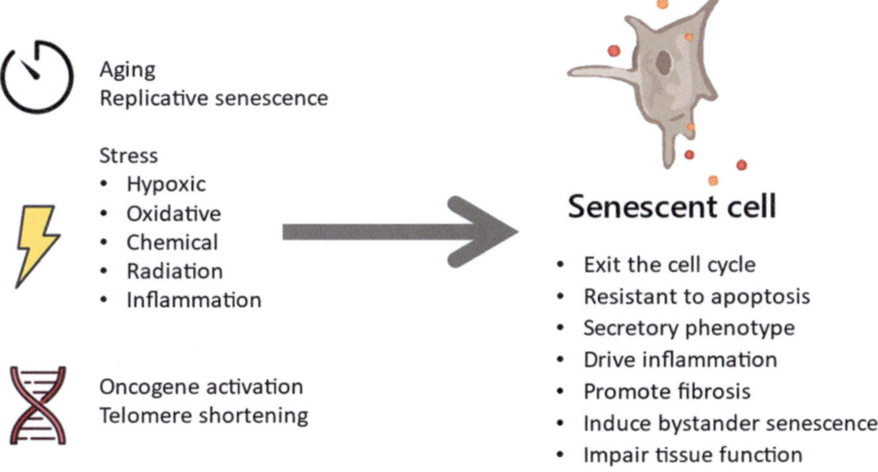

Fig. 3.2 Key drivers of senescence and characteristics of senescent cells

staining for the senescence-associated β-galactosidase (SA-β-gal), p21 and/or p16 and accumulation of p53 [15].

p53 (also known as the guardian of the genome and many other names) is a master regulator of cell cycling. It programs cell fate, e.g., senescence in the context of short telomeres, apoptosis in the context of irreparable DNA damage, etc. p53 undergoes unique posttranslational modifications in senescent cells that confer resistance to the apoptosis fate [16]. The resistance of senescent cells to apoptosis is a key characteristic and results in the accumulation and persistence of senescent cells in tissue.

The Senescence-Associated Secretory Phenotype (SASP)

Another key characteristic of senescent cells is the distinct set of bioactive substances (soluble proteins, lipids, nucleic acids, and miRNAs) they secrete into the extracellular space. Collectively, these molecules are described as the senescence-associated secretory phenotype (SASP) [17]. The composition or signature of the SASP varies depending on the cell of origin, the stimulus, and the time that has elapsed since induction of the senescent phenotype. There are over 200 documented proteins in the SASP [18], and Fig. 3.3 gives an overview of the broad effects of the SASP in vivo with examples of responsible components.

Combinations of these components explain the great heterogeneity of SASP signatures, datasets so large that researchers are turning to computer-based '-omics' methodologies to handle their size and for in silico deconvolutional analyses to assign pathway functionality. SASP bioactive proteins, like the soluble cytokines

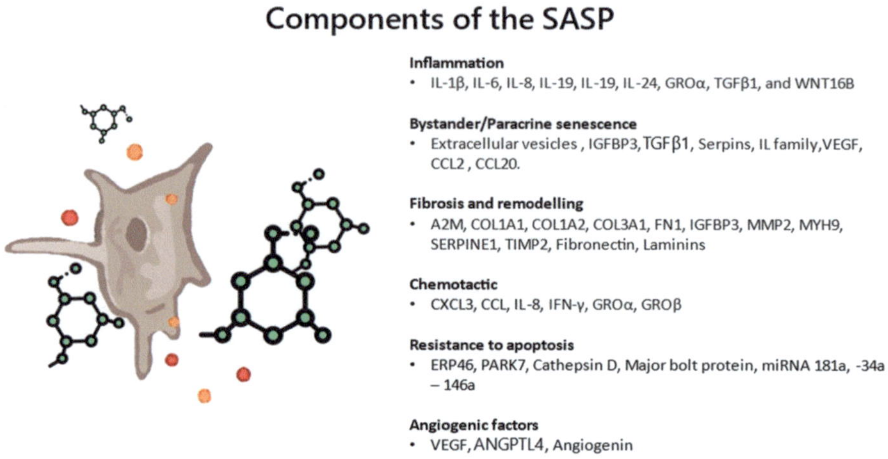

Fig. 3.3 The SASP is responsible for propagation of senescence in tissues, inflammation and remodeling. A selection of some key SASP components and associated pathways are presented

interleukin (IL)-6, IL-8, and transforming growth factor (TGF)-β, act in both a paracrine and autocrine fashion, leading to inflammation and propagation of the senescent state in the cell's environmental niche [19]. SASP bioactive molecules trigger a wide array of biological effects, e.g., lipid prostaglandin E2 suppresses anti-tumor immunity in certain contexts, etc. [20].

The heterogeneity of SASP signatures conceals deep redundancy, with different SASPs replicating functions that are highly conserved across contexts. Such conserved functions include induction of pro-inflammatory pathways (e.g., immune cell attraction and activation), modulation of the regulation of cell proliferation, wound healing, and an incompletely understood role in post-injury fibrosis and tissue repair [21–24].

Senescent cells may not replicate but they do have capacity to remodel their environmental niche via SASP-mediated paracrine effects, a phenomenon known as bystander senescence [25, 26]. Bystander senescence is observed in human bronchial epithelial cells (↑ SA-β-gal, ↑ p21) exposed to the serum from patients with chronic obstructive pulmonary disease [27]. In vitro murine tumor cell line studies show that docetaxel-induced senescence results in the classic combination of growth arrest, SA-β-gal staining, increase of the cyclin-dependent kinase inhibitor p21 and a SASP signature that induces bystander senescence [28]. T helper 1 cytokines (interferon (IFN)-γ and tumor necrosis factor (TNF)-α) added to the cultures do not alter the characteristic features of cellular senescence (i.e., proliferation arrest, morphological changes and increased p21), but do interrupt bystander senescence. The senescent cells retain the starter malignant phenotype and are able to subsequently form tumors in vivo [28]. A landmark 2018 paper reported bystander senescence can be transplanted, using senescent preadipocytes injected into mice, resulting in physical dysfunction and decreased survival [29].

Collectively, these findings highlight that the senescent phenotype is preserved across cell lines/models and senescence inducers. Importantly, the authors of the landmark paper also provide proof-of-concept evidence that senolytic agents (i.e., dasatanib and quercetin), cell therapy that selectively eliminates senescent cells, prevents the emergence of the bystander senescence phenomenon in transplanted hosts [29].

Aging and Senescence Reciprocity in the Kidney

The pathobiology of aging of the kidney is a maze of multiple and redundant processes of complex cellular/molecular check-points, like the cell cycle regulators, senescence-associated pathways, etc. [30]. The morphological changes of aging in the kidney include a decline in the total size and number of the basic functional units of the kidney, the nephron-rarefaction of endothelial cells, glomerulosclerosis, and tubulointerstitial changes [31–34]. The latter two represent the loss of specialized kidney cells and the accumulation of fibrosis. As nephrons drop out, the glomerular filtration rate (GFR) declines. Age-related decline in GFR is of the order of 0.5–1.5 mL/min/1.73m^2 body surface area per annum [30, 35]. Other nephron functions, like free water clearance, homeostatic control of electrolytes, metabolic bone balance, erythropoiesis functions, etc., begin to decline as GFR drops below 60 mL/min/1.73m^2, irrespective of the cause of loss of GFR [30, 36]. Collectively, these age-related structural and functional alterations result in less robust survival responses and increased susceptibility to subsequent injury inducers, leading to acute kidney injury (AKI) and chronic kidney disease (CKD) in the older kidney [30, 37, 38].

Senescent cells accumulate in the kidney, particularly in the cortex, in response to both aging and injury. The senescent cell burden and expression of the p16^{INK4a} and p53 biomarkers correlate with the age-related histopathological alterations of glomerulosclerosis, interstitial fibrosis, and tubular atrophy and with functional decline, resulting in poor clinical outcomes [18, 39–41]. p16^{INK4a} is expressed by almost all cell types of the cortex of the aging human kidney (tubular, glomerular, interstitial, vascular cells), but expression is highest in tubular cells [40].

The mitochondrial-rich tubular epithelium is a preferred epicenter of kidney senescence, exquisitely responsive to hypoxia and oxidative stressors delivered through pathways like age-related vascular changes [42]. A seminal 2016 study deleting p16^{INK4a}-positive cells by transgenic engineering to produce INK-ATTAC transgenic mice [43] is compelling. The investigators show age-related senescence localized to the proximal tubules. Moreover, they suggest that senescent tubular cells propagate pathological changes in the associated environmental niches, encompassing glomeruli (i.e., glomerulosclerosis), via production of SASP signatures that hyperactivate the local renin-angiotensin-aldosterone system [43]. The propagation of SASP-mediated bystander senescence throughout the tubulointerstitial compartment is confirmed in a mouse allogeneic transplant model where senescent (irradiated) tubular cells injected systemically into healthy recipients engraft into the kidneys that then develop higher burdens of inflammation, microvascular dropout and fibrosis [44].

Case 2 Senescence in the Diseased Kidney

A 65-year-old woman underwent left nephrectomy for renal cell carcinoma discovered after investigations for hematuria. Her kidney function measured by eGFR was 72 mL/min/1.73m^2 pre-operatively. Histology of the lesion was consistent with encapsulated clear cell renal cell carcinoma with no vascular nor lymphatic invasion. eGFR was 30 mL/min/1.73m^2 post-operatively and, when it had not improved by 6 months, the tissue samples were re-examined. Kidney parenchyma away from the tumor showed arteriosclerosis, interstitial fibrosis in 30% of the cortex, and tubular atrophy (IFTA). The tissue was entered into a local research project and SA-β-gal special staining and p21/p16^{ink4a} immunofluorescence was performed. Her kidney was found to have increased numbers of senescent tubular, endothelial, and mesangial cells relative to aged-matched control kidneys.

The increased age-disproportionate burden of senescent cells in the kidney in this case may explain the failure of kidney hypertrophy and recovery of eGFR after nephrectomy.

Senescence in Kidney Disease

The cellular senescence pathway has been described in the pathobiology of various experimental animal models of kidney diseases and observational studies in human kidney tissue. Senescent cells (SA-β-gal$^+$, p16^{INK4a+} and/or p21$^+$ cells) accumulate in damaged kidneys, predominantly in the cortex. The cell source is usually tubular, but glomerular, interstitial and vascular cells also transition to the senescent state [42]. The type and localization of senescent cells are dependent on the pathophysiological context, the mode of injury and pattern of kidney disease. Typical markers used to identify senescent cells, such as positive p21 staining and SA-β-gal staining, are demonstrated in Fig. 3.4.

Glomerulonephritis

The senescence-associated biomarker p16^{INK4a} is increased in human kidneys with the immune deposition glomerular diseases of membranous nephropathy, IgA nephropathy, and focal segmental glomerular sclerosis (FSGS) compared to age-matched controls [45]. Double senescent biomarker staining (p16^{INK4a+}, SA-β-gal$^+$) is reported in glomerular, interstitial, and tubular cells in patients

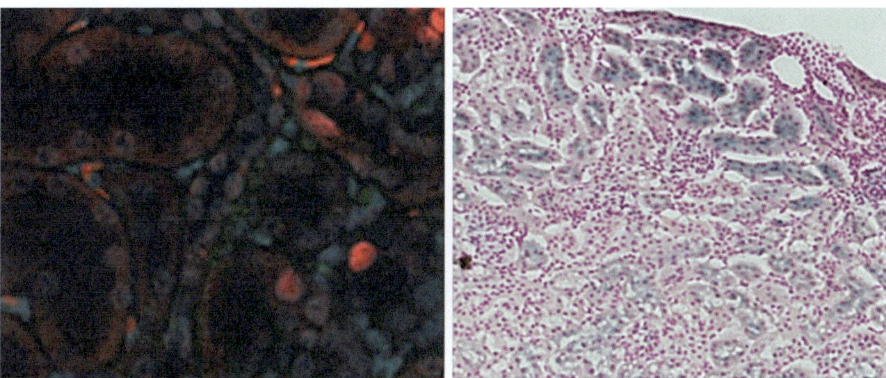

Fig. 3.4   (left) Immunofluorescence demonstrating p21$^+$ nuclei (red) in the tubular epithelium in an aged murine kidney—DAPI = blue, COL1 = green. (right) SA-β-gal staining (blue) of a murine kidney following reversed unilateral ureteric obstructive injury

with minimal change disease (no immune deposits) as well as membranous nephropathy and FSGS, i.e., not dependent on immune deposition pathobiological signaling [46, 47]. p16^{INK4a} expression is higher in the nuclei of glomerular and interstitial cells in human kidneys with glomerular diseases as compared to kidneys with normal aging or tubulointerstitial nephritis [46]. Moreover, increased tubular expression of p16^{INK4a} at the time of initial biopsy is an independent predictor of progression to end-stage kidney failure in the glomerular pattern of FSGS [47]. The data support the concept of senescence triggered by glomerular inflammatory diseases and the accumulation of senescent cells in glomeruli.

Diabetic Kidney Disease

Kidney cellular senescence is also observed in patients with metabolic diseases like diabetes. p16^{INK4a} and SA-β-gal are upregulated in predominantly tubular cells and to a lesser extent podocytes in kidney biopsies of adults with type 2 diabetic kidney disease (DKD) compared to age-matched controls [48]. The increased tubular SA-β-gal correlates with body mass index and blood glucose levels, both systemic drivers of aging as well as cellular senescence. The findings are reproducible in vitro, with proximal tubule cells cultured under high glucose conditions displaying a similar senescent phenotype (↑ p16^{INK4a}, ↑ SA-β-gal) [48]. Mechanisms of senescence were interrogated in streptozotocin-induced diabetic mice, with in vivo evidence that hyperglycaemia causes tubular senescence via a sodium-glucose co-transporter-2 (SGLT2) and p21-dependent pathway [49]. This 2014 finding has a fresh impact on small molecule blockers of the sodium-glucose co-transporter family (SGLT2) pathways now licensed for clinical use.

Kidney Vascular Disease

Vascular disease is one of the most common causes of advanced kidney disease in first-world countries and increasingly across the globe.

The kidney vasculature is a preferential target of acquired cellular senescence. The accumulation of senescent vascular smooth muscle cells (VSMC) in atherosclerotic plaques and areas of calcification correlates with impaired vascular flow and kidney disease progression [50, 51]. Reactive oxygen species (ROS)-mediated Lamin B1 accumulation is posited to be the key mechanistic driver of chronic kidney disease-associated VSMC senescence [52]. A rat model of radiation-induced kidney damage reported prominent senescent biomarker staining (increased p16[+], SA-β-gal activity, p53[+], p21[+] and SASP, particularly IL-6) in vascular endothelial cells [53]. The data expands the evolving maps of the pathobiology in specific patterns of kidney vascular disease to include senescent signaling pathways.

Allograft Nephropathy

Pre- and post-transplant human kidney biopsies offer time-lapsed insights into the role of senescent cells in allograft rejection. As for other kidney diseases, markers of cellular senescence in pre-transplant biopsies (i.e., p16^{INK4a}) predict graft dysfunction and poor long-term outcomes [54, 55]. Similarly, the presence of senescent cells (↑ p16^{INK4a} or SA-β-gal) in post-transplant biopsies significantly correlates with chronic allograft nephropathy (CAN—now defined as "interstitial fibrosis and tubular atrophy without evidence of specific etiology") [45, 56, 57]. Cellular senescence burden in CAN exceeds levels predicted for normal aging, demonstrating CAN is associated with accelerated senescence [45]. The observation of accelerated senescence with CAN is confirmed in experimental animal models. Mice receiving kidney transplants from p16^{INK4a} knock-out mice (i.e., kidneys with a reduced capacity to induce cellular senescence) exhibit lower senescent cell burden, less pathological tubulointerstitial changes, and improved allograft survival compared with wild-type control donor kidneys [58].

Targeting the senescence pathway to inhibit premature senescence in kidney transplantation is a promising therapeutic strategy to prolong graft survival.

Polycystic Kidney Disease

In contrast, autosomal dominant polycystic kidney disease (ADPKD) demonstrates the importance of kidney cellular senescence for organ health. The expression of cell cycle inhibitor and senescence marker p21 is *decreased* in kidneys of people with ADPKD and also in a non-transgenic rat model of ADPKD, resulting in dysregulated tubular epithelial cell proliferation expressed morphologically as expanding cysts [59]. Treatment with the cyclin-dependent kinase inhibitor roscovitine restores p21 expression levels both in vitro and in vivo and attenuates disease progression in a mouse model of ADPKD [59–61]. These findings demonstrate the protective role of senescence in editing excess tissue, in this case tubular cell proliferation, and preventing ADPKD progression in ex utero life. This kidney disease illustrates that not all senescence is deleterious.

Therapeutic Targeting of Cellular Senescence in the Kidney

With some exceptions, current therapeutics that target cellular senescence fail to prevent adverse outcomes across a range of kidney diseases. Best-performing drugs target the hemodynamics of glomerular filtration. The newest of these, the SGLT2 inhibitors, are also thought to act via glomerular hemodynamics, and reduction of insulin levels which mimic a fasting state, but an additional benefit of this drug class is inhibition of the senescence pathway.

Senescent cells are emerging as novel therapeutic targets in diseases characterized by propagation of the phenotype. Pharmacological agents that target senescent cells or senescence-associated pathways are collectively known as "senotherapies" (Fig. 3.5). Senotherapies are broadly divided into two categories: (1) those that selectively eliminate senescent cells (senolytics); and (2) those that suppress pathogenic elements of SASPs (senostatics) [62].

Senolytics: Elimination of Senescent Cells

Senescent cells share the cancer cell characteristics of activation of anti-apoptotic/ pro-survival signaling pathways that resist cell death [63]. Therefore, repurposing existing anticancer drugs that reprogram the apoptotic cell death pathway is a promising approach to eliminating senescent cells in kidney diseases [18]. Senolytic agents that have been used to target senescent cells in vivo and in vitro include: (1) ABT-263 (Navitoclax), an inhibitor of the anti-apoptotic BCL family members BCL-2, BCL-xL, and BCL-W, in ischemia reperfusion injury (IRI), unilateral ureteric injury (UUO), reversed unilateral ureteric injury (R-UUO), aged kidneys, and irradiation-induced injury [64, 65]; (2) Combinational treatment with quercetin and dasatinib that together inhibit a broad spectrum of protein kinases and tyrosine kinases and been shown to reduce senescence in human diabetic kidney disease as well as murine IRI, and cisplatin-induced injury [66, 67]; and (3) The FOXO4-D-Retro-Inverso (FOXO4-DRI) peptide that competes with normal anti-apoptotic FOXO4-p53 binding and depletes senescent cells in aged murine models [68].

Translation of these drugs to the injured or aging kidney is still in its infancy. Allograft nephropathy is one of the kidney diseases where senolytics may offer

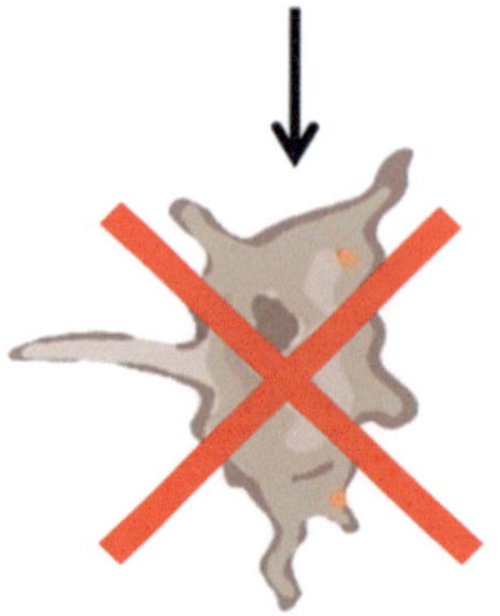

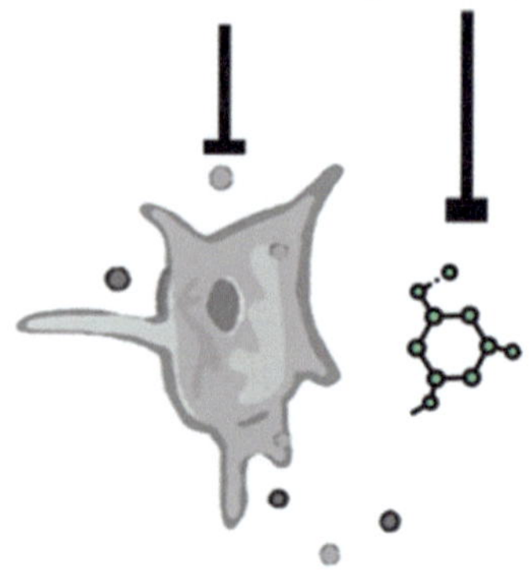

Fig. 3.5 The key difference between senolytics and senostatics with examples of each

significant therapeutic benefits. Treatment of kidney donors with senolytic agents prior to explanting the organ or, alternatively, perfusing the kidney with senolytics after removal may attenuate the accumulation of senescent cells and improve allograft survival [18]. Given that the accumulation of senescent cells depends on the mode of injury [69], senolytic efficacy will need to be examined for each discrete kidney disease pattern.

Gene expression and SASP signatures of individual cells within senescent populations are highly variable [70] and a combined drug approach may be required. The benefits of senolytics extend beyond the specific disease with growing evidence that pharmacological depletion of senescent cells also prevents/delays tissue dysfunction in animal models of aging [11, 68, 71]. Senolytics are an emerging therapeutic field, with the dual benefits of targeting senescent cells and supporting healthy kidney aging.

Modulation of SASP

The disadvantage of the senolytic approach is the lack of reversibility once senescent cells (and associated SASPs) are eliminated. Some bioactive molecules of the SASPs are in fact desirable, as in wound healing post-transplantation [72]. Thus, the clinical need is precision senostatics—agents which target specific deleterious molecule/s of the SASP signature but leave beneficial SASP molecules active. SASP-modulating agents of this order of precision are generally inhibitors of the pro-inflammatory signaling pathways that promote further senescence and fibrosis, including the nuclear factor (NF)-κB, c-Jun N-terminal kinase (JNK), or p38 mitogen-activated protein kinase (MAPK) pathways [73]. A pan-JNK inhibitor (SP600125) reduces the burden of senescent tubular cells, titers of pro-fibrotic TGF-β and the development of fibrosis in a mouse model of ischemic injury [74]. Beyond this publication, experimental assessment of senostatics in the injured or aged kidney remain limited.

The role of senescence as either a cause or consequence or enabler/amplifier of age-related kidney pathology remains a fundamental question. The answers are important because they will direct us to either senotherapeutics and/or molecules targeting other pathobiological signaling pathways in the pursuit of preserving kidney function post-injury and with aging.

Conclusions and Future Directions

In conclusion, senescence and aging are distinct. Aging is a global term used to describe the phenotype of cells, tissues, organ systems, and the organism holistically. Its discriminatory characteristic appears to be telomere length. Senescence, biologically, is limited to cells and its discriminatory characteristic is an irreversible exit from cell cycling. The two pathobiological processes are tightly interconnected. Telomere shortening converts the host cell to a senescent phenotype. A depleted stem cell pool is a shared characteristic of both processes. The two processes have biomarkers in common, e.g., increased p16^{INK4a} expression, SASPs. In the kidney, at least, tissue phenotype is similar, with glomerulosclerosis, vascular endothelial rarefaction and tubulointerstitial atrophy/fibrosis associated with both pathobiological processes. Aging may be viewed as the aggregate of multiple signaling pathways, of which senescence is one.

The mechanism of how the senescent cell burden models surrounding tissue remains incompletely understood, limiting the development of specific therapies. Complicating matters, in vitro studies report senescent cells are highly heterogenous and exhibit varying phenotypes at any given time point and in response to different modes of senescence induction. Even within a tissue, senescent cells express different markers, secrete variable SASP signatures and use different anti-apoptotic escape pathways, suggesting drug combinations are likely more efficacious than single agents.

Despite these barriers, the evidence that pharmacological depletion of senescent cells leads to improved organ function in animal models of aging and disease is growing. Senescence is an exciting field of biology which is increasingly generating enormous funding and research interest. Beyond the hyperbolic headlines, enthusiastic investors and evermore biotech start-ups are filling a field with immense therapeutic potential to help millions of patients.

Acknowledgments The authors would like to thank Marie Docherty, University of Edinburgh, for supplying the immunofluorescence images in Fig. 3.4.

Funding The work was funded by Pathology Queensland and a National Health and Medical Research Council (NHMRC) Project Grant (GNT1161319).

Conflict of Interest The authors declare that they have no conflict of interest.

References

1. Flatt T. A new definition of aging? Front Genet. 2012;3:148.
2. Williams G. Pleiotropy, natural selection, and the evolution of senescence. Evolution (NY). 1957;11:398–411.
3. Di Micco R, Krizhanovsky V, Baker D, d'Adda di Fagagna F. Cellular senescence in ageing: from mechanisms to therapeutic opportunities. Nat Rev Mol Cell Biol. 2021;22(2):75–95.
4. Kim WY, Sharpless NE. The regulation of INK4/ARF in cancer and aging. Cell. 2006;127(2):265–75.
5. Hornsby PJ. Cellular senescence and tissue aging in vivo. J Gerontol A Biol Sci Med Sci. 2002;57(7):B251–6.
6. Vilas JM, Carneiro C, Da Silva-Alvarez S, Ferreiros A, Gonzalez P, Gomez M, et al. Adult Sox2+ stem cell exhaustion in mice results in cellular senescence and premature aging. Aging Cell. 2018;17(5):e12834.
7. Molofsky AV, Slutsky SG, Joseph NM, He S, Pardal R, Krishnamurthy J, et al. Increasing p16INK4a expression decreases forebrain progenitors and neurogenesis during ageing. Nature. 2006;443(7110):448–52.
8. Janzen V, Forkert R, Fleming HE, Saito Y, Waring MT, Dombkowski DM, et al. Stem-cell ageing modified by the cyclin-dependent kinase inhibitor p16INK4a. Nature. 2006;443(7110): 421–6.
9. Krishnamurthy J, Ramsey MR, Ligon KL, Torrice C, Koh A, Bonner-Weir S, et al. p16INK4a induces an age-dependent decline in islet regenerative potential. Nature. 2006;443(7110):453–7.
10. Baker DJ, Perez-Terzic C, Jin F, Pitel KS, Niederlander NJ, Jeganathan K, et al. Opposing roles for p16Ink4a and p19Arf in senescence and ageing caused by BubR1 insufficiency. Nat Cell Biol. 2008;10(7):825–36.
11. Baker DJ, Wijshake T, Tchkonia T, LeBrasseur NK, Childs BG, van de Sluis B, et al. Clearance of p16Ink4a-positive senescent cells delays ageing-associated disorders. Nature. 2011;479(7372):232–6.
12. Schafer MJ, Zhang X, Kumar A, Atkinson EJ, Zhu Y, Jachim S, et al. The senescence-associated secretome as an indicator of age and medical risk. JCI Insight. 2020;5(12):e133668.
13. Munoz-Espin D, Canamero M, Maraver A, Gomez-Lopez G, Contreras J, Murillo-Cuesta S, et al. Programmed cell senescence during mammalian embryonic development. Cell. 2013;155(5):1104–18.
14. Storer M, Mas A, Robert-Moreno A, Pecoraro M, Ortells MC, Di Giacomo V, et al. Senescence is a developmental mechanism that contributes to embryonic growth and patterning. Cell. 2013;155(5):1119–30.
15. Bringold F, Serrano M. Tumor suppressors and oncogenes in cellular senescence. Exp Gerontol. 2000;35(3):317–29.

16. Webley K, Bond JA, Jones CJ, Blaydes JP, Craig A, Hupp T, et al. Posttranslational modifications of p53 in replicative senescence overlapping but distinct from those induced by DNA damage. Mol Cell Biol. 2000;20(8):2803–8.
17. Coppe JP, Desprez PY, Krtolica A, Campisi J. The senescence-associated secretory phenotype: the dark side of tumor suppression. Annu Rev Pathol. 2010;5:99–118.
18. Sturmlechner I, Durik M, Sieben CJ, Baker DJ, van Deursen JM. Cellular senescence in renal ageing and disease. Nat Rev Nephrol. 2017;13(2):77–89.
19. van Deursen JM. The role of senescent cells in ageing. Nature. 2014;509(7501):439–46.
20. Loo TM, Kamachi F, Watanabe Y, Yoshimoto S, Kanda H, Arai Y, et al. Gut microbiota promotes obesity-associated liver cancer through PGE2-mediated suppression of antitumor immunity. Cancer Discov. 2017;7(5):522–38.
21. Jun JI, Lau LF. The matricellular protein CCN1 induces fibroblast senescence and restricts fibrosis in cutaneous wound healing. Nat Cell Biol. 2010;12(7):676–85.
22. Krizhanovsky V, Yon M, Dickins RA, Hearn S, Simon J, Miething C, et al. Senescence of activated stellate cells limits liver fibrosis. Cell. 2008;134(4):657–67.
23. Freund A, Orjalo AV, Desprez PY, Campisi J. Inflammatory networks during cellular senescence: causes and consequences. Trends Mol Med. 2010;16(5):238–46.
24. Coppe JP, Kauser K, Campisi J, Beausejour CM. Secretion of vascular endothelial growth factor by primary human fibroblasts at senescence. J Biol Chem. 2006;281(40):29568–74.
25. Hubackova S, Krejcikova K, Bartek J, Hodny Z. IL1-and TGFbeta-Nox4 signaling, oxidative stress and DNA damage response are shared features of replicative, oncogene-induced, and drug-induced paracrine 'bystander senescence'. Aging (Albany NY). 2012;4(12):932–51.
26. Nelson G, Wordsworth J, Wang C, Jurk D, Lawless C, Martin-Ruiz C, et al. A senescent cell bystander effect: senescence-induced senescence. Aging Cell. 2012;11(2):345–9.
27. Kuznar-Kaminska B, Mikula-Pietrasik J, Witucka A, Romaniuk A, Konieczna N, Rubis B, et al. Serum from patients with chronic obstructive pulmonary disease induces senescence-related phenotype in bronchial epithelial cells. Sci Rep. 2018;8(1):12940.
28. Sapega O, Mikyskova R, Bieblova J, Mrazkova B, Hodny Z, Reinis M. Distinct phenotypes and 'bystander' effects of senescent tumour cells induced by docetaxel or immunomodulatory cytokines. Int J Oncol. 2018;53(5):1997–2009.
29. Xu M, Pirtskhalava T, Farr JN, Weigand BM, Palmer AK, Weivoda MM, et al. Senolytics improve physical function and increase lifespan in old age. Nat Med. 2018;24(8):1246–56.
30. O'Sullivan ED, Hughes J, Ferenbach DA. Renal aging: causes and consequences. J Am Soc Nephrol. 2017;28(2):407–20.
31. Tan H, Xu J, Liu Y. Ageing, cellular senescence and chronic kidney disease: experimental evidence. Curr Opin Nephrol Hypertens. 2022;31(3):235–43.
32. Newbold KM, Sandison A, Howie AJ. Comparison of size of juxtamedullary and outer cortical glomeruli in normal adult kidney. Virchows Arch A Pathol Anat Histopathol. 1992;420(2):127–9.
33. Nyengaard JR, Bendtsen TF. Glomerular number and size in relation to age, kidney weight, and body surface in normal man. Anat Rec. 1992;232(2):194–201.
34. Hommos MS, Glassock RJ, Rule AD. Structural and functional changes in human kidneys with healthy aging. J Am Soc Nephrol. 2017;28(10):2838–44.
35. Lindeman RD, Tobin J, Shock NW. Longitudinal studies on the rate of decline in renal function with age. J Am Geriatr Soc. 1985;33(4):278–85.
36. Glassock RJ, Winearls C. Ageing and the glomerular filtration rate: truths and consequences. Trans Am Clin Climatol Assoc. 2009;120:419–28.
37. Stevens LA, Viswanathan G, Weiner DE. Chronic kidney disease and end-stage renal disease in the elderly population: current prevalence, future projections, and clinical significance. Adv Chronic Kidney Dis. 2010;17(4):293–301.
38. Schmitt R, Cantley LG. The impact of aging on kidney repair. Am J Physiol Renal Physiol. 2008;294(6):F1265–72.
39. Ferenbach DA, Bonventre JV. Mechanisms of maladaptive repair after AKI leading to accelerated kidney ageing and CKD. Nat Rev Nephrol. 2015;11(5):264–76.

40. Melk A, Schmidt BM, Takeuchi O, Sawitzki B, Rayner DC, Halloran PF. Expression of p16INK4a and other cell cycle regulator and senescence associated genes in aging human kidney. Kidney Int. 2004;65(2):510–20.
41. Chkhotua AB, Gabusi E, Altimari A, D'Errico A, Yakubovich M, Vienken J, et al. Increased expression of p16(INK4a) and p27(Kip1) cyclin-dependent kinase inhibitor genes in aging human kidney and chronic allograft nephropathy. Am J Kidney Dis. 2003;41(6):1303–13.
42. Valentijn FA, Falke LL, Nguyen TQ, Goldschmeding R. Cellular senescence in the aging and diseased kidney. J Cell Commun Signal. 2018;12(1):69–82.
43. Baker DJ, Childs BG, Durik M, Wijers ME, Sieben CJ, Zhong J, et al. Naturally occurring p16(Ink4a)-positive cells shorten healthy lifespan. Nature. 2016;530(7589):184–9.
44. Kim SR, Jiang K, Ferguson CM, Tang H, Chen X, Zhu X, et al. Transplanted senescent renal scattered tubular-like cells induce injury in the mouse kidney. Am J Physiol Renal Physiol. 2020;318(5):F1167–F76.
45. Melk A, Schmidt BM, Vongwiwatana A, Rayner DC, Halloran PF. Increased expression of senescence-associated cell cycle inhibitor p16INK4a in deteriorating renal transplants and diseased native kidney. Am J Transplant. 2005;5(6):1375–82.
46. Sis B, Tasanarong A, Khoshjou F, Dadras F, Solez K, Halloran PF. Accelerated expression of senescence associated cell cycle inhibitor p16INK4A in kidneys with glomerular disease. Kidney Int. 2007;71(3):218–26.
47. Verzola D, Saio M, Picciotto D, Viazzi F, Russo E, Cipriani L, et al. Cellular senescence is associated with faster progression of focal segmental glomerulosclerosis. Am J Nephrol. 2020;51(12):950–8.
48. Verzola D, Gandolfo MT, Gaetani G, Ferraris A, Mangerini R, Ferrario F, et al. Accelerated senescence in the kidneys of patients with type 2 diabetic nephropathy. Am J Physiol Renal Physiol. 2008;295(5):F1563–73.
49. Kitada K, Nakano D, Ohsaki H, Hitomi H, Minamino T, Yatabe J, et al. Hyperglycemia causes cellular senescence via a SGLT2-and p21-dependent pathway in proximal tubules in the early stage of diabetic nephropathy. J Diabetes Complicat. 2014;28(5):604–11.
50. Matthews C, Gorenne I, Scott S, Figg N, Kirkpatrick P, Ritchie A, et al. Vascular smooth muscle cells undergo telomere-based senescence in human atherosclerosis: effects of telomerase and oxidative stress. Circ Res. 2006;99(2):156–64.
51. Kovacic JC, Moreno P, Hachinski V, Nabel EG, Fuster V. Cellular senescence, vascular disease, and aging: part 1 of a 2-part review. Circulation. 2011;123(15):1650–60.
52. Wang X, Bi X, Yang K, Huang Y, Liu Y, Zhao J. ROS/p38MAPK-induced Lamin B1 accumulation promotes chronic kidney disease-associated vascular smooth muscle cells senescence. Biochem Biophys Res Commun. 2020;531(2):187–94.
53. Aratani S, Tagawa M, Nagasaka S, Sakai Y, Shimizu A, Tsuruoka S. Radiation-induced premature cellular senescence involved in glomerular diseases in rats. Sci Rep. 2018;8(1):16812.
54. McGlynn LM, Stevenson K, Lamb K, Zino S, Brown M, Prina A, et al. Cellular senescence in pretransplant renal biopsies predicts postoperative organ function. Aging Cell. 2009;8(1):45–51.
55. Koppelstaetter C, Schratzberger G, Perco P, Hofer J, Mark W, Ollinger R, et al. Markers of cellular senescence in zero hour biopsies predict outcome in renal transplantation. Aging Cell. 2008;7(4):491–7.
56. Ferlicot S, Durrbach A, Ba N, Desvaux D, Bedossa P, Paradis V. The role of replicative senescence in chronic allograft nephropathy. Hum Pathol. 2003;34(9):924–8.
57. Halloran PF, Melk A, Barth C. Rethinking chronic allograft nephropathy: the concept of accelerated senescence. J Am Soc Nephrol. 1999;10(1):167–81.
58. Braun H, Schmidt BM, Raiss M, Baisantry A, Mircea-Constantin D, Wang S, et al. Cellular senescence limits regenerative capacity and allograft survival. J Am Soc Nephrol. 2012;23(9):1467–73.
59. Park JY, Schutzer WE, Lindsley JN, Bagby SP, Oyama TT, Anderson S, et al. p21 is decreased in polycystic kidney disease and leads to increased epithelial cell cycle progression: roscovitine augments p21 levels. BMC Nephrol. 2007;8:12.

60. Park JY, Park SH, Weiss RH. Disparate effects of roscovitine on renal tubular epithelial cell apoptosis and senescence: implications for autosomal dominant polycystic kidney disease. Am J Nephrol. 2009;29(6):509–15.
61. Bukanov NO, Smith LA, Klinger KW, Ledbetter SR, Ibraghimov-Beskrovnaya O. Long-lasting arrest of murine polycystic kidney disease with CDK inhibitor roscovitine. Nature. 2006;444(7121):949–52.
62. Childs BG, Durik M, Baker DJ, van Deursen JM. Cellular senescence in aging and age-related disease: from mechanisms to therapy. Nat Med. 2015;21(12):1424–35.
63. Zhu Y, Tchkonia T, Pirtskhalava T, Gower AC, Ding H, Giorgadze N, et al. The Achilles' heel of senescent cells: from transcriptome to senolytic drugs. Aging Cell. 2015;14(4):644–58.
64. Mylonas KJ, O'Sullivan ED, Humphries D, Baird DP, Docherty MH, Neely SA, et al. Cellular senescence inhibits renal regeneration after injury in mice, with senolytic treatment promoting repair. Sci Transl Med. 2021;13(594):eabb0203.
65. O'Sullivan ED, Mylonas KJ, Bell R, Carvalho C, Baird DP, Cairns C, et al. Single cell analysis of senescent epithelia reveals targetable mechanisms promoting fibrosis. bioRxiv. 2022:2022.03.21.485189.
66. Li C, Shen Y, Huang L, Liu C, Wang J. Senolytic therapy ameliorates renal fibrosis postacute kidney injury by alleviating renal senescence. FASEB J. 2021;35(1):e21229.
67. Hickson LJ, Langhi Prata LGP, Bobart SA, Evans TK, Giorgadze N, Hashmi SK, et al. Senolytics decrease senescent cells in humans: preliminary report from a clinical trial of Dasatinib plus quercetin in individuals with diabetic kidney disease. EBioMedicine. 2019;47:446–56.
68. Baar MP, Brandt RMC, Putavet DA, Klein JDD, Derks KWJ, Bourgeois BRM, et al. Targeted apoptosis of senescent cells restores tissue homeostasis in response to Chemotoxicity and aging. Cell. 2017;169(1):132–47 e16.
69. Hernandez-Segura A, de Jong TV, Melov S, Guryev V, Campisi J, Demaria M. Unmasking transcriptional heterogeneity in senescent cells. Curr Biol. 2017;27(17):2652–60 e4.
70. Wiley CD, Flynn JM, Morrissey C, Lebofsky R, Shuga J, Dong X, et al. Analysis of individual cells identifies cell-to-cell variability following induction of cellular senescence. Aging Cell. 2017;16(5):1043–50.
71. Chang J, Wang Y, Shao L, Laberge RM, Demaria M, Campisi J, et al. Clearance of senescent cells by ABT263 rejuvenates aged hematopoietic stem cells in mice. Nat Med. 2016;22(1):78–83.
72. Demaria M, Ohtani N, Youssef SA, Rodier F, Toussaint W, Mitchell JR, et al. An essential role for senescent cells in optimal wound healing through secretion of PDGF-AA. Dev Cell. 2014;31(6):722–33.
73. Docherty MH, Baird DP, Hughes J, Ferenbach DA. Cellular senescence and Senotherapies in the kidney: current evidence and future directions. Front Pharmacol. 2020;11:755.
74. Yang L, Besschetnova TY, Brooks CR, Shah JV, Bonventre JV. Epithelial cell cycle arrest in G2/M mediates kidney fibrosis after injury. Nat Med. 2010;16(5):535–43, 1p following 143.

Chapter 4
Mental Health Disorders: An Overlooked Aspect of Chronic Kidney Disease in Older Adults

Antonio Gabriel D. Corona, Linda G. Wang, and Maureen E. Brogan

A 65-year-old male was referred to the nephrology clinic by his primary care provider (PCP) for further evaluation and management of chronic kidney disease (CKD). He has a known past medical history of hypertension, type 2 diabetes mellitus, hyperlipidemia and arthritis. When asked about his kidney history, the patient shared he had been told his kidney function progressively worsened the past few years and is now at stage four.

The patient reports that over the past year, he has felt a general sense of fatigue and decrease in motivation to "live his life". He does not feel like his "usual self" most of the time, and his wife and friends have pointed this out to him as well. As an example, the patient says he used to be an avid hiker. However, his last hike was over 6 months ago which is very unusual. He attributes this fatigue to inadequate rest at night, which leaves him feeling tired throughout the day. When asked if he thinks he is depressed, the patient replies, "Maybe."

A. G. D. Corona (✉)
Nephrology/Palliative Medicine, Department of Nephrology, Montefiore Medical Center, Bronx, NY, USA
e-mail: ancorona@montefiore.org

L. G. Wang
Department of Internal Medicine Division of Geriatric and Palliative Medicine, Michigan Medicine, Ann Arbor, MI, USA

M. E. Brogan
Nephrology, Montefiore Medical Center, Bronx, NY, USA
e-mail: Mbrogan@Montefiore.org

H. Kramer et al. (eds.), *Kidney Disease in the Elderly*,
https://doi.org/10.1007/978-3-031-68460-9_4

Introduction

Mental health disorders (MHD) are common in adults with CKD. Approximately 1 in 4 patients suffer from any psychiatric illness with more than 7% of cases classified as "serious", which is associated with significant functional impairment [1]. Because of its associations with poorer health outcomes and quality of life [2], MHD is an under-recognized complication of kidney disease and should be regarded as a growing public health concern.

Data on MHD within the context of CKD remains inadequate due to the heterogeneity of MHD psychiatric definitions and the difficulties disentangling mental health symptoms vs disease vs. the metabolic effects of CKD. Insomnia, for example, is a recognized precursor to and manifestation of psychiatric disorders, but it can also exist as a primary psychiatric diagnosis. Sleeping patterns can also be influenced by uremic factors in CKD.

Regardless, numerous descriptive studies have found associations of comorbid MHD in CKD with increased morbidity and mortality. Depression is a common reported disorder in this population [3] and is closely linked with an increased risk of hospitalizations and death [4]. Schizophrenia, anxiety, and substance abuse disorders are also implicated as potential factors leading to more adverse events [5, 6]. One possible explanation for these poor outcomes of MHD in CKD is non-adherence to treatment plans, which applies not only to dialytic therapies [7], but also to medications [8]and diet [9]. Moreover, poorly controlled psychiatric disorders can preclude access to kidney transplantation [10].

A Prominent Issue in Older Adults

MHD remains an important concern for older populations. By the year 2040, more than 20% of the general population will be age 65 years and older and both CKD and MHD are diseases of older individuals. Physiologically, glomerular filtration rate begins to decline consistently after age 30 as part of the normal process of aging [11]. In the same manner, senescence itself presents many risk factors for developing MHD including neurovascular and structural changes in later life [12].

There's a plethora of MHD present in CKD. Diagnosis and management remain challenging for various reasons relevant to the older adult population:

1. Symptoms like fatigue are very pervasive in this cohort [13] and may mask, or even divert from the detection of, signs and symptoms of MHD.
2. The older person with CKD is at risk for adverse pharmacologic effects.
3. Lack of time with and access to providers limits access to mental health services and comprehensive wellness care [14].

Table 4.1 General approach to manage

Therapy must be initiated for the purpose of promoting an improvement in well-being and avoiding negative effects	– The exercise of balancing the benefits of the drug and the unintended side effects must be done constantly throughout the course of treatment – The patient should be involved throughout the therapeutic decision-making process, as therapy should be contextual to the patient's goals of treatment
Dosis sola facit venenum or "the dose makes the poison"	– Treatment should be started low and slow: Using the lowest effective dose possible and with sufficient time between dose up-titration – Subsequent dose changes should be done with caution
The interdisciplinary team is an integral part of the management plan	– Referral to mental health wellness experts for supportive care is recommended especially for more complicated cases – Patient quality of care is shown to be enhanced with this approach [18]

Pharmacologic Beneficence and Non-maleficence

Older adults with CKD are vulnerable to the effects of polypharmacy, especially due to the reduced kidney clearance of psychopharmacologic medications [15]. Since most drugs are eliminated through the kidneys, reductions in glomerular filtration, tubular secretion, and reabsorption affect the pharmacokinetic and pharmacodynamic properties of these medications, and thereby increase the risk of serious drug reactions [16]. The hazards of polypharmacy in older persons are known, but unfortunately, it is not uncommon for older individuals with CKD to take more than ten medications daily [17].

These risks should not completely preclude treatment for MHD if a patient's condition warrants medication use. Instead, presence of MHD should alert cliniicans on heightened need for medication stewardship. The general approach to manage patients with MHD are outlined in Table 4.1.

Case Continued

You investigate his symptoms further and find that the patient has had persistent feelings of being sad and irritable for the past year. He feels tremendous guilt and disappointment in himself for not controlling his diabetes adequately and it has caused his kidneys to fail. After going through an immersive symptom checklist, you screen the patient for a depressive disorder.

Depression

Depression and CKD co-exist due to biological and socioeconomic factors affecting our patients. The brain-kidney axis is an evolving concept and knowledge continues to evolve [3]. These two organ systems, the kidney and brain, are linked via vascular, neurohormonal, and immunologic pathways that seem to operate bidirectionally when it comes to depression and CKD. Patients with depression are found to have an increased incidence of CKD, and patients with CKD are found to have an increased incidence of depression [19].

A major theory of how CKD leads to depression centers on derangements in the immune system that arise from the inflammatory milieu that results from increased cytokine production and reduced cytokine clearance with reduced glomerular filtration rate [20]. Elevated levels of inflammatory molecules and upregulation of gene expression of inflammatory pathways in depressive conditions can affect dopaminergic neurons in the central nervous system [21]. Immunosenescence and inflammation are prominent findings in aging [22].

Lower household income, lower educational levels, and unemployment, factors seen more frequently in CKD [23], are associated with an increased risk of depression [24]. Adverse health-related behaviors such as smoking and sedentarism are common in depression and may lead to CKD progression [25]. Contrarily, CKD is associated with multiple lifestyle changes such as more restrictive diets and increased time in healthcare settings. Patients with advanced kidney disease also have a significant burden and impaired functionality, which is more pronounced in older individuals [26]. These factors can play a critical role in the development of depression in the setting of CKD.

Diagnosing Depression

The diagnosis of depression can be challenging in older adults, especially in the setting of CKD. The many potential obstacles for proper evaluation of patients (Fig. 4.1) with depression should be recognized. One of the most concerning barriers is masked or misattributed symptoms of depression, which can be due to the presence of fatigue, polypharmacy, and cognitive impairments.

Fatigue is a shared experience in CKD and older adults and difficult to define and even more difficult to measure. Fatigue can be considered as a group of symptoms such as weakness, tiredness, and exhaustion that coalesce into a burdensome condition [27]. Kidney dysfunction and conditions that affect older adults share many factors that contribute to fatigue: anemia, hypogonadism, deconditioning, malnutrition, and even pain [13, 28]. While fatigue and depression overlap and may coincide with each other, patients should be screened for depression after a complete medical workup for other possible illnesses.

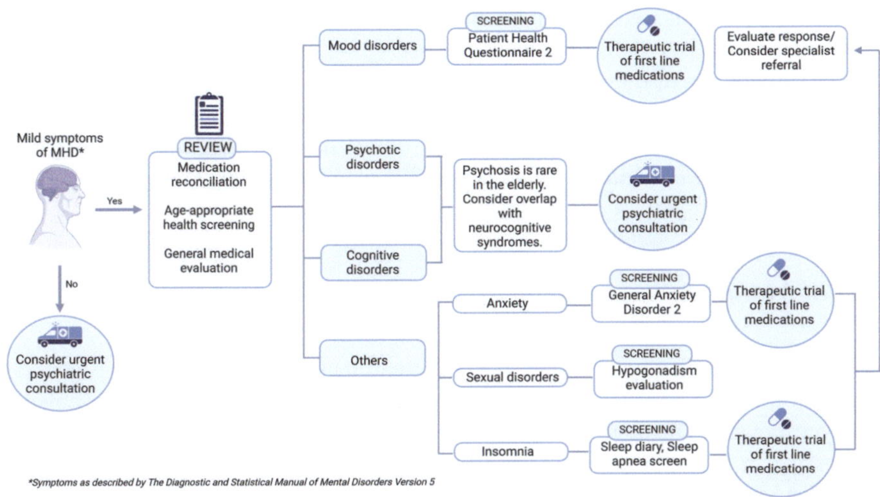

Fig. 4.1 Biorender diagram

Polypharmacy is also associated with an increased risk of depression [29]. Most notably, beta blockers have been implicated in causing depressive symptoms, but more recent literature suggests this relationship may be based on protopathic bias [30]. Nevertheless, a number of drugs used in general medical practice are potentially depressogenic [31] and may muddy the evaluation of a patient with an underlying mood disorder.

Finally, our brains undergo structural and neurovascular changes during senescence and with decline of kidney function that can progress to cognitive impairment [32]. Clinically, it is difficult to differentiate between symptoms of cognitive impairment, especially in earlier stages, to those of cognitive impairment associated with depression [33]. With the development of neurologic deficits affecting attention, memory and higher executive functions, the diagnosis may become even more complicated [34].

Ultimately, what is needed for prompt diagnosis is an increased level of vigilance of depressive symptoms while caring for our patients. The selection of the most appropriate screening tool for patients with CKD is controversial. The Beck Depression Inventory II is the most studied tool [4] but it has its limitations. Notably, it has 21 items and can be intimidating or tedious for both patients and clinicians to use.

An interdisciplinary approach to managing depression can enhance the quality of care delivered [18]. Timely referrals to mental health wellness experts, after our primary assessment, are recommended for more comprehensive, subspecialized care. For our purposes, the Patient Health Questionnaire-2 (PHQ-2), which is arguably the most used depression screening in clinical settings, can be a useful screening tool. Although the PHQ-2 does not have robust literature backing its use in perons with CKD, it has utility in the initial assessment of our patients and is easily incorporated into our visits (Table 4.2).

The patient scores a four on the PHQ-2. You discuss starting him on an antidepressant. He is hesitant at first because he has never been on any of these medications in the past. Additionally, he worries about some of the side effects of the "uppers" he has heard about. He asks you if they will affect his kidneys.

Initial Management of Depression

A number of studies have shown that the treatment of depression in the general population improves psychosocial and medical outcomes. However, improvements in psycosocial and medical outcomes have not been demonstrated with treatment of depression in the setting of CKD and end-stage kidney disease (ESKD) [36]. This lack of evidence may be due to most studies requiring a higher level of glomerular filtration rate for their inclusion criteria. Regardless, the lack of data should not dissuade us from treating our patients.

What we can extrapolate from existing research is that a combination of psychotherapy and antidepressants is more efficacious than either by itself [36] and this emphasizes the need for multidisciplinary and comprehensive care for our patients with depression.

Antidepressant medication stewardship is challenging in older patients with CKD for a number of reasons (Fig. 4.1) [37]. First, protein-binding capacity is reduced in CKD leading to a larger volume of distribution, possibly due to a uremic milieu [38]. This higher protein-binding capacity can affect antidepressant medications like tricyclic antidepressants.

Secondly, phosphate binders, which are commonly prescribed in CKD, may affect the absorption of other medications [39]. Not much has been studied but the recommendation is that patients should take their other medications separately to prevent any interference in drug absorption.

Third, the pill burden in the older adult population with advanced CKD is one of the highest among all conditions [40]. Due to the number of medications this cohort is prescribed to take on a daily basis, adherence has remained a persistent problem [41].

Last, there is unfortunately a scarcity of data to aid in the management of depression in an older individual with CKD [42]. Additionally, most depression studies

Table 4.2 Patient Health Questionnaire [35]

Over the last 2 weeks, how often have you been bothered by the following problems?	Not at all	Several days	More than half the days	Nearly everyday
Little interest or pleasure doing things	0	1	2	3
Feeling down, depressed or hopeless	0	1	2	3

Scores of 3 or greater suggest a major depressive disorder is likely

focus on younger age groups. Because of this, there is apprehension to provide therapeutics due to safety concerns.

Choice of Antidepressant

The choice of initial antidepressant should rely on the patient's medical history, other medications, and the drug's safety profile. Limited efficacy should also be considered by providers when choosing the initial therapy. Selective serotonin reuptake inhibitors (SSRIs) and serotonin and norepinephrine reuptake inhibitors (SNRIs) are the most widely-used class of antidepressants for older patients with kidney disease. Tricyclic antidepressants (TCAs) are less preferred agents because of their anticholinergic and cardiovascular side effects. Furthermore, TCAs are highly protein-bound and their pharmacokinetics may be greatly affected by hypoalbuminemic, uremic or edematous states.

SSRIs are relatively more well-tolerated than SNRIs because they do not significantly affect blood pressure, while the latter has been shown to modestly increase systolic and diastolic pressures at higher doses [43]. The syndrome of inappropriate ADH secretion is not exclusive to SSRIs as it is also caused by SNRIs [44]. Both classes can cause drowsiness, insomnia, dry mouth, constipation and sexual dysfunction.

Among the SSRIs, Sertraline at 50 mg daily has been studied in CKD with mixed findings [36, 45] but ultimately, offers the most potential benefits as a starting point of therapy, including improving intradialytic hypotension [46], fatigue [47] and uremic pruritus [48]. Fluoxetine is not recommended as first-line treatment because of its long half-life and potential for multiple CYP450-mediated drug-drug interactions [49]. Additionally, paroxetine has the greatest anticholinergic potential and should be avoided in older adults [50]. Citalopram and escitalopram are safe to use in older adults and have very low potential to inhibit cytochrome enzymes, reducing the risk of drug-drug interactions. Citalopram is linked to QT interval prolongation but no significant adverse cardiac outcomes have been associated with its use [51]. Both drugs can be considered as initial agents, although data regarding dosage guidance is scarce. SNRIs have the additional advantage of being used as an adjunct for chronic pain [52]. Venlafaxine is an attractive choice for the older adult group because of its limited interactions with other drugs and its relatively safer side-effect profile [53]. Dose adjustment is needed in CKD due to accumulation of the parent drug and its metabolite. A starting dose of 18.75 mg daily is recommended. Duloxetine is not recommended for use in patients with creatinine clearance of less than 30 ml/min [54].

Mirtazapine, a noradrenergic and specific serotonergic antidepressant, is commonly prescribed for depression. There is limited pharmacologic data to guide its use in older adults and those with CKD. Dose reduction is likely necessary to reduce its hypnotic and sedating effects [54]. It may have the added benefit of being an effective orexigenic in anorexia and cachexia syndromes.

As you discuss your management plan for CKD further with the patient, you notice that he starts fidgeting restlessly when you bring up the topic of hemodialysis. He asks you if hemodialysis is an unavoidable outcome. He says his father was a hemodialysis patient and that he remembers the burden it was on his family, including the repeated admissions to the hospital. The patient says he is afraid he will end up on a similar path and this worries him constantly since he realized the severity of his condition.

Anxiety

Anxiety is prevalent in patients with CKD and frequency and symptoms do differ by CKD stages [55]. The high prevalence of anxiety in CKD mirrors the anxiety prevalence in older adults [56] and comorbid anxiety, which is anxiety associated with medical conditions, is common in the older adult population as well [57]. Comorbid anxiety is often mistakenly attributed to an adjustment disorder, especially if the patient starts dialytic therapies, but both anxiety and an adjustment disorder can co-exist. Adjustment disorders have multiple phenotypes that present with anxiety that extends beyond the scope of the stressor. Historical clues that may warrant additional workup or early psychiatric evaluation include irritability, excessive worrying, difficulty concentrating, and fear of separation from home or close attachments. Several screening tests may be used for anxiety, but none are validated in the presence of CKD. Studies have used The Beck Anxiety Inventory, a 21-item self-report questionnaire which has been validated for use in the older patient population [58]. The General Anxiety Disorder 7 and the abbreviated General Anxiety Disorder 2 (GAD-2) has also been studied in the older patient population [59]. With the primary assessment of psychiatric conditions, other medical issues must also be ruled out by the clinician, including thyroid disorders, dysrhythmias or underlying cardiac issues, and substance use disorders.

There are extremely few studies outlining the initial therapeutic strategies for anxiety. Benzodiazepines and beta blockers should be avoided in older adults as first-line medications. The former can increase risk of falls and hip fractures [60], while the latter will not be as efficacious as other available anxiolytics and can cause depression and fatigue [61]. SSRIs and mirtazapine are safe first-line agents to use in older patients with CKD. Cognitive behavioral therapy should also be offered to patients with anxiety or depression as it has been shown to reduce psychiatric symptoms in those with CKD [62].

On review of systems, the patient also complains of poor sleep. He has trouble initiating sleep and staying asleep. There is a component of anxiety to his insomnia, but even during times he feels generally well, he wakes up multiple times in the evening and has trouble going back to bed. This usually leaves him very tired throughout the day. The patient takes long naps after lunch to keep him refreshed.

Insomnia

Insomnia is one of the most common complaints among patients, with over five million office visits per year in the US [63]. Insomnia and poor sleep quality are especially common among patients with CKD. A systematic review and meta-analysis found that 46–68% of patients with advanced CKD but without kidney replacement therapy as well as patients receiving kidney replacement therapy and kidney transplant patients had poor sleep quality. Insomnia was also significantly more prevalent in patients >60 years old [64].

Multiple underlying factors contribute to insomnia, such as psychiatric disorders, neurological disorders, medical conditions and medications, or other substances. Older adults with CKD have a higher incidence of geriatric syndromes, such as polypharmacy, dementia, urinary incontinence, and malnutrition; all underlying conditions that can contribute to poor sleep [65]. The biological effects of CKD itself can impact sleep quality. Autonomic reflex function impairment can cause hyperactivity of the sympathetic nervous system and decreased vagal tone [66]. High levels of parathyroid hormone, which is often associated with bone pain and pruritis, are linked with prevalence of insomnia in patients on hemodialysis. Not surprisingly, patients with more time spent on hemodialysis are at significantly higher risk of insomnia. Patients dialyzed during the morning shift also had an increased risk of insomnia compared to those dialyzed in the afternoon [67].

Diagnosis of insomnia is primarily a clinical diagnosis, with information obtained from the patient and collateral information obtained from family and caregivers. Physical examination and laboratory studies have limited value in diagnosing insomnia, however, it may lead to diagnosis of other underlying medical conditions that contribute to insomnia. Polysomnography is not required unless evaluating for underlying sleep disorders such as obstructive sleep apnea or restless leg syndrome. Evaluation for insomnia requires a comprehensive approach, as insomnia is usually a symptom of other comorbid medical conditions. Assessment should include a detailed sleep history to describe the sleep problem, a review of comorbid conditions, lifestyle components, and current medication use and timing of use. Reporting of specific symptoms occurring during sleep may lead to diagnosis of other underlying sleep disorders. Due to the complex nature of diagnosing insomnia and the heavy reliance on patient-reported information, a sleep diary is a useful tool to record data on symptoms and their fluctuation or progression, sleep habits, medication use, etc. A sleep diary helps keep information more objective, formal and consistent, thus reducing recall bias [68]. Validated screening tools for insomnia, such as the Pittsburgh Sleep Quality Index [69] or the Insomnia Severity Index [70] can be useful in obtaining objective information.

Data on treatment of insomnia in patients with CKD remain limited and more research is needed to support specific treatments, especially pharmacological interventions. Treatment of insomnia, like diagnosis, requires a comprehensive and multifactorial approach. The goal of treatment is to improve sleep, both subjectively and objectively, as well as improve quality of life. General approach to treatment of insomnia should focus on treating any reversible underlying conditions (e.g., medical conditions, psychiatric conditions, substance abuse, acute stressors, polypharmacy, and medication side effects). This may include optimizing treatment for kidney disease, optimizing kidney replacement therapy, or even kidney transplant [71].

Ideally, treatment of insomnia in older adults with CKD should emphasize non-pharmacological treatment over pharmacologic treatment. Multiple studies have shown the efficacy of cognitive behavioral therapy in treating insomnia (CBT-I) compared to pharmacological therapy. CBT-I has longer-lasting benefits, lower adverse effects, and increased efficacy in the treatment of insomnia in patients with coexisting medical and psychiatric conditions [72]. Studies have also shown that CBT-I is effective in treating insomnia in patients with CKD as well [73].

Physical exercise has beneficial effects on many aspects of health, including slowing the decline of kidney function [74], maintaining cognitive function [75], and improving quality of sleep in older adults within the general population [76]. Evidence of physical exercise on improving the quality of sleep in patients with CKD is scant, but a couple of systematic reviews have found that physical exercise can improve sleep quality, improve fatigue, and improve symptoms of depression [77].

Pharmacological treatment of insomnia in older adults with CKD should start with evaluation for polypharmacy and consideration of medication side effects that contribute to insomnia. Therefore, deprescribing unnecessary medications will reduce medication side effects and decrease pill burden. If certain medications cannot be discontinued, then consideration of reducing medication dosages can also reduce medication side effects [78]. Initiating pharmacological treatment for insomnia is not first-line treatment and requires individualized tailoring, especially in older adults. The use of hypnotic benzodiazepines and non-benzodiazepine receptor agonist (nonBZRAs) hypnotics ((e.g., zolpidem, eszopiclone, zaleplon) in CKD patients are associated with increased mortality [79]. In addition, many of the medications commonly prescribed to treat insomnia are on the Beers Criteria, which lists potentially inappropriate medication use in older adults [80]. Medications such as TCAs are highly anticholinergic; hypnotic benzodiazepines (e.g. temazepam, quazepam, triazolam) and nonBZRAs hypnotics are highly sedating, worsen cognitive impairment, are deliriogenic, and increase risk for dependence and abuse. Sedating antipsychotics are also highly sedating, causing increased risk for falls, and there is a black box warning that antipsychotics in older adults increase mortality.

Melatonin is a common over-the-counter medication that is prescribed for treatment of insomnia. Ramelteon is a melatonin receptor agonist that has a similar mechanism of action as melatonin. Both can help facilitate sleep on set and manage circadian rhythm disorders. Melatonin and ramelteon have low medication side effects and are generally well-tolerated. Systematic reviews of melatonin and ramelteon use in the treatment of insomnia have shown modest improvement in reducing sleep latency and increasing total sleep time [81]. Patients with CKD have low nocturnal melatonin secretion as well as lack the circadian rhythm in melatonin secretion [82]. Therefore, exogenous melatonin supplementation has been shown to be beneficial in improving sleep quality [83]. Melatonin is also the first-line treatment for insomnia associated with rapid eye movement sleep behavior disorder, found in neurodegenerative diseases such as dementia with Lewy bodies and Parkinson's disease [84].

If a medication is required to treat insomnia, and melatonin is ineffective, a nonBZRA hypnotic would be recommended as a first-choice medication, especially for the treatment of acute insomnia. NonBZRA hypnotics are FDA-approved for the treatment of insomnia; it has a relatively short half-life, and it does not need to be dose adjusted for kidney impairment or dialysis. However, its use should be limited to less than 4 weeks and in cases of chronic insomnia, concurrent use of a nonBZRA hypnotic can be used initially while patients receive CBT-I treatment, with the intention of weaning off the nonBZRA hypnotic. If pharmacologic treatment with non-preferred medications, such as sedating antipsychotics or benzodiazepines, is required due to difficult-to-manage behavioral disturbances from underlying cognitive impairment/dementia, the patient should receive co-management from a geriatric psychiatrist for additional medication management. Other agents such as over-the-counter sleep aids and antihistamines are not recommended for use in treatment of insomnia. Be aware that some medications have a lower maximum dose recommendation for older adults compared to younger patients, and always dose-adjust based on kidney function. As is true for initiation of all medications in older adults, the adage "start low and go slow" (i.e., start with the lowest dose and increase the dose slowly) also applies to the initiation of medications to treat insomnia.

Lastly, the patient is initially reluctant to address the questions regarding his sexual history. He volunteers that he has been having problems getting erections, which has caused him embarrassment. Because of this, he has tried to avoid initiating intercourse with his wife, which he admits has caused some strain on their relationship.

Sexual Dysfunction

Based on observational studies using validated and unvalidated screening tools, sexual dysfunction (SD) appears common among females and males with chronic kidney disease [85, 86]. Trying to separate SD into medical or psychiatric etiologies has made standardization of the definition difficult. SD seems to rise as GFR (Glomerular Filtration Rate) declines, however, most studies explored sexual dysfunction in later stages of kidney disease. Sexual health in patients with CKD adversely affects well-being indicated by dialysis health-related quality of life (HRQoL) scores.

The etiology of sexual dysfunction is multifactorial. The multiple comorbidities that patients with CKD possess, including diabetes, hypertension, anemia and vascular disease, and their treatment side effects compound the problem. Sexual dissatisfaction may also be related to fatigue and depressed mood affecting lack of interest. Toorians et al. point out that lack of libido may be the main cause of SD [87]. The prevalence of depression among patients with CKD could be as high as 25–30% and this can be a strong factor linked to sexual dysfunction [88]. Other barriers to achieving optimal sexual health specific to CKD patients include difficulty discussing their illness and required treatments with a partner and negative self-image related to dialysis access [89]. Despite being a frequent problem, sexual dysfunction among patients with CKD is not well defined, and there is little research on mechanism and treatment for this important contributor to a patient's life quality.

Sexual Dysfunction

Declining kidney function in male patients with CKD affects the hypothalamic-pituitary-gonadal axis causing hypogonadism. CKD is associated with low total and free testosterone and hyperprolactinemia [90]. Testosterone levels decline as the GFR declines [91]. Medications routinely used for patients with CKD may also lower androgen levels such as renin-angiotensin system blockers and calcineurin inhibitors [92]. Hypogonadism is also a risk factor in patients with ESKD (end-stage kidney disease) from their other comorbidities: older age, diabetes and obesity. Most men with ESKD and hypogonadism have sexual dysfunction. The most common complaint is erectile dysfunction [92]. Testosterone replacement, in small studies, may improve sexual function but it does not come without potential susceptibly of prostate cancer and cardiovascular risks [91]. Medication to treat hypertension such as central-acting agents and beta blockers contribute to sexual dysfunction [93]. Phosphodiesterase inhibitors can be prescribed to appropriate patients with erectile dysfunction not taking nitrates. Kidney transplantation does not completely reverse the hypogonadism caused by uremia. Peritoneal dialysis may be associated with a lower prevalence of SD, but residual kidney function is preserved longer with this modality.

While there is a paucity of data on sexual dysfunction in females, it is known that female patients with CKD have hormonal imbalances such as high prolactin levels and low estrogen, which cause anovulation, menstrual irregularities and low sex drive. Low estrogen levels also lead to early menopause and side effects include vaginal dryness and dyspareunia.

Luckily, hormonal imbalances are not permanent. Erythropoiesis Stimulating Agents (ESA), intensive dialysis and kidney transplantation can improve sexual well-being. ESA, however, comes with its side effects including increasing cardiovascular outcomes, thrombosis, and risk of cancer. Nocturnal hemodialysis, in small studies, may also help control hormonal irregularities and may be an option for those who are waitlisted or unable to get a kidney transplant. Proper education and counseling are required of the transplant team.

SD among patients with CKD and is often caused by a complex array of overlapping illnesses, medication side effects, psychosocial factors, and primary and secondary hormonal imbalances. Fortunately, most dialysis units have adopted patient-centered approaches to preferences and treatment. Multidisciplinary teams may be useful in providing counseling and support with nonpharmacological approaches [85]. Discussions about sexual health or lack of should become routine. Providing proper clearance at dialysis, treatment of anemia and careful medication review for side effects are some easily modified practices that can be instituted. Hormone replacement may be an option for low libido in the appropriate patient. Patients should be aware kidney transplantation can reverse some of the symptoms of SD.

The prevalence of SD among patients with CKD should be evaluated using validated screening tools and updated definitions. SD should be distinguished from lack of sexual interest and activity [94]. Patients' perceptions and the impact of gender identity should be considered in future questionnaires [95]. Since the incidence of CKD requiring kidney replacement therapy will double by 2030, modifiable risk factors and iatrogenic causes need to be addressed to improve sexual health.

References

1. Wilk AS, Hu JC, Chehal P, Yarbrough CR, Ji X, Cummings JR. National estimates of mental health needs among adults with self-reported CKD in the United States. Kidney Int Rep. 2022;7(7):1630–42. https://doi.org/10.1016/j.ekir.2022.04.088. PMID: 35812303; PMCID: PMC9263246.
2. Vaingankar JA, Chong SA, Abdin E, et al. Understanding the relationships between mental disorders, self-reported health outcomes and positive mental health: findings from a national survey. Health Qual Life Outcomes. 2020;18:55. https://doi.org/10.1186/s12955-020-01308-0.
3. Simões E Silva AC, Miranda AS, Rocha NP, Teixeira AL. Neuropsychiatric disorders in chronic kidney disease. Front Pharmacol. 2019;10:932. https://doi.org/10.3389/fphar.2019.00932. PMID: 31474869; PMCID: PMC6707423.
4. Hedayati SS, Minhajuddin AT, Afshar M, Toto RD, Trivedi MH, Rush AJ. Association between major depressive episodes in patients with chronic kidney disease and initiation of dialysis, hospitalization, or death. JAMA. 2010;303(19):1946–53. https://doi.org/10.1001/jama.2010.619. PMID: 20483971; PMCID: PMC3217259.
5. Loosman WL, Rottier MA, Honig A, et al. Association of depressive and anxiety symptoms with adverse events in Dutch chronic kidney disease patients: a prospective cohort study. BMC Nephrol. 2015;16:155. https://doi.org/10.1186/s12882-015-0149-7.
6. Kimmel PL, Fwu CW, Abbott KC, Moxey-Mims MM, Mendley S, Norton JM, Eggers PW. Psychiatric illness and mortality in hospitalized ESKD dialysis patients. Clin J Am Soc Nephrol. 2019;14(9):1363–71. https://doi.org/10.2215/CJN.14191218. Epub 2019 Aug 22. PMID: 31439538; PMCID: PMC6730507.
7. Kauric-Klein Z. Depression and medication adherence in patients on hemodialysis. Curr Hypertens Rev. 2017;13(2):138–43. https://doi.org/10.2174/1573402113666171129182611. PMID: 29205118.
8. Fotaraki ZM, Gerogianni G, Vasilopoulos G, Polikandrioti M, Giannakopoulou N, Alikari V. Depression, adherence, and functionality in patients undergoing hemodialysis. Cureus. 2022;14(2):e21872. https://doi.org/10.7759/cureus.21872. PMID: 35273844; PMCID: PMC8901145.
9. Gebrie MH, Ford J. Depressive symptoms and dietary non-adherence among end stage renal disease patients undergoing hemodialysis therapy: systematic review. BMC Nephrol.

2019;20(1):429. https://doi.org/10.1186/s12882-019-1622-5. PMID: 31752741; PMCID: PMC6873524.

10. Cahn-Fuller KL, Parent B. Transplant eligibility for patients with affective and psychotic disorders: a review of practices and a call for justice. BMC Med Ethics. 2017;18(1):72. https://doi.org/10.1186/s12910-017-0235-4. PMID: 29216883; PMCID: PMC5721543.

11. Bitzer M, Wiggins J. Aging biology in the kidney. Adv Chronic Kidney Dis. 2016;23(1):12–8. https://doi.org/10.1053/j.ackd.2015.11.005. PMID: 26709058.

12. Alexopoulos GS. Mechanisms and treatment of late-life depression. Transl Psychiatry. 2019;9:188. https://doi.org/10.1038/s41398-019-0514-6.

13. Gregg LP, Bossola M, Ostrosky-Frid M, Hedayati SS. Fatigue in CKD: epidemiology, pathophysiology, and treatment. Clin J Am Soc Nephrol. 2021;16(9):1445–55. https://doi.org/10.2215/CJN.19891220. Epub 2021 Apr 15. PMID: 33858827; PMCID: PMC8729574.

14. McQuoid J, Jowsey T, Talaulikar G. Contextualising renal patient routines: everyday space-time contexts, health service access, and wellbeing. Soc Sci Med. 2017;183:142–50. https://doi.org/10.1016/j.socscimed.2017.04.043. Epub 2017 Apr 27. PMID: 28482275; PMCID: PMC5512548.

15. Mair A, Wilson M, Dreischulte T. Addressing the challenge of polypharmacy. Annu Rev Pharmacol Toxicol. 2020;60:661–81. https://doi.org/10.1146/annurev-pharmtox-010919-023508. Epub 2019 Oct 7. PMID: 31589822.

16. Lea-Henry TN, Carland JE, Stocker SL, Sevastos J, Roberts DM. Clinical pharmacokinetics in kidney disease: fundamental principles. Clin J Am Soc Nephrol. 2018;13(7):1085–95.

17. Secora A, Alexander GC, Ballew SH, Coresh J, Grams ME. Kidney function, polypharmacy, and potentially inappropriate medication use in a community-based cohort of older adults. Drugs Aging. 2018;35(8):735–50.

18. Heip T, Van Hecke A, Malfait S, Van Biesen W, Eeckloo K. The effects of interdisciplinary bedside rounds on patient centeredness, quality of care, and team collaboration: a systematic review. J Patient Saf. 2022;18(1):e40–4.

19. Zheng X, Wu W, Shen S. Prospective bidirectional associations between depression and chronic kidney diseases. Sci Rep. 2022;12(1):10903. https://doi.org/10.1038/s41598-022-15212-8. PMID: 35764693; PMCID: PMC9240037.

20. Jayakumar S, Jennings S, Halvorsrud K, Clesse C, Yaqoob MM, Carvalho LA, Bhui K. A systematic review and meta-analysis of the evidence on inflammation in depressive illness and symptoms in chronic and end-stage kidney disease. Psychol Med. 2022;53(12):5839–51. https://doi.org/10.1017/S0033291722003099. PMID: 36254747.

21. Beurel E, Toups M, Nemeroff CB. The bidirectional relationship of depression and inflammation: double trouble. Neuron. 2020;107(2):234–56. https://doi.org/10.1016/j.neuron.2020.06.002. Epub 2020 Jun 17. PMID: 32553197; PMCID: PMC7381373.

22. Buford TW. Hypertension and aging. Ageing Res Rev. 2016;26:96–111.

23. Nicholas SB, Kalantar-Zadeh K, Norris KC. Socioeconomic disparities in chronic kidney disease. Adv Chronic Kidney Dis. 2015;22:6–15. https://doi.org/10.1053/j.ackd.2014.07.002.

24. Fischer MJ, Xie D, Jordan N, Kop WJ, Krousel-Wood M, Kurella Tamura M, et al. Factors associated with depressive symptoms and use of antidepressant medications among participants in the Chronic Renal Insufficiency Cohort (CRIC) and Hispanic-CRIC Studies. Am J Kidney Dis. 2012;60:27–38. https://doi.org/10.1053/j.ajkd.2011.12.033.

25. Katon WJ. Epidemiology and treatment of depression in patients with chronic medical illness. Dialogues Clin Neurosci. 2011;13:7–23.

26. Fried LF, Lee JS, Shlipak M, Chertow GM, Green C, Ding J, Harris T, Newman AB. Chronic kidney disease and functional limitation in older people: health, aging and body composition study. J Am Geriatr Soc. 2006;54(5):750–6. https://doi.org/10.1111/j.1532-5415.2006.00727.x. PMID: 16696739.

27. Artom M, Moss-Morris R, Caskey F, Chilcot J. Fatigue in advanced kidney disease. Kidney Int. 2014;86(3):497–505. https://doi.org/10.1038/ki.2014.86. Epub 2014 Apr 2. PMID: 24694985.

28. Torossian M, Jacelon CS. Chronic illness and fatigue in older individuals: a systematic review. Rehabil Nurs. 2021;46(3):125–36. https://doi.org/10.1097/RNJ.0000000000000278. PMID: 32657851; PMCID: PMC7935454.
29. Cheng C, Bai J. Association between polypharmacy, anxiety, and depression among chinese older adults: evidence from the chinese longitudinal healthy longevity survey. Clin Interv Aging. 2022;17:235–44. https://doi.org/10.2147/CIA.S351731. PMID: 35283629; PMCID: PMC8909463.
30. Bornand D, Reinau D, Jick SS, Meier CR. β-Blockers and the risk of depression: a matched case-control study. Drug Saf. 2022;45(2):181–9. https://doi.org/10.1007/s40264-021-01140-5. Epub 2022 Jan 19. PMID: 35044637; PMCID: PMC8857000.
31. Celano CM, Freudenreich O, Fernandez-Robles C, Stern TA, Caro MA, Huffman JC. Depressogenic effects of medications: a review. Dialogues Clin Neurosci. 2011;13(1):109–25. https://doi.org/10.31887/DCNS.2011.13.1/ccelano. PMID: 21485751; PMCID: PMC3181967.
32. Xie Z, Tong S, Chu X, Feng T, Geng M. Chronic kidney disease and cognitive impairment: the kidney-brain axis. Kidney Dis (Basel). 2022;8(4):275–85. https://doi.org/10.1159/000524475. PMID: 36157262; PMCID: PMC9386403.
33. Perini G, Cotta Ramusino M, Sinforiani E, Bernini S, Petrachi R, Costa A. Cognitive impairment in depression: recent advances and novel treatments. Neuropsychiatr Dis Treat. 2019;15:1249–58. https://doi.org/10.2147/NDT.S199746. PMID: 31190831; PMCID: PMC6520478.
34. Marvel CL, Paradiso S. Cognitive and neurological impairment in mood disorders. Psychiatr Clin North Am. 2004;27(1):19–36, vii–viii. https://doi.org/10.1016/S0193-953X(03)00106-0. PMID: 15062628; PMCID: PMC2570029.
35. Kroenke K, Spitzer RL, Williams JB. The Patient Health Questionnaire-2: validity of a two-item depression screener. Med Care. 2003;41(11):1284–92. https://doi.org/10.1097/01.MLR.0000093487.78664.3C.
36. Hedayati SS, Gregg LP, Carmody T, Jain N, Toups M, Rush AJ, Toto RD, Trivedi MH. Effect of sertraline on depressive symptoms in patients with chronic kidney disease without dialysis dependence: the CAST randomized clinical trial. JAMA. 2017;318(19):1876–90. https://doi.org/10.1001/jama.2017.17131. PMID: 29101402; PMCID: PMC5710375.
37. Shirazian S, Grant CD, Aina O, Mattana J, Khorassani F, Ricardo AC. Depression in chronic kidney disease and end-stage renal disease: similarities and differences in diagnosis, epidemiology, and management. Kidney Int Rep. 2016;2(1):94–107. https://doi.org/10.1016/j.ekir.2016.09.005. PMID: 29318209; PMCID: PMC5720531.
38. Klammt S, Wojak H-J, Mitzner A, Koball S, Rychly J, Reisinger EC, Mitzner S. Albumin-binding capacity (ABiC) is reduced in patients with chronic kidney disease along with an accumulation of protein-bound uraemic toxins. Nephrol Dial Transplant. 2012;27(6):2377–83. https://doi.org/10.1093/ndt/gfr616.
39. Chan S, Au K, Francis RS, Mudge DW, Johnson DW, Pillans PI. Phosphate binders in patients with chronic kidney disease. Aust Prescr. 2017;40(1):10–4. https://doi.org/10.18773/austprescr.2017.002. Epub 2017 Feb 1. PMID: 28246429; PMCID: PMC5313253.
40. Roux-Marson C, Baranski JB, Fafin C, et al. Medication burden and inappropriate prescription risk among elderly with advanced chronic kidney disease. BMC Geriatr. 2020;20:87. https://doi.org/10.1186/s12877-020-1485-4.
41. Chiu YW, Teitelbaum I, Misra M, de Leon EM, Adzize T, Mehrotra R. Pill burden, adherence, hyperphosphatemia, and quality of life in maintenance dialysis patients. Clin J Am Soc Nephrol. 2009;4(6):1089–96. https://doi.org/10.2215/CJN.00290109. Epub 2009 May 7. PMID: 19423571; PMCID: PMC2689877.
42. Nagler EV, Webster AC, Vanholder R, Zoccali C. Antidepressants for depression in stage 3-5 chronic kidney disease: a systematic review of pharmacokinetics, efficacy and safety with recommendations by European Renal Best Practice (ERBP). Nephrol Dial Transplant.

2012;27(10):3736–45. https://doi.org/10.1093/ndt/gfs295. Epub 2012 Aug 1. PMID: 22859791.

43. Zhong Z, Wang L, Wen X, Liu Y, Fan Y, Liu Z. A meta-analysis of effects of selective serotonin reuptake inhibitors on blood pressure in depression treatment: outcomes from placebo and serotonin and noradrenaline reuptake inhibitor controlled trials. Neuropsychiatr Dis Treat. 2017;13:2781–96. https://doi.org/10.2147/NDT.S141832. PMID: 29158677; PMCID: PMC5683798.

44. De Picker L, Van Den Eede F, Dumont G, Moorkens G, Sabbe BG. Antidepressants and the risk of hyponatremia: a class-by-class review of literature. Psychosomatics. 2014;55(6):536–47. https://doi.org/10.1016/j.psym.2014.01.010. Epub 2014 Apr 21. PMID: 25262043.

45. Atalay H, Solak Y, Biyik Z, et al. Sertraline treatment is associated with an improvement in depression and health related quality of life in chronic peritoneal dialysis patients. Int Urol Nephrol. 2010;42:527–36.

46. Razeghi E, Dashti-Khavidaki S, Nassiri S, Abolghassemi R, Khalili H, Hashemi Nazari SS, Mansournia MA, Taraz M. A randomized crossover clinical trial of sertraline for intradialytic hypotension. Iran J Kidney Dis. 2015;9(4):323–30. PMID: 26174461.

47. Gandotra K, Jaskiw G, Fuller M, Vaidya P, Chiang A, Konicki E, Strohl KP. Sertraline as an adjunctive treatment for insomnia comorbid with other mental health disorders. J Affect Disord Rep. 2022;10:100389. https://doi.org/10.1016/j.jadr.2022.100389.

48. Shakiba M, Sanadgol H, Azmoude HR, Mashhadi MA, Sharifi H. Effect of sertraline on uremic pruritus improvement in ESRD patients. Int J Nephrol. 2012;2012:363901. https://doi.org/10.1155/2012/363901. Epub 2012 Aug 29. PMID: 22973512; PMCID: PMC3437632.

49. Deodhar M, Rihani SBA, Darakjian L, Turgeon J, Michaud V. Assessing the mechanism of fluoxetine-mediated CYP2D6 inhibition. Pharmaceutics. 2021;13(2):148. https://doi.org/10.3390/pharmaceutics13020148. PMID: 33498694; PMCID: PMC7912198.

50. Nevels RM, Gontkovsky ST, Williams BE. Paroxetine-the antidepressant from hell? Probably not, but caution required. Psychopharmacol Bull. 2016;46(1):77–104. PMID: 27738376; PMCID: PMC5044489.

51. McCarrell JL, Bailey TA, Duncan NA, Covington LP, Clifford KM, Hall RG, Blaszczyk AT. A review of citalopram dose restrictions in the treatment of neuropsychiatric disorders in older adults. Ment Health Clin. 2019;9(4):280–6. https://doi.org/10.9740/mhc.2019.07.280. PMID: 31293848; PMCID: PMC6607952.

52. Robinson C, Dalal S, Chitneni A, Patil A, Berger AA, Mahmood S, Orhurhu V, Kaye AD, Hasoon J. A look at commonly utilized serotonin noradrenaline reuptake inhibitors (SNRIs) in chronic pain. Health Psychol Res. 2022;10(3):32309. https://doi.org/10.52965/001c.32309. PMID: 35774919; PMCID: PMC9239373.

53. Staab JP, Evans DL. Efficacy of venlafaxine in geriatric depression. Depress Anxiety. 2000;12(Suppl 1):63–8. https://doi.org/10.1002/1520-6394(2000)12:1+<63::AID-DA8>3.0.CO;2-T. PMID: 11098416.

54. Eyler RF, Unruh ML, Quinn DK, Mary Vilay A. Psychotherapeutic agents in end-stage renal disease. Semin Dial. 2015;28(4):417–26.

55. Lee YJ, Kim MS, Cho S, Kim SR. Association of depression and anxiety with reduced quality of life in patients with predialysis chronic kidney disease. Int J Clin Pract. 2013;67:363–8. https://doi.org/10.1111/ijcp.12020.

56. Bryant C, Jackson H, Ames D. The prevalence of anxiety in older adults: methodological issues and a review of the literature. J Affect Disord. 2008;109(3):233–50. https://doi.org/10.1016/j.jad.2007.11.008. Epub 2007 Dec 26. PMID: 18155775.

57. Fung AWT, Lam LCW. A cross-sectional study on clinical correlates of anxiety disorders in 613 community living older adults in Hong Kong. Int J Geriatr Psychiatry. 2017;32(7):742–9. https://doi.org/10.1002/gps.4516. Epub 2016 Jun 9. PMID: 27280741.

58. Balsamo M, Cataldi F, Carlucci L, Fairfield B. Assessment of anxiety in older adults: a review of self-report measures. Clin Interv Aging. 2018;13:573–93. https://doi.org/10.2147/CIA.S114100. PMID: 29670342; PMCID: PMC5896683.

59. Wild B, Eckl A, Herzog W, Niehoff D, Lechner S, Maatouk I, Schellberg D, Brenner H, Müller H, Löwe B. Assessing generalized anxiety disorder in elderly people using the GAD-7 and GAD-2 scales: results of a validation study. Am J Geriatr Psychiatry. 2014;22(10):1029–38. https://doi.org/10.1016/j.jagp.2013.01.076. Epub 2013 Jun 12. PMID: 23768681.
60. Gage SBD, Moride Y, Ducruet T, Kurth T, Verdoux H, Tournier M, Pariente A, Begaud B. Benzodiazepine use and risk of Alzheimer's disease: case-control study. BMJ. 2014;349:g5205. https://doi.org/10.1136/bmj.g5205.
61. Crocco EA, Jaramillo S, Cruz-Ortiz C, Camfield K. Pharmacological management of anxiety disorders in the elderly. Curr Treat Options Psychiatry. 2017;4(1):33–46. https://doi.org/10.1007/s40501-017-0102-4. Epub 2017 Feb 10. PMID: 28948135; PMCID: PMC5609714.
62. Valsaraj BP, Bhat SM, Latha KS. Cognitive behaviour therapy for anxiety and depression among people undergoing haemodialysis: a randomized control trial. J Clin Diagn Res. 2016;10(8):VC06–10. https://doi.org/10.7860/JCDR/2016/18959.8383. Epub 2016 Aug 1. PMID: 27656536; PMCID: PMC5028450.
63. Ford ES, et al. Trends in outpatient visits for insomnia, sleep apnea, and prescriptions for sleep medications among US adults: findings from the National Ambulatory Medical Care survey 1999–2010. Sleep. 2014;37(8):1283–93.
64. Tan LH, et al. Insomnia and poor sleep in CKD: a systematic review and meta-analysis. Kidney Med. 2022;4(5):100458.
65. Soysal P, et al. Prevalence and co-incidence of geriatric syndromes according to glomerular filtration rate in older patients. Int Urol Nephrol. 2022;55(2):469–76.
66. Neumann J, et al. Sympathetic hyperactivity in chronic kidney disease: pathogenesis, clinical relevance, and treatment. Kidney Int. 2004;65(5):1568–76.
67. Sabbatini M, et al. Insomnia in maintenance haemodialysis patients. Nephrol Dial Transplant. 2002;17(5):852–6.
68. Carney CE, et al. The consensus sleep diary: standardizing prospective sleep self-monitoring. Sleep. 2012;35(2):287–302.
69. Buysse DJ, et al. The Pittsburgh Sleep Quality Index: a new instrument for psychiatric practice and research. Psychiatry Res. 1989;28(2):193–213.
70. Espie CA, et al. The Sleep Condition Indicator: a clinical screening tool to evaluate insomnia disorder. BMJ Open. 2014;4(3):e004183.
71. Russcher M, et al. The effects of kidney transplantation on sleep, melatonin, circadian rhythm and quality of life in kidney transplant recipients and living donors. Nephron. 2015;129(1):6–15.
72. Sateia MJ, et al. Clinical practice guideline for the pharmacologic treatment of chronic insomnia in adults: an American Academy of Sleep Medicine clinical practice guideline. J Clin Sleep Med. 2017;13(2):307–49.
73. Trauer JM, et al. Cognitive behavioral therapy for chronic insomnia: a systematic review and metaanalysis. Ann Intern Med. 2015;163(3):191–204.
74. Shlipak MG, et al. Effect of structured, moderate exercise on kidney function decline in sedentary older adults: an ancillary analysis of the LIFE study randomized clinical trial. JAMA Intern Med. 2022;182(6):650–9.
75. Blondell SJ, Hammersley-Mather R, Veerman JL. Does physical activity prevent cognitive decline and dementia?: a systematic review and meta-analysis of longitudinal studies. BMC Public Health. 2014;14:510.
76. Yang PY, et al. Exercise training improves sleep quality in middle-aged and older adults with sleep problems: a systematic review. J Physiother. 2012;58(3):157–63.
77. Song YY, et al. Effects of exercise training on restless legs syndrome, depression, sleep quality, and fatigue among hemodialysis patients: a systematic review and meta-analysis. J Pain Symptom Manage. 2018;55(4):1184–95.
78. Mohottige D, Manley HJ, Hall RK. Less is more: deprescribing medications in older adults with kidney disease: a review. Kidney360. 2021;2(9):1510–22.

79. Weich S, et al. Effect of anxiolytic and hypnotic drug prescriptions on mortality hazards: retrospective cohort study. BMJ. 2014;348:g1996.
80. By the 2019 American Geriatrics Society Beers Criteria® Update Expert Panel. American Geriatrics Society 2019 updated AGS Beers Criteria® for potentially inappropriate medication use in older adults. J Am Geriatr Soc. 2019;67(4):674–94.
81. Marupuru S, et al. Use of melatonin and/on ramelteon for the treatment of insomnia in older adults: a systematic review and meta-analysis. J Clin Med. 2022;11(17):5138.
82. Karasek M, et al. Decreased melatonin nocturnal concentrations in hemodialyzed patients. Neuro Endocrinol Lett. 2005;26(6):653–6.
83. Koch BC, et al. The effects of melatonin on sleep-wake rhythm of daytime haemodialysis patients: a randomized, placebo-controlled, cross-over study (EMSCAP study). Br J Clin Pharmacol. 2009;67(1):68–75.
84. Zhang W, et al. Exogenous melatonin for sleep disorders in neurodegenerative diseases: a meta-analysis of randomized clinical trials. Neurol Sci. 2016;37(1):57–65.
85. Harrison TG, Skrtic M, Verdin NE, Lanktree MB, Elliott MJ. Improving sexual function in people with chronic kidney disease: a narrative review of an unmet need in nephrology research. Can J Kidney Health Dis. 2020;7:2054358120952202. https://doi.org/10.1177/2054358120952202. PMID: 32953127; PMCID: PMC7485155.
86. Navaneethan SD, Vecchio M, Johnson DW, Saglimbene V, Graziano G, Pellegrini F, Lucisano G, Craig JC, Ruospo M, Gentile G, Manfreda VM, Querques M, Stroumza P, Torok M, Celia E, Gelfman R, Ferrari JN, Bednarek-Skublewska A, Dulawa J, Bonifati C, Hegbrant J, Wollheim C, Jannini EA, Strippoli GF. Prevalence and correlates of self-reported sexual dysfunction in CKD: a meta-analysis of observational studies. Am J Kidney Dis. 2010;56(4):670–85. https://doi.org/10.1053/j.ajkd.2010.06.016. PMID: 20801572.
87. Toorians AW, Janssen E, Laan E, Gooren LJ, Giltay EJ, Oe PL, Donker AJ, Everaerd W. Chronic renal failure and sexual functioning: clinical status versus objectively assessed sexual response. Nephrol Dial Transplant. 1997;12(12):2654–63. https://doi.org/10.1093/ndt/12.12.2654. PMID: 9430867.
88. Vecchio M, Palmer SC, Tonelli M, Johnson DW, Strippoli GF. Depression and sexual dysfunction in chronic kidney disease: a narrative review of the evidence in areas of significant unmet need. Nephrol Dial Transplant. 2012;27(9):3420–8. https://doi.org/10.1093/ndt/gfs135. PMID: 22942174.
89. Dumanski SM, Eckersten D, Piccoli GB. Reproductive health in chronic kidney disease: the implications of sex and gender. Semin Nephrol. 2022;42(2):142–52. https://doi.org/10.1016/j.semnephrol.2022.04.005. PMID: 35718362.
90. Kuczera P, Więcek A, Adamczak M. Impaired fertility in women and men with chronic kidney disease. Adv Clin Exp Med. 2022;31(2):187–95. https://doi.org/10.17219/acem/141188. PMID: 35178904.
91. Garibotto G, Esposito P, Picciotto D, Verzola D. Testosterone disorders and male hypogonadism in kidney disease. Semin Nephrol. 2021;41(2):114–25. https://doi.org/10.1016/j.semnephrol.2021.03.006. PMID: 34140090.
92. Chou J, Kiebalo T, Jagiello P, Pawlaczyk K. Multifaceted sexual dysfunction in dialyzing men and women: pathophysiology, diagnostics, and therapeutics. Life (Basel). 2021;11(4):311. https://doi.org/10.3390/life11040311. PMID: 33918412; PMCID: PMC8065963.
93. Palmer BF. Sexual dysfunction in uremia. J Am Soc Nephrol. 1999;10(6):1381–8. https://doi.org/10.1681/ASN.V1061381. PMID: 10361878.
94. Mor MK, Sevick MA, Shields AM, Green JA, Palevsky PM, Arnold RM, Fine MJ, Weisbord SD. Sexual function, activity, and satisfaction among women receiving maintenance hemodialysis. Clin J Am Soc Nephrol. 2014;9(1):128–34. https://doi.org/10.2215/CJN.05470513. Epub 2013 Dec 19. PMID: 24357510; PMCID: PMC3878703.
95. Finkelstein FO, Finkelstein SH. Sexual Inactivity among hemodialysis patients: the patients' perspective. Clin J Am Soc Nephrol. 2014;9(1):6–7. https://doi.org/10.2215/CJN.11831113. Epub 2013 Dec 19. PMID: 24357511; PMCID: PMC3878711.

Chapter 5
Geriatric 5Ms in Patients with Kidney Disease

Nitzy N. Muñoz Casablanca, Ko Harada, and Yuji Yamada

Mind

Dementia

The first M in the 5Ms of Geriatric care is Mind. Previous epidemiologic data suggest that patients at any stage of CKD have a higher risk of developing cognitive disorders and dementia. For instance, in studies of patients receiving maintenance hemodialysis, the prevalence of cognitive impairment has ranged from 30% to 60% [1] and is attributed to a high prevalence of both symptomatic and asymptomatic ischemic cerebrovascular lesions. Other potential mechanisms include direct neuronal injury by uremic toxins and cerebral microbleeds [1]. Furthermore, alternate etiologies such as Alzheimer's disease may also contribute. The US Preventive Services Task Force currently does not recommend for or against routine screening for dementia in older adults due to insufficient evidence that earlier detection will improve outcomes [2]. However, observed cognitive difficulty during a patient encounter should prompt an initial cognitive assessment and appropriate consultation as needed because early interventions are critical to slow down the progression

N. N. Muñoz Casablanca (✉)
Department of Medicine, Division of Nephrology, Elmhurst Hospital Center, Queens, New York, USA

K. Harada
Department of Medicine, Icahn School of Medicine at Mount Sinai Beth Israel, NY, New York, USA
e-mail: ko.harada@mountsinai.org

Y. Yamada
Brookdale Department of Geriatrics and Palliative Medicine, Icahn School of Medicine at Mount Sinai, NY, New York, USA
e-mail: yuji.yamada@mssm.edu

H. Kramer et al. (eds.), *Kidney Disease in the Elderly*,
https://doi.org/10.1007/978-3-031-68460-9_5

of cognitive decline and/or allow the addition of pharmacologic agents. Moreover, cognitive impairment may interfere with the overall capacity for self-care and hinder the capacity for informed decision-making [3].

There are several cognitive tools available for clinicians to assess cognition including MMSE, MoCA, and Mini-Cog.

Mini-Mental State Examination (MMSE)

The MMSE is the best-known and most frequently used test worldwide. It is a 30-point cognitive function test consisting of 11 items: time registration, place registration, immediate and delayed playback of three words, calculation, object naming, sentence recitation, three levels of verbal commands, written commands, written writing, and graphic imitation [4]. A score of 23 or below is suspicious for dementia.

The MMSE was originally developed as a method to identify cognitive impairment of various etiologies in patients admitted to psychiatric wards [4]. However, it has since been primarily used for outpatient screening and has been validated for this purpose. The MMSE exhibits a pooled sensitivity of 81% and a pooled specificity of 89% for identifying dementia. When used to assess patients for mild cognitive impairment (MCI), the MMSE was reported to have a sensitivity of 62.7% and a specificity of 63.3% [5].

The MMSE score is unique in that it is composed of three major components: verbal, memory, and construction abilities. For this reason, the MMSE is considered best suited to identify patients with mild to moderate Alzheimer's disease who are characterized by these impairments [6].

Montreal Cognitive Assessment (MoCA)

The MoCA is another well-known screening tool specifically designed to detect mild cognitive impairment. Like the MMSE, the MoCA is scored on a 30-point scale with items that assess delayed word recall (5 points), visuospatial/executive function (7 points; includes clock drawing), language (6 points), attention/concentration (6 points), and orientation (6 points).

The MoCA exhibits a pooled sensitivity of 89% and a pooled specificity of 75% for identifying MCI. Similarly, it has a pooled sensitivity of 91% and a pooled specificity of 81% for identifying dementia.

Mini-Cog™

The Mini-Cog is a screening test that combines immediate and delayed playback of three unrelated words with clock drawing [7]. Patient receives 1 point for each word spontaneously recalled without cueing, and 2 points for a normal clock depiction.

Clock drawing is assessed dichotomously as either normal with all numbers appearing in the correct order and the hands correctly indicating the given time, or abnormal. A cut point of <3 with failure to recall all three words, or failure to recall one to two words and abnormal clock drawing, is considered suspicious for cognitive dysfunction. Conversely, if the patient can recall all three words or if the clock drawing is normal with recall of one to two words, the patient is considered to be free of cognitive impairment.

When compared to other existing screening methods like the MMSE, the Mini-Cog is unique in that it is considered a language-independent assessment. It was initially tested on 249 subjects, of whom 124 were non-English speakers and the Mini-Cog assessment proved accurate in these subjects as well [8]. Since its validation, a series of study reports used the Mini-Cog have been published. While the Mini-Cog has been reported to have sufficient sensitivity (91%) to identify patients with dementia in primary care settings, its specificity is relatively low (54–86%) [5, 9]. The assessment is also not suitable for identifying patients with MCI (sensitivity 39–84%, specificity 73–88%). These data suggest that the Mini-Cog is suited to rule out dementia over a short period of time (approximately 3 min), but may be an inadequate assessment for other purposes (Table 5.1).

Delirium

Delirium is characterized by an acute, transient, and potentially reversible change in cognition. Causes of delirium that are relevant for patients with CKD include the following [3]:

1. Uremic encephalopathy.
2. Electrolyte disturbances.
3. Medications.
4. Hypotension during dialysis.

Table 5.1 Comparison of cognitive assessment tools for identifying dementia [5]

	Time	Sensitivity[a]	Specificity[a]	Characteristics
MMSE	5–10 min	81%	89%	Most widely used assay in clinical practice worldwide. Relatively low sensitivity. Use is restricted by copyright
Mini-cog	3 min	91%	86%	Can be performed in a short time, even in a busy outpatient setting, and has sensitivity and specificity comparable to MMSE. Not suitable for follow-up
MoCA	10 min	91%	81%	Originally developed to screen for mild cognitive impairment (MCI), it shows strength in the assessment of MCI. Freely accessible for clinical use at the MoCA website

[a]Pooled sensitivity and specificity for identifying dementia are shown

5. Cerebrovascular disease.
6. Dialysis disequilibrium syndrome.

Delirium and dementia can coexist, making it difficult to distinguish between these disorders. The Confusion Assessment Method (CAM) is a standardized evidence-based tool used to identify delirium in clinical settings. The CAM consists of four criteria, namely (1) a change in mental status with an acute onset and/or fluctuating course, (2) inattention, (3) disorganized thinking and/or (4) altered level of consciousness. The diagnosis of delirium by CAM requires the presence of features 1 and 2 and either 3 or 4. The tool has been found to have high sensitivity and specificity (both >90%) [10].

The 3D-CAM [11], which stands for "3-minute diagnostic interview for CAM defined delirium", is depicted below (Table 5.2). Among the criteria, confirmation of inattention by the clinician is particularly important since the other two criteria are easy to confirm based on nurses' report. Confirmation of inattention is usually achieved by asking patients to do one of the following: (1) recite days of the week backward, (2) recite months of the year backward, and (3) counting 30 to 1 backward.

Depression

Another issue for Mind, the first M in the 5 Ms of Geriatrics is depression because the most common psychiatric disorder observed in patients treated with dialysis is unipolar major depression (major depressive disorder) [12]. Depression is associated with reduced adherence to treatment for ESKD, as well as increased hospitalization and mortality regardless of dialysis adequacy [13]. Risk of depression increases with age and late-life depression often goes undetected and may have a

Table 5.2 3D-CAM [11]

Type of assessment	Acute, fluctuating	Inattention	Disorganized thinking	Altered level of consciousness
Patient responses	Ask if patient experienced the following in the past day: Being confused; Thinking that they are not in the hospital; Seeing things that are not really there	Ask patient to say days of the week or months of the year backward	Ask patient to state the current year, the day of the week, and the type of place	None
Interviewer observations	Fluctuations in the level of consciousness, attention, thinking, or speech	Trouble keeping track of the interview	Unclear or illogical flow of idea; Rambling or Limited speech	Sleepy, Stuporous or comatose; Hypervigilant

Table 5.3 The five-item Geriatric Depression Scale [15]

1	Are you basically satisfied with your life?
2	Do you often get bored?
3	Do you often feel helpless?
4	Do you prefer to stay at home rather than going out and doing new things?
5	Do you feel pretty worthless the way you are now?

Two out of five depressive responses including "no" to question 1 or "yes" to question 2 through 5 suggests a diagnosis of depression

significant adverse impact on patients' quality-of-life [14]. Several screening tools have been developed for depression, but the five-item Geriatric Depression Scale (GDS) has been most frequently studied among older adults in multiple settings [15]. This instrument consists of the following five questions (Table 5.3).

Another available screening tool to identify depression is the Patient Health Questionnaire (PHQ-9). The PHQ-9 has been validated in adult patients with kidney failure on maintenance dialysis and deemed to performed best for a depressive diagnosis at a value of 10 or greater among the cohort with both sensitivity and specificity of 92% [16].

Mobility

Falls Assessment

The second M in the 5 Ms of Geriatric care is mobility. Impaired mobility and falls are common in older adults. Falls are a major clinical concern among older adults due to their association with increased risk of serious injuries and hospitalization. In addition, falls represent a significant cost burden for the health care system overall. Fall assessment is very relevant in patients with CKD since this population is more susceptible to falls, fall-related fractures, hospitalizations, and death [17].

Screening for fall risk is an essential initial step in fall prevention. Initial screening involves asking patients the following three questions [18]:

1. Have you had two or more falls within the past 12 months?
2. Have you had a fall with injury?
3. Do you have any problems with gait or balance?

Patients who answer "yes" to any of the screening questions need further evaluation to determine their fall risk. Having fallen in the past year is a strong predictor of future falls. Nevertheless, older persons reporting only a single fall and reporting or demonstrating no difficulty or unsteadiness during the evaluation of gait and balance do not require a fall risk assessment [18].

The Timed Up and Go test (TUG) is another helpful tool to assess mobility and fall risk. It measures how long it takes a person to rise from a chair, walk three meters, turn, walk back, and sit down again (Table 5.4). An older adult who takes ≥ 12 seconds to complete the TUG is also at risk of falling [19, 20]. These initial assessments must be followed by a comprehensive evaluation and the formulation of a strategy to address identified risk factors. The likelihood of falling increases significantly as the number of risk factors rises.

Frailty Assessment

Frailty is a major inhibitor for mobility. Frailty is characterized by multisystem dysregulations that result in a loss of dynamic homeostasis and diminished physiologic reserve, which may in turn lead to adverse health outcomes, increased

Table 5.4 Timed Up and Go test

Directions	
	Patients wear their regular footwear and can use an assistive device, if needed. Begin by having the patient sit back in a standard armchair and identify a line 3 meters, or 10 feet away, on the floor
Instruct the patient	
	Stand up from the chair
	Walk to the line on the floor at your normal pace
	Turn
	Walk back to the chair at your normal pace
	Sit down again
Timing	
	On the word "go," begin timing. Stop timing after the patient sits back down. Record time
Factors to note	
	Sitting balance
	Transfers from sitting to standing
	Pace and stability of walking
	Ability to turn without staggering
Modified qualitative scoring	
No fall risk	Well-coordinated movements, without walking aid
Low fall risk	Controlled, but adjusted movements
Some fall risk	Uncoordinated movements
High fall risk	Supervision necessary
Very high fall risk	Physical support of stand by, physical support necessary

healthcare costs, and shorter survival [21]. While there is an association between mobility impairment and frailty, the latter entails the cumulative effect of medical, functional, and psychosocial deficits.

The prevalence of frailty among older adults living in the community is estimated to be 11%, and it is frequently seen among those with CKD [22]. Previous studies have reported a frailty prevalence of more than 60% in patients receiving maintenance dialysis [23, 24]. In addition, frailty is independently associated with unfavorable clinical outcomes in all stages of CKD, with a higher risk of mortality and hospitalization [25].

When selecting a frailty screening instrument, there are varieties of options available. The most frequently cited tool for assessing frailty is the Fried frailty phenotype, which defines frailty as the presence of five components: weakness, slowness, exhaustion, low physical activity, and unintentional weight loss [26]. Individuals can be classified as robust, pre-frail, or frail depending on the number of components scored (0 components, 1–2 components, or $\geq$ 3 components, respectively).

A clinical frailty scale (CFS) was proposed in an effort to produce a simple worldwide assessment of frailty for screening purposes [27]. The CFS identifies eight categories with increasing degrees of frailty and a ninth category for terminally ill patients (Table 5.5). In comparison to other measures for diagnosing frailty, the CFS's simplicity is its best feature. In addition, the CFS permits the monitoring of changes in the severity of frailty over time. It has been demonstrated that the CFS has similar predictive properties to the Fried frail phenotype in the general population and a higher CFS score is associated with an increased risk of mortality in patients with pre-dialysis CKD as well as those on dialysis [28, 29].

Medications

The third M in Geriatric care is medications because polypharmacy is common in older adults with all stages of CKD, including those receiving maintenance dialysis. Patients with CKD at stages 2–5 take an average of eight different medications, while those on dialysis take an average of 10–12 [29–32]. In the older adult population with CKD/ESRD, several factors like age-related physiological changes, inadequate nutritional status, and kidney disease-related abnormalities alter the pharmacokinetics and pharmacodynamic properties of drugs. These physiologic deviances along with the increased prevalence of multimorbidity and the "prescribing cascade" (i.e. the prescription of one drug to treat the side effects of another) increase the risk of medication-related complications [33, 34]. Previous studies have reported that 13– 96% of prescriptions for patients with impaired renal function contain errors such as inappropriate doses or intervals, contraindications, or precautions related to renally inappropriate medications [34, 35]. Furthermore, it is estimated that the overall incidence of adverse drug reactions is 3–10 times higher in older adults with CKD than in those without it [36]. Polypharmacy and the

Table 5.5 Clinical Frailty Scale

1	Very fit	People who are robust, active, energetic, and motivated. They tend to exercise regularly and are among the fittest for their age
2	Fit	People who have no active disease symptoms, but are less fit than category 1. They exercise or are very active occasionally, e.g., seasonally
3	Managing well	People whose medical problems are well controlled, even if occasionally symptomatic, but often are not regularly active beyond routine walking
4	Living with very mild frailty	Previously "vulnerable", this category marks early transition from complete independence. While not dependent on others for daily help, symptoms often limit activities. A common complaint is being "slowed up" and/or being tired during the day
5	Living with mild frailty	People who often have more evident slowing, and need help with high order instrumental activities of daily living (finances, transportation, heavy housework). Typically, mild frailty progressively impairs shopping and walking outside alone, meal preparation, taking medications appropriately, and begins to restrict light housework
6	Living with moderate frailty	People who need help with all activities outside and with managing a household. In the home, they often have problems with stairs and need help with bathing and might need minimal assistance (cuing, standby) with dressing
7	Living with severe frailty	Completely dependent for personal care, from whatever cause (physical or cognitive). Even so, they seem stable and not at high risk of dying (within ~6 months)
8	Living with very severe frailty	Completely dependent for personal care and approaching end of life. Typically, they could not recover even from a minor illness
9	Terminally ill	Approaching the end of life. This category applies to people with a life expectancy <6 months, who are not otherwise living with severe frailty. (Many terminally ill people can still exercise until very close to death.)

prescription of potentially inappropriate medications (PIM) in older adults also have associations with increased risk of falls, nonadherence, healthcare costs, and death [37–41].

Recognition of the multilayered impact of medication utilization has refocused the designation of polypharmacy beyond the traditional numerical cutoff of ≥ 5 medications to incorporate the appropriateness and safety of therapy. Several strategies have been developed to reduce the risk of medication-related complications, especially in susceptible individuals. The American Geriatrics Society Beers Criteria® for Potentially Inappropriate Medication Use in Older Adults [42] is a readily available compendium of medications that should be used with caution or avoided in older people due to evidenced-based unfavorable balance of benefits and harms. The recommendations, first developed in 1991 and last updated in 2023, are graded by quality and strength of evidence, and divided into categories according to considerations such as medications that should be dosed differently or should be avoided in reduced kidney function/estimated creatinine clearance. A recent retrospective observational study conducted in US assessed the risk of PIM, as defined by Beers Criteria, in adults with CKD participating in the Chronic Renal Insufficiency

Cohort. About 80% of the cohort reported use of PIM, with increasing prevalence in the older participants. The most frequently prescribed PIMs in older adults were proton pump inhibitors and α-blockers [37]. Another cross-sectional study conducted in Japan extended the Beers Criteria to older adult patients on hemodialysis and, similarly, found that prescription of PIM was common, and the three most frequently prescribed PIMs were H_2 blockers, antiplatelet agents, and α-blockers [43].

There are other helpful tools and interventions that may be used in conjunction with the Beers Criteria for guiding treatment decisions and improving medication safety. The Screening Tool of Older Persons' Potentially Inappropriate Prescriptions (STOPP) and the Screening Tool to Alert doctors to Right Treatment (START) are a set of criteria used in the clinical setting to determine appropriateness of initial prescribing and evaluate existing medication regimens including potential prescribing omissions (PPO) [34]. While the tools were developed to evaluate medication use in older patients and not in specific disease populations, a study conducted by Parker et al. showed effectiveness of using STOPP/START criteria to identify PIM and reduce the number of PPO in older adults with CKD [44]. Lastly, multiple studies suggest that collaboration with pharmacists helps reduce polypharmacy because they can assist with medication reconciliation, identify PIM use, promote deprescribing, and counsel patients [45–47].

Multi-Complexity

The first three Ms in the 5Ms of Geriatric care focused on individual issues but the fourth M targets multi-complexity or embracing the whole person and integrating their biopsychosocial heterogeneity. The concept of multi-complexity encompasses the presence and burden of multiple comorbidities, geriatric syndromes, and serious illnesses [48]. It also includes the assessment of social concerns such as financial issues and social isolation while gauging the impact of cognitive changes in health outcomes and highlighting the management of complex psychosocial needs.

When caring for older adults with CKD/ESKD, a nephrologist must consider the implications related to age and disease. Older adults with CKD are at increased risk for serious complications like cardiovascular disease, anemia, malnutrition, and infections [49–51]. When older adults with CKD develop medical comorbidities, they tend to have limited treatment options as decreased kidney function often makes it difficult to select renally-excreted drugs and increases the risk of medication side effects [52] . These issues complicate care planning for this population. Moreover, patients may have psychological and social complexities that limit treatment strategies. Providing comprehensive care for older adults with CKD can be challenging in busy practices, but implementing age-friendly strategies can be achieved with integration of interdisciplinary teams.

Multidisciplinary Team Approach

The multi-complexity of older adults with CKD requires a multidisciplinary team approach. Older adults have a wide variety of complex needs, ranging from variations in physical agility and abilities to conduct daily activities to impairments in mental health, and variable levels of social support. Therefore, it is critical to use a multidisciplinary team approach when caring for older adults, especially those with CKD. Several studies have evaluated the benefits of multidisciplinary care in CKD, particularly in the outpatient setting, and found evidence of improved patient outcomes when compared to traditional nephrology care delivery models. Improvements in care with a multidisciplinary approach were demonstrated in fistula rates, hospitalization, CKD progression, and mortality [53].

Transition of Care

Multi-complexity also requires caution when transitioning care. The term 'Transition of Care' refers to the coordination process that aims to ensure adequate continuity of care for patients as they transition to a different level of care or between facilities. When caring for patients with CKD, attention to care transitions is critically important. For example, randomized trials have shown that education and psychosocial support result in the delayed need for dialysis and improved survival after dialysis initiation when provided to patients as their kidney disease progresses and they prepare to transition to dialysis [54]. Likewise, older age and CKD at any stage are associated with hospitalizations. To prevent errors of omission or commission during the inpatient/outpatient transitions of care, a thorough medication reconciliation should be performed. Optimal management of care transitions should also include proactive discharge planning, patient education, clear communication among providers, especially verbal patient handoff, proper follow-up, and timely completion of discharge summaries to prevent negative health outcomes [55].

Matters Most

Finally, the last M of the 5Ms of Geriatric care is attention to what matters most. Matters most refers to an individuals' own meaningful health outcomes and care preferences based on their values, and priorities. Advance care planning (ACP) is the process by which patients, caregivers, and clinicians share disease-related information, discuss what matters most, and document future medical management based on shared decisions. ACP is an important part of the comprehensive care of older adults and adults with serious illness, yet it is estimated to occur in only 6–49% of patients with advance CKD [56, 57].

Studies evaluating patients' perspectives on ACP have shown that patients with advanced CKD/ESRD would prefer to have goals-of-care discussions early in the disease course because such conversation may impact decision-making. In older patients, this is of particular significance because for some individuals, dialysis offers marginal survival benefit, and the procedure has significant quality-of-life and quality-of-death implications [57–60]. During ACP conversations, patients may evaluate options such as a time-limited trial of dialysis or acknowledge that withdrawal from dialysis is a choice at any given time. Moreover, conservative kidney management may be an alternate and proactive multidisciplinary approach to address physical symptoms and psychosocial needs for those who do not wish or would not benefit from dialysis [61–63].

While ACP discussions have numerous advantages, there are challenges to holding this type of conversation and evidence suggests that nephrologists tend not to engage in ACP. Some of the identified barriers to conducting goals-of-care conversations include discordant views about who is responsible for engaging in ACP, prognostic uncertainty, time constrains, concerns about culturally sensitive approaches, and limited training in communications skills that help sustain difficult conversations [64–66].

Many stepwise communication frameworks have been developed to help healthcare providers navigate challenging goals-of-care conversations. REMAP is one such framework that structures the key components in goals-of-care conversations (Table 5.6) [67]. The "talking map" incorporates the ask-tell-ask collaborative method which assist clinicians in (1) identifying existing knowledge, learning what the patient wants to know, and determining readiness to initiate/continue ACP, and (2) recognizing the patient's health literacy and respecting their autonomy and cultural context. The discussion can combine open-ended questions, rating scales, narratives, and/or decision analysis. Regardless of the style chosen, the practice of exploring patient's perspective and perception surrounding high-stakes decisions inevitably elicits emotions. While display of emotion often hinders the clinician from continuing the discussion, studies indicate that serious illness conversations do not increase patient distress. Instead, using empathic communication skills like NURSE statements (Table 5.7) helps to build trust, increases patient satisfaction, decreases anxiety, and improves information recall [68].

It is widely recognized that palliative care principles should be integrated into the routine care of patients with advanced CKD/ESRD. In fact, initiatives such as Kidney Disease Improving Global Outcomes (KDIGO) have endorsed the use of supportive care and recommended that treatment care teams engage in ACP discussions [69, 70]. To enhance provider's education and confidence in leading such discussions, several training programs including NephroTalk Conservative Care Curriculum, VitalTalk, and Coalition for Supportive Care of Kidney Patients are available [71].

Table 5.6 REMAP [67]

REMAP	Notes	Examples
Reframe the situation	1. Preparation phase: Review patient's chart, identify risk/ prognostic factor, discuss with other physicians as necessary 2. Assess patient's understanding of the illness, current health status, disease trajectory 3. Determine readiness for participation in ACP 4. Use a preamble and share the headline (new information and its meaning in the context of the bigger picture). Share this in a succinct way with simple language 5. Address emotions and, if the patient is willing, explore their views	"I'd like to take some time to discuss your illness and what's important to you" "What have you heard from the doctors so far?", "what have you heard about dialysis?" "Would it be ok if I share what we know/some updates?" "We are concern that the symptoms you are experiencing are related to the progression of your kidney disease. For some patients with similar health conditions, dialysis can be associated with side effects and burdens, so I would like to learn more about what is important to you to understand if dialysis or conservative therapy is right for you"
Expect emotions and empathize	Watch for emotional cues and attend to patients' needs. May use NURSE statements and allow strategic silence	See NURSE statements (Table 5.7)
Map out patient's goals	Answer questions in regard to illness trajectory and management options (dialysis vs conservative kidney management); then assess values, goals, and preferences	"Given the news about your illness, what's most important to you?" – If deemed adequate, the physician can give options. For example: "Try dialysis and live as long as possible", "try dialysis, but stop if suffering or marginal benefits (timed-limited dialysis)", "focus on comfort with non-dialytic interventions", "unsure." "As you think about the future, what concerns you?" "What would be an unacceptable quality-of-life for you?" "Has anyone else in your life been on dialysis?" "What gives you strength?"

(continued)

Table 5.6 (continued)

REMAP	Notes	Examples
Align with goals	Reflect and summarize the patient's values, goals, and preferences	"It sounds like the most important things are…" "I hear you saying you want to avoid…"
Propose a plan	1. Ask for permission to give recommendation 2. Share values-concordant recommendations among feasible options 3. Outline a care plan that identifies milestones and specific setbacks for potential withdrawal of dialysis 4. Check in with patient and care partner	"Would it be helpful if I offer a recommendation based on what you told me?" "Based on…, I would recommend that we…" "We will monitor if dialysis is working for you (name milestones) and be alert of situations when dialysis should be readdressed like (name setbacks). How does that sound to you?"

Table 5.7 NURSE [68]

NURSE	Notes	Examples
Naming	Name the emotion	"I can see how this is upsetting/frustrating you"
Understanding	Acknowledging the situation or emotion	"I can't imagine how hard this must be for you" "I can see that this is a difficult conversation"
Respecting	Showing respect and praising efforts	"I admire how you have been dealing with the disease" "I can see how hard you've worked"
Supporting	Showing partnership	"We will continue to meet" "I will be here for you"
Exploring	Exploring feelings or viewpoints	"Can you tell me more about…"

Geriatric Comanagement

Geriatric comanagement is defined as a shared responsibility and collaborative decision-making between a treating physician and a geriatrician who provides complementary medical care to prevent or manage geriatric-oriented problems. Although systematic reviews have demonstrated that geriatric comanagement reduces functional decline, complications, length of hospital stay, and mortality rates [72, 73], the impact of geriatric comanagement in patients with kidney disease is not well established.

Globally, the population with ESKD is growing fastest among patients over 65 years of age. Patients aged 65–74, and 75 years or older constitute 24% and 34%, respectively, of the population receiving maintenance dialysis in the United States [74]. Dialysis, while a lifesaving treatment, carries its own side effects and complications. The decision-making process should thus incorporate several viewpoints, including those of the patient, caregiver/family, and, ideally, a geriatrician-nephrologist collaborative team. The comanagement team should be established early in the disease progression to align the patient's care with their goals and assist in identifying cognitive, functional, and psychosocial issues as the disease progresses. Due to age-related physiological changes, medical comorbidities, and presence of geriatric syndromes, the risk profile of dialysis in older adults is worse than in younger counterparts. Recognizing the complexity of geriatric nephrology should trigger planning for potential problems and prompt counseling on appropriate treatment options based on what matters most to patients and family members.

Geriatric comanagement may help decision-making regarding kidney transplantation as well. A systematic review showed that 1 in 6 kidney transplant recipients is frail before transplantation, and that frailty is significantly associated with advancing age, lower rate of pre-emptive transplantation, longer duration of delayed graft function, and length of hospital stay [75]. The influence of frailty on mortality in older transplant recipients is still poorly understood, and there are no guidelines indicating at which level of frailty a patient should be excluded from a waiting list [74]. Assessing frailty and cognitive impairment has the potential to improve decisions about who among the many older transplant candidates should proceed with transplantation.

In this chapter, we proposed the GERIATRIC 5Ms framework as a tool to assess geriatric concerns in older adults with CKD. The systematic approach may facilitate nephrology practices in providing the comprehensive care needed for this population. Recognizing the complexity and heterogeneity in care, we also suggest the integration of an interdisciplinary team, namely geriatric comanagement, in efforts to positively impact health outcomes.

References

1. Bugnicourt JM, Godefroy O, Chillon JM, Choukroun G, Massy ZA. Cognitive disorders and dementia in CKD: the neglected kidney-brain Axis. J Am Soc Nephrol. 2013;24:353–63.
2. Owens DK, Davidson KW, Krist AH, et al. Screening for cognitive impairment in older adults: US preventive services task force recommendation statement. JAMA. 2020;323:757–63.
3. Tamura MK, Yaffe K. Dementia and cognitive impairment in ESRD: diagnostic and therapeutic strategies. Kidney Int. 2011;79:14–22.
4. Folstein MF, Folstein SE, McHugh PR. 'Mini-mental state'. A practical method for grading the cognitive state of patients for the clinician. J Psychiatr Res. 1975;12:189–98.
5. Tsoi KKF, Chan JYC, Hirai HW, Wong SYS, Kwok TCY. Cognitive tests to detect dementia: a systematic review and meta-analysis. JAMA Intern Med. 2015;175:1450–8.
6. Tombaugh TN, McIntyre NJ. The mini-mental state examination: a comprehensive review. J Am Geriatr Soc. 1992;40:922–35.
7. Borson S, Scanlan JM, Chen P, Ganguli M. The mini-cog as a screen for dementia: validation in a population-based sample. J Am Geriatr Soc. 2003;51:1451–4.
8. Borson S, Scanlan J, Brush M, Vitaliano P, Dokmak A. The mini-cog: a cognitive 'vital signs' measure for dementia screening in multi-lingual elderly. Int J Geriatr Psychiatry. 2000;15:1021–7.

9. Lin JS, O'Connor E, Rossom RC, Perdue LA, Eckstrom E. Screening for cognitive impairment in older adults: a systematic review for the U.S. preventive services task force. Ann Intern Med. 2013;159:601–12.

10. Inouye SK, Van Dyck CH, Alessi CA, Balkin S, Siegal AP, Horwitz RI. Clarifying confusion: the confusion assessment method: a new method for detection of delirium. Ann Intern Med. 1990;113:941–8.

11. Marcantonio ER, Ngo LH, O'Connor M, et al. 3D-CAM: derivation and validation of a 3-minute diagnostic interview for CAM-defined delirium: a cross-sectional diagnostic test study. Ann Intern Med. 2014;161:554–61.

12. King-Wing Ma T, Kam-Tao LP. Depression in dialysis patients. Nephrology (Carlton). 2016;21:639–46.

13. Kimmel PL, Fwu CW, Abbott KC, et al. Psychiatric illness and mortality in hospitalized ESKD dialysis patients. Clin J Am Soc Nephrol. 2019;14:1363–71.

14. Hybels CF, Blazer DG. Epidemiology of late-life mental disorders. Clin Geriatr Med. 2003;19:663–96.

15. Rinaldi P, Mecocci P, Benedetti C, et al. Validation of the five-item geriatric depression scale in elderly subjects in three different settings. J Am Geriatr Soc. 2003;51:694–8.

16. Watnick S, Wang PL, Demadura T, Ganzini L. Validation of 2 depression screening tools in dialysis patients. Am J Kidney Dis. 2005;46(5):919–24. https://doi.org/10.1053/j.ajkd.2005.08.006. PMID: 16253733.

17. Papakonstantinopoulou K, Sofianos I. Risk of falls in chronic kidney disease. J Frailty Sarcopenia Falls. 2017;2(2):33–8. PMID: 32300681; PMCID: PMC7155375.

18. Panel on Prevention of Falls in Older Persons, American Geriatrics Society and British Geriatrics Society. Summary of the updated American Geriatrics Society/British geriatrics society clinical practice guideline for prevention of falls in older persons. J Am Geriatr Soc. 2011;59(1):148–57. https://doi.org/10.1111/j.1532-5415.2010.03234.x. PMID: 21226685.

19. Fleming KC, Evans JM, Weber DC, Chutka DS. Practical functional assessment of elderly persons: a primary-care approach. Mayo Clin Proc. 1995;70(9):890–910. https://doi.org/10.1016/S0025-6196(11)63949-9. PMID: 7643645.

20. Nordin E, Lindelöf N, Rosendahl E, Jensen J, Lundin-Olsson L. Prognostic validity of the timed up-and-go test, a modified get-up-and-go test, staff's global judgement and fall history in evaluating fall risk in residential care facilities. Age Ageing. 2008;37(4):442–8. https://doi.org/10.1093/ageing/afn101. Epub 2008 May 30. PMID: 18515291.

21. Hoogendijk EO, Afilalo J, Ensrud KE, Kowal P, Onder G, Fried LP. Frailty: implications for clinical practice and public health. Lancet. 2019;394(10206):1365–75. https://doi.org/10.1016/S0140-6736(19)31786-6. PMID: 31609228.

22. Collard RM, Boter H, Schoevers RA, Oude Voshaar RC. Prevalence of frailty in community-dwelling older persons: a systematic review. J Am Geriatr Soc. 2012;60(8):1487–92. https://doi.org/10.1111/j.1532-5415.2012.04054.x. Epub 2012 Aug 6. PMID: 22881367.

23. Bao Y, Dalrymple L, Chertow GM, Kaysen GA, Johansen KL. Frailty, dialysis initiation, and mortality in end-stage renal disease. Arch Intern Med. 2012;172(14):1071–7. https://doi.org/10.1001/archinternmed.2012.3020. PMID: 22733312; PMCID: PMC4117243.

24. Johansen KL, Chertow GM, Jin C, Kutner NG. Significance of frailty among dialysis patients. J Am Soc Nephrol. 2007;18(11):2960–7. https://doi.org/10.1681/ASN.2007020221. Epub 2007 Oct 17. PMID: 17942958.

25. Shen Z, Ruan Q, Yu Z, Sun Z. Chronic kidney disease-related physical frailty and cognitive impairment: a systemic review. Geriatr Gerontol Int. 2017;17(4):529–44. https://doi.org/10.1111/ggi.12758. Epub 2016 May 31. PMID: 27240548.

26. Fried LP, Tangen CM, Walston J, Newman AB, Hirsch C, Gottdiener J, Seeman T, Tracy R, Kop WJ, Burke G, McBurnie MA. Cardiovascular health study collaborative research group. Frailty in older adults: evidence for a phenotype. J Gerontol A Biol Sci Med Sci. 2001;56(3):M146–56. https://doi.org/10.1093/gerona/56.3.m146. PMID: 11253156.

27. Rockwood K, Song X, MacKnight C, Bergman H, Hogan DB, McDowell I, Mitnitski A. A global clinical measure of fitness and frailty in elderly people. CMAJ. 2005;173(5):489–95. https://doi.org/10.1503/cmaj.050051. PMID: 16129869; PMCID: PMC1188185.
28. Pugh J, Aggett J, Goodland A, Prichard A, Thomas N, Donovan K, Roberts G. Frailty and comorbidity are independent predictors of outcome in patients referred for pre-dialysis education. Clin Kidney J. 2016;9(2):324–9. https://doi.org/10.1093/ckj/sfv150. Epub 2016 Jan 29. PMID: 26985387; PMCID: PMC4792625.
29. Alfaadhel TA, Soroka SD, Kiberd BA, Landry D, Moorhouse P, Tennankore KK. Frailty and mortality in dialysis: evaluation of a clinical frailty scale. Clin J Am Soc Nephrol. 2015;10(5):832–40. https://doi.org/10.2215/CJN.07760814. Epub 2015 Mar 4. PMID: 25739851; PMCID: PMC4422241.
30. Bhattarai M. Geriatric issues in older dialysis patients. R I Med J. 2016;99(7):15–8. PMID: 27379352.
31. Hayward S, Hole B, Denholm R, Duncan P, Morris JE, SDS F, Payne RA, Roderick P, Chesnaye NC, Wanner C, Drechsler C, Postorino M, Porto G, Szymczak M, Evans M, Dekker FW, Jager KJ, Caskey FJ, EQUAL Study investigators. International prescribing patterns and polypharmacy in older people with advanced chronic kidney disease: results from the European quality study. Nephrol Dial Transplant. 2021;36(3):503–11. https://doi.org/10.1093/ndt/gfaa064. PMID: 32543669.
32. Molnar AO, Bota S, Jeyakumar N, McArthur E, Battistella M, Garg AX, Sood MM, Brimble KS. Potentially inappropriate prescribing in older adults with advanced chronic kidney disease. PLoS One. 2020;15(8):e0237868. https://doi.org/10.1371/journal.pone.0237868. PMID: 32818951; PMCID: PMC7444541.
33. Secora A, Alexander GC, Ballew SH, Coresh J, Grams ME. Kidney function, polypharmacy, and potentially inappropriate medication use in a community-based cohort of older adults. Drugs Aging. 2018;35(8):735–50. https://doi.org/10.1007/s40266-018-0563-1. PMID: 30039344; PMCID: PMC6093216.
34. Gallieni M, Cancarini G. Drugs in the elderly with chronic kidney disease: beware of potentially inappropriate medications. Nephrol Dial Transplant. 2015;30(3):342–4. https://doi.org/10.1093/ndt/gfu191. Epub 2014 Jun 12. PMID: 24923769.
35. Wong NA, Jones HW. An analysis of discharge drug prescribing amongst elderly patients with renal impairment. Postgrad Med J. 1998;74(873):420–2. https://doi.org/10.1136/pgmj.74.873.420.
36. Qato D, Caleb G, Johnson M, Schumm P, Tessler LS. Use of prescription and over-the-counter medications and dietary supplements among older adults in the United States. JAMA. 2008;300(24):2867. https://doi.org/10.1001/jama.2008.892.
37. Hall RK, Blumenthal JB, Doerfler RM, Chen J, Diamantidis CJ, Jaar BG, Kusek JW, Kallem K, Leonard MB, Navaneethan SD, Sha D, Sondheimer JH, Wagner LA, Yang W, Zhan M, Fink JC, CRIC Study Investigators. Risk of Potentially Inappropriate Medications in Adults With CKD: Findings From the Chronic Renal Insufficiency Cohort (CRIC) Study. Am J Kidney Dis. 2021;78(6):837–845.e1. https://doi.org/10.1053/j.ajkd.2021.03.019. Epub 2021 May 23. PMID: 34029681; PMCID: PMC8608689.
38. Fick DM, Waller JL, Maclean JR. Potentially inappropriate medication use in a Medicare managed care population: association with higher costs and utilization. J Manag Care Pharm. 2001;7(5):407–13.
39. Fick DM, Mion LC, Beers MH, Waller JL. Health outcomes associated with potentially inappropriate medication use in older adults. Res Nurs Health. 2008;31(1):42–51. https://doi.org/10.1002/nur.20232. PMID: 18163447; PMCID: PMC2247370.
40. Muhlack DC, Hoppe LK, Weberpals J, Brenner H, Schöttker B. The Association of Potentially Inappropriate Medication at older age with cardiovascular events and overall mortality: a systematic review and meta-analysis of cohort studies. J Am Med Dir Assoc. 2017;18(3):211–20. https://doi.org/10.1016/j.jamda.2016.11.025. Epub 2017 Jan 26. PMID: 28131719.

41. Hyttinen V, Jyrkkä J, Valtonen H. A systematic review of the impact of potentially inappropriate medication on health care utilization and costs among older adults. Med Care. 2016;54(10):950–64. https://doi.org/10.1097/MLR.0000000000000587. PMID: 27367864.
42. By the 2019 American Geriatrics Society Beers Criteria® Update Expert Panel. American Geriatrics Society 2019 Updated AGS beers criteria® for potentially inappropriate medication use in older adults. J Am Geriatr Soc. 2019;67(4):674–94. https://doi.org/10.1111/jgs.15767. Epub 2019 Jan 29. PMID: 30693946.
43. Kondo N, Nakamura F, Yamazaki S, Yamamoto Y, Akizawa T, Akiba T, Saito A, Kurokawa K, Fukuhara S. Prescription of potentially inappropriate medications to elderly hemodialysis patients: prevalence and predictors. Nephrol Dial Transplant. 2015;30(3):498–505. https://doi.org/10.1093/ndt/gfu070. Epub 2014 Apr 28. PMID: 24777993.
44. Parker K, Bull-Engelstad I, Benth JŠ, Aasebø W, von der Lippe N, Reier-Nilsen M, Os I, Stavem K. Effectiveness of using STOPP/START criteria to identify potentially inappropriate medication in people aged ≥65 years with chronic kidney disease: a randomized clinical trial. Eur J Clin Pharmacol. 2019;75(11):1503–11. https://doi.org/10.1007/s00228-019-02727-9. Epub 2019 Jul 29. PMID: 31359099.
45. Triantafylidis LK, Hawley CE, Perry LP, Paik JM. The role of Deprescribing in older adults with chronic kidney disease. Drugs Aging. 2018;35(11):973–84. https://doi.org/10.1007/s40266-018-0593-8. PMID: 30284120; PMCID: PMC8150926.
46. McIntyre C, McQuillan R, Bell C, Battistella M. Targeted Deprescribing in an outpatient hemodialysis unit: a quality improvement study to decrease polypharmacy. Am J Kidney Dis. 2017;70(5):611–8. https://doi.org/10.1053/j.ajkd.2017.02.374. Epub 2017 Apr 14. PMID: 28416321.
47. Kim AJ, Lee H, Shin EJ, Cho EJ, Cho YS, Lee H, Lee JY. Pharmacist-led collaborative medication Management for the Elderly with chronic kidney disease and polypharmacy. Int J Environ Res Public Health. 2021;18(8):4370. https://doi.org/10.3390/ijerph18084370. PMID: 33924094; PMCID: PMC8074256.
48. Tip Sheet: The 5Ms of Geriatricsl. HealthInAging.org. https://www.healthinaging.org/tools-and-tips/tip-sheet-5ms-geriatrics. Accessed 10 Sept 2022.
49. Snyder JJ, Collins AJ. Association of preventive health care with atherosclerotic heart disease and mortality in CKD. J Am Soc Nephrol. 2009;20:1614–22.
50. Astor BC, Muntner P, Levin A, Eustace JA, Coresh J. Association of kidney function with anemia: the third National Health and nutrition examination survey (1988-1994). Arch Intern Med. 2002;162:1401–8.
51. Dalrymple LS, Katz R, Kestenbaum B, et al. The risk of infection-related hospitalization with decreased kidney function. Am J Kidney Dis. 2012;59:356–63.
52. Cardone KE, Bacchus S, Assimon MM, Pai AB, Manley HJ. Medication-related problems in CKD. Adv Chronic Kidney Dis. 2010;17:404–12.
53. Collister D, Pyne L, Cunningham J, Donald M, Molnar A, Beaulieu M, Levin A, Brimble KS. Multidisciplinary chronic kidney disease clinic practices: a scoping review. Can J Kidney Health Dis. 2019;6:2054358119882667. https://doi.org/10.1177/2054358119882667. PMID: 31666978; PMCID: PMC6801876.
54. Devins GM, Mendelssohn DC, Barré PE, Taub K, Binik YM. Predialysis psychoeducational intervention extends survival in CKD: a 20-year follow-up. Am J Kidney Dis. 2005;46(6):1088–98. https://doi.org/10.1053/j.ajkd.2005.08.017. PMID: 16310575.
55. Zurlo A, Zuliani G. Management of care transition and hospital discharge. Aging Clin Exp Res. 2018;30:263–70.
56. Sellars M, Clayton JM, Morton RL, Luckett T, Silvester W, Spencer L, Pollock CA, Walker RG, Kerr PG, Tong A. An interview study of patient and caregiver perspectives on advance care planning in ESRD. Am J Kidney Dis. 2018;71(2):216–24. https://doi.org/10.1053/j.ajkd.2017.07.021. Epub 2017 Nov 11. PMID: 29132946.

57. Mandel EI, Bernacki RE, Block SD. Serious Illness Conversations in ESRD. Clin J Am Soc Nephrol. 2017;12(5):854–63. https://doi.org/10.2215/CJN.05760516. Epub 2016 Dec 28. PMID: 28031417; PMCID: PMC5477207.

58. Ramer SJ, McCall NN, Robinson-Cohen C, Siew ED, Salat H, Bian A, Stewart TG, El-Sourady MH, Karlekar M, Lipworth L, Ikizler TA, Abdel-Kader K. Health outcome priorities of older adults with advanced CKD and concordance with their nephrology Providers' perceptions. J Am Soc Nephrol. 2018;29(12):2870–8. https://doi.org/10.1681/ASN.2018060657. Epub 2018 Nov 1. PMID: 30385652; PMCID: PMC6287864.

59. Kurella Tamura M, Montez-Rath ME, Hall YN, Katz R, O'Hare AM. Advance directives and end-of-life care among nursing home residents receiving maintenance dialysis. Clin J Am Soc Nephrol. 2017;12(3):435–42. https://doi.org/10.2215/CJN.07510716. Epub 2017 Jan 5. PMID: 28057703; PMCID: PMC5338713.

60. Stallings TL, Temel JS, Klaiman TA, Paasche-Orlow MK, Alegria M, O'Hare A, O'Connor N, Dember LM, Halpern SD, Eneanya ND. Integrating conservative kidney management options and advance care planning education (COPE) into routine CKD care: a protocol for a pilot randomised controlled trial. BMJ Open. 2021;11(2):e042620. https://doi.org/10.1136/bmjopen-2020-042620. PMID: 33619188; PMCID: PMC7903110.

61. Verberne WR, Geers AB, Jellema WT, Vincent HH, van Delden JJ, Bos WJ. Comparative survival among older adults with advanced kidney disease managed conservatively versus with dialysis. Clin J Am Soc Nephrol. 2016;11(4):633–40. https://doi.org/10.2215/CJN.07510715. Epub 2016 Mar 17. PMID: 26988748; PMCID: PMC4822664.

62. Raghavan D, Holley JL. Conservative Care of the Elderly CKD patient: a practical guide. Adv Chronic Kidney Dis. 2016;23(1):51–6. https://doi.org/10.1053/j.ackd.2015.08.003. PMID: 26709063.

63. Saeed F, Adams H, Epstein RM. Matters of life and death: why do older patients choose conservative management? Am J Nephrol. 2020;51(1):35–42. https://doi.org/10.1159/000504692. Epub 2019 Nov 27. PMID: 31775149.

64. Ladin K, Neckermann I, D'Arcangelo N, Koch-Weser S, Wong JB, Gordon EJ, Rossi A, Rifkin D, Isakova T, Weiner DE. Advance care planning in older adults with CKD: patient, care partner, and clinician perspectives. J Am Soc Nephrol. 2021;32(6):1527–35. https://doi.org/10.1681/ASN.2020091298. Epub 2021 Apr 7. PMID: 33827902; PMCID: PMC8259659.

65. Schell JO, Patel UD, Steinhauser KE, Ammarell N, Tulsky JA. Discussions of the kidney disease trajectory by elderly patients and nephrologists: a qualitative study. Am J Kidney Dis. 2012;59(4):495–503. https://doi.org/10.1053/j.ajkd.2011.11.023. Epub 2012 Jan 4. PMID: 22221483; PMCID: PMC3626427.

66. Baddour NA, Siew ED, Robinson-Cohen C, Salat H, Mason OJ, Stewart TG, Karlekar M, El-Sourady MH, Lipworth L, Abdel-Kader K. Serious illness treatment preferences for older adults with advanced CKD. J Am Soc Nephrol. 2019;30(11):2252–61. https://doi.org/10.1681/ASN.2019040385. Epub 2019 Sep 11. PMID: 31511360; PMCID: PMC6830783.

67. Childers JW, Back AL, Tulsky JA, Arnold RM. REMAP: a framework for goals of care conversations. J Oncol Pract. 2017;13(10):e844–50. https://doi.org/10.1200/JOP.2016.018796. Epub 2017 Apr 26. PMID: 28445100.

68. van Vliet LM, Lindenberger E, van Weert JC. Communication with older, seriously ill patients. Clin Geriatr Med. 2015;31(2):219–30. https://doi.org/10.1016/j.cger.2015.01.007. Epub 2015 Feb 18. PMID: 25920057.

69. Davison SN, Levin A, Moss AH, Jha V, Brown EA, Brennan F, Murtagh FE, Naicker S, Germain MJ, O'Donoghue DJ, Morton RL. Obrador GT; kidney disease: improving global outcomes. Executive summary of the KDIGO controversies conference on supportive care in chronic kidney disease: developing a roadmap to improving quality care. Kidney Int. 2015;88(3):447–59. https://doi.org/10.1038/ki.2015.110. Epub 2015 Apr 29. PMID: 25923985.

70. Davison SN. Advance care planning in patients with chronic kidney disease. Semin Dial. 2012;25(6):657–63. https://doi.org/10.1111/sdi.12039.PMID: 23173893

71. Schell JO, Arnold RM. NephroTalk: communication tools to enhance patient-centered care. Semin Dial. 2012;25(6):611–6. https://doi.org/10.1111/sdi.12017. Epub 2012 Oct 19. PMID: 23078102.
72. Van Grootven B, Flamaing J, Dierckx de Casterlé B, Dubois C, Fagard K, Herregods MC, Hornikx M, Laenen A, Meuris B, Rex S, Tournoy J, Milisen K, Deschodt M. Effectiveness of in-hospital geriatric co-management: a systematic review and meta-analysis. Age Ageing. 2017;46(6):903–10. https://doi.org/10.1093/ageing/afx051. PMID: 28444116.
73. Van Grootven B, Mendelson DA, Deschodt M. Impact of geriatric co-management programmes on outcomes in older surgical patients: update of recent evidence. Curr Opin Anaesthesiol. 2020;33(1):114–21. https://doi.org/10.1097/ACO.0000000000000815. PMID: 31789902.
74. Segall L, Nistor I, Pascual J, Mucsi I, Guirado L, Higgins R, Van Laecke S, Oberbauer R, Van Biesen W, Abramowicz D, Gavrilovici C, Farrington K, Covic A. Criteria for and appropriateness of renal transplantation in elderly patients with end-stage renal disease: a literature review and position statement on behalf of the European renal association-European dialysis and transplant association Descartes working group and European renal best practice. Transplantation. 2016;100(10):e55–65. https://doi.org/10.1097/TP.0000000000001367. PMID: 27472096.
75. Quint EE, Zogaj D, Banning LBD, Benjamens S, Annema C, Bakker SJL, Nieuwenhuijs-Moeke GJ, Segev DL, McAdams-DeMarco MA, Pol RA. Frailty and kidney transplantation: a systematic review and meta-analysis. Transplant Direct. 2021;7(6):e701. https://doi.org/10.1097/TXD.0000000000001156. PMID: 34036171; PMCID: PMC8133203.

Further Readings

Centers for Disease Control and Prevention. Chronic Kidney Disease in the United States, 2021. Atlanta, GA: US Department of Health and Human Services, Centers for Disease Control and Prevention; 2021.
McCullough KP, Morgenstern H, Saran R, Herman WH, Robinson BM. Projecting ESRD Incidence and Prevalence in the United States through 2030. J Am Soc Nephrol. 2019;30(1):127–35. https://doi.org/10.1681/ASN.2018050531. Epub 2018 Dec 17. PMID: 30559143; PMCID: PMC6317596.
Molnar F, Frank CC. Optimizing geriatric care with the GERIATRIC 5*M*s. Can Fam Physician. 2019;65(1):39. PMID: 30674512; PMCID: PMC6347324.
United States Renal Data System. 2021 USRDS annual data report: epidemiology of kidney disease in the United States. Bethesda, MD: National Institutes of Health, National Institute of Diabetes and Digestive and Kidney Diseases; 2021.
US Census Bureau. "Population characteristics release updates." Censusgov, 19 July 2022. https://www.census.gov/library/visualizations/interactive/vintage-2021-population-estimates.html.

Chapter 6
Urinary Symptoms in Older Adults with Chronic Kidney Disease

Emily Janak and Holly Kramer

Case

An 81-year-old male with chronic kidney disease (CKD) stage 3B due to type 2 diabetes mellitus presents for routine follow-up. His medications include losartan 100 mg daily and amlodipine 10 mg daily. The clinic blood pressure is 148/63 mmHg. His exam reveals decreased sensation to vibration in both feet and 1+ pitting edema in both lower extremities. The serum creatinine is stable at 2.2 mg/dL but a random urine albumin-to-creatinine ratio has increased from 177 mg/g 4 months ago to 675 mg/g at this visit. The clinician discusses initiation of a sodium-glucose cotransporter 2 inhibitor (SGLT2i) and outlines the potential risks of this medication class including groin infections. The patient then relates his struggles with urinary incontinence for the past 6 years. He states that urinary incontinence occurs when he develops an urge to urinate and cannot make it to the bathroom fast enough. Over the past year, urinary incontinence has become so frequent that he is now wearing adult briefs almost continuously.

E. Janak
Medicine, Maywood, IL, USA

H. Kramer (✉)
Department of Public Health Sciences and Medicine, Loyola University Chicago, Maywood, IL, USA
e-mail: hkramer@lumc.edu

H. Kramer et al. (eds.), *Kidney Disease in the Elderly*,
https://doi.org/10.1007/978-3-031-68460-9_6

Introduction

Urinary tract symptoms (LUTS) include a wide variety of voiding or obstructive symptoms such as hesitancy, poor and/or intermittent stream, straining, and feeling of incomplete bladder emptying and dribbling. LUTS also include storage or irritative symptoms such as urinary frequency, urgency, incontinence, and nocturia. These bothersome urinary symptoms affect a large percentage of older adults [1–6]. The frequency of LUTS generally increases with age and is higher among adults with diabetes. Despite the high prevalence of LUTS in older adults, most will never discuss urinary symptoms with their physician and seek or receive treatment due to embarrassment and or belief that LUTS is a normal process of aging.

For the nephrologist, LUTS may complicate the treatment of kidney diseases and associated comorbidities such as hypertension and heart failure. For example, patients may not take diuretic medications as prescribed due to worsening of LUTS. Use of SGLT2i may be contraindicated due to risk of groin and urinary tract infections from incontinence. Lack of attention to LUTS could potentially lead to suboptimal outcomes from poor compliance with medications [4] and increased risk of hospitalizations. Incontinence is also associated with the need for assistance with daily tasks of living and unmet care needs. Thus, identifying LUTS, especially incontinence and nocturia, may help discern patients who require more social support and assistance with disease self-management.

Diabetes remains a major cause of CKD globally and SGLT2is are indicated for the treatment of diabetes to slow CKD progression and reduce risk of cardiovascular disease. Older adults with diabetes may be a group with highest risk of LUTS and LUTS severity. Chronic hyperglycemia damages the autonomic nervous system innervation of the bladder. Bladder pathology in diabetes may progress from deceased sensation to bladder hypotonicity, whereby patients go to the bathroom less frequently leading to higher bladder capacity. This chronic stretching of the bladder then progresses to poor bladder emptying due to bladder wall stress and nerve damage. Thus, LUTS in a person with diabetes may begin with urinary urgency due to a distended bladder, progress to urgency incontinence and then further progress to overflow incontinence. Patients may also have other comorbidities that can cause stress incontinence such as obesity or prior pelvic floor trauma from pregnancies. Approximately half of all adults with diabetes mellitus will suffer with some form of LUTS and generally symptoms may be more severe in this group [7, 8].

In this chapter, we review the definitions and epidemiology of specific urinary symptoms which encompass LUTS. The chapter also provides sample questions which may be used to query presence of LUTS and assist with diagnosis. Finally, management strategies are discussed specifically for older adults with non-dialysis dependent kidney disease.

Overactive Bladder

The patient's complaint of a sudden urge to urinate with or without involuntary urinary leakage when rushing to the toilet is known as overactive bladder syndrome (OAB) [5, 9, 10]. OAB is common and affects approximately 10% of adults over the age of 50 years but risk of OAB increases with age [5, 6]. OAB, especially if incontinence is present, can reduce quality of life due to social isolation [10]. Individuals may fear leaving the house due to the frequent and sudden urge to urinate and need to find a bathroom. Despite the psychological stress and personal burden of OAB, most will not seek treatment. In addition, LUTS are not routinely queried by primary physicians or nephrologists due to competing demands to address other healthcare issues. Lack of discussion of LUTS during clinic visits translates to underdiagnosis and under-treatment of OAB.

Lack of attention to OAB may influence cardiovascular disease (CVD) risk due to the connection between bladder function, the autonomic nervous system and blood pressure (BP). Several studies have shown that individuals with OAB have higher sympathetic activity relative to parasympathetic activity which may heighten bladder sensitivity and lead to detrusor muscle contraction at lower bladder volumes, urinary urgency, and even urinary incontinence [11, 12]. Higher sympathetic activity relative to parasympathetic activity can also heighten blood pressure [13]. In a cross-sectional study of older men and women, presence of OAB was associated with significantly higher BP and lower odds of hypertension control but these associations were limited to men [13]. According to the American Heart Association Scientific Statement on BP measurement, measurement of BP should not occur in patients with a full bladder [14].

Incontinence

Urinary incontinence is defined as the involuntary loss of urine and the urine loss may range from just a few drops to a large amount. Up to 1 in every 3 women and 1 in 10 men are affected by urinary incontinence which may negatively affect quality of life [5, 6]. The economic burden of urinary incontinence is substantial and likely exceeds 80 billion per year with the bulk of expenditures on pads and briefs, items not covered by Medicare or private insurance [15]. Urinary incontinence is categorized into three main groups: stress, urgency or mixed. Stress incontinence is defined as loss of urine with coughing, laughing or physical activity. In general, the risk of stress urinary incontinence alone does not increase with advancing age and is the least prevalent of all incontinence types among older adults [1, 5, 6]. Any condition that weakens the pelvic floor muscles such as chronic coughing or straining, pelvic floor damage after vaginal birth, or heavy lifting can lead to stress incontinence.

The most common risk factor for stress incontinence is overweight and obesity, which heightens risk for all forms of incontinence due to the increased pressure on the bladder and surrounding muscles [16]. Obesity actually doubles the risk of urinary incontinence and severity among women [16]. Among men, stress incontinence may occur after a radical prostatectomy for the treatment of cancer [17, 18]. Stress incontinence alone accounts for half of all cases of incontinence but only a smaller percentage of incontinence among older age groups due to the increasing risk of urgency incontinence with advancing age.

In older adults, stress incontinence is often complicated by urgency incontinence and the combination of stress and urgency incontinence is defined as mixed urinary incontinence. Urgency incontinence is a common and burdensome condition that affects up to 1 in every 2 older women and 1 in every 3 older men [1, 2, 5, 6, 19]. Urgency incontinence is defined as loss of urine accompanied by the urgency to urinate. Typically, the individual feels the need to void but cannot rush to the toilet fast enough before urinating. Functional limitations such as frailty and/or arthritis can lead to or exacerbate urgency urinary incontinence due to difficulties with getting to the bathroom promptly. Difficulties with ambulation alone leading to incontinence are termed functional urinary incontinence.

Multiple factors can lead to urgency urinary incontinence and likely the development of bladder dysfunction due to a combination of factors as shown in Fig. 6.1. Low physical activity can not only contribute to obesity but can also lead to

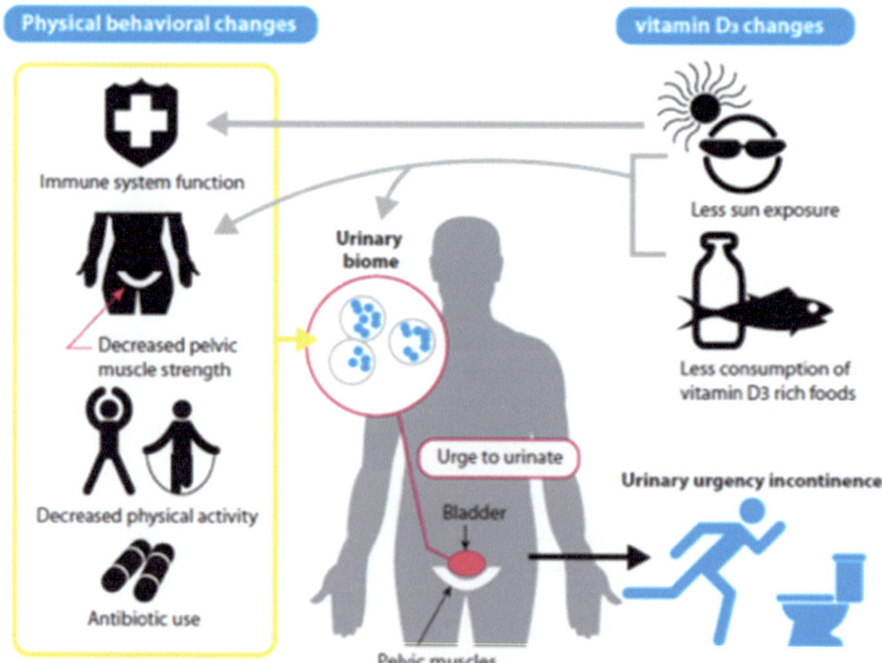

Fig. 6.1 Proposed schema of factors that may influence urgency urinary incontinence

decreased pelvic floor muscle strength. Vitamin D deficiency can contribute to decreased pelvic muscle strength. Use of antibiotics can in theory disrupt the urinary microbiome. Importantly, frequent urinary tract infections could cause scarring and inflammation and alter bladder distension and relaxation.

Overflow urinary incontinence is characterized by spilling, usually small amounts, of urine after completing urination due to incomplete bladder emptying. Overflow urinary incontinence is caused by detrusor muscle underactivity or bladder outlet obstruction, and typically presents with continuous urinary leakage or dribbling in the setting of incomplete bladder emptying. Associated symptoms can include weak or intermittent urinary stream, hesitancy, frequency and nocturia. When the bladder is very full, stress urinary leakage can occur or low amplitude bladder contractions can be triggered resulting in symptoms similar to stress and/or urgency urinary incontinence.

Nocturia

Nocturia is one of the most prevalent components of LUTS and often goes unnoticed in a clinical setting. Lack of attention to nocturia is especially problematic for older persons with kidney disease because nocturia is very frequent in this population and can interrupt sleep and negatively impact quality of life [20–22]. Nocturia is defined as awakening from sleep at least once due to the need to urinate. Urinating two more times per night is generally associated with a high reported rate of bother by the patient and is considered clinically important [23]. The majority of older adults age 65+ years void at least two or more times per night. The prevalence and severity of nocturia may even be higher among older adults with CKD, depending on the CKD stage [24, 25]. Older adults with nocturia should be counseled on the risk of nocturnal falls, which can lead to fractures. Patients should be encouraged to remove all loose rugs in the pathway from the bed to the bathroom and to use a nightlight.

Normally most urine production occurs during activity and decreases during sleep. All of the factors that influence urine formation follow a circadian rhythm including renal plasma flow, vasopressin release, and even the osmotic corticomedullary pressure [26]. Disruption of any of these circadian rhythms can disrupt the circadian rhythm of urine production and output. Normally, increased nocturnal release of Arginine vasopressin (AVP) from the hypothalamus reduces nighttime urine production. [27] With aging, the circadian rhythm of AVP release is altered and nighttime release of AVP declines and shifts more urine production during nocturnal sleep time [28, 29]. Normally, less than 25% of 24-h urine occurs during sleep [29] and total volume of urine during sleep exceeding 30% of urine output in 24 h is classified as nocturnal polyuria. Nocturnal polyuria can also be due to excessive fluid intake, especially with caffeinated or alcoholic beverages, before bedtime. Individuals with volume overload and edema such as heart failure and CKD may mobilize fluid during sleep due to supine position alleviating the gravitation pull of fluid into the lower extremities. The mobilization of fluid at night then stimulates release of atrial natriuretic peptide (ANP) which increases glomerular filtration rate and natriuresis [30]. In sleep apnea, an individual may awaken from sleep due to choking or coughing and then get out of bed to urinate. However, urine production may increase with severe sleep apnea because hypoxia upregulates genetic expression of ANP and its release [31]. Successful treatment of sleep apnea has been shown to markedly improve or cure nocturia [32]. Patients with CKD often lack dipping of nocturnal blood pressure, which is also associated with nocturia [33].

While lack of concentrating ability in CKD has been described as a risk factor for nocturia, most nocturia in this population is due to osmotic diuresis [30]. Use of compression stockings during the day or staggered use of diuretics early may reduce the number of nocturnal voids [34]. Individuals should also be counseled to reduce fluid intake several hours before bedtime and avoid caffeinated and alcoholic beverages. Presence of sleep apnea should be elucidated and treated as clinically indicated.

Regardless of presence of nocturnal polyuria, bladder dysfunction often contributes or is the cause of bothersome nocturia. Heightened sensitivity to bladder filling may occur with chronic bladder outlet obstruction from benign prostatic hyperplasia or increased pressure on the bladder from obesity. Basically, any factor that can reduce the amount of urine storage in the bladder can lead to frequent nocturnal urination, especially if urine production is high. Diagnosis and treatment of nocturia due to overactive bladder should include urodynamic testing and measurement of post-void residual to assess bladder capacity [30].

Bladder Function

A discussion of the complex process of micturition illustrates why neurologic diseases and diabetes are frequently complicated by urgency urinary incontinence or other LUTS. Micturition involves the somatic and autonomic nervous system and requires contraction of the detrusor muscles with simultaneous relaxation of the urethral sphincter. Postganglionic parasympathetic nerves stimulate muscarinic (M3) stretch receptors via acetylcholine. Thus, when these nerves are stretched, the M3 receptors are stimulated leading to detrusor muscle contraction [35].

Micturition requires coordination of detrusor muscle contraction with simultaneous relaxation of the urethral sphincter and this relaxation occurs due to signals from pelvic neurons that inhibit interneurons in the sacral spinal cord [35]. The inhibition of the sacral spinal cord interneurons blocks signals to the pudendal motor neurons which innervate the periurethral striated muscles. Pudendal nerves can be consciously activated (somatic nervous system) to prevent urethral relaxation and urination. Conscious activation of the pudendal nerves occurs when an individual feels the urge to urinate but holds the urine in their bladder until they reach the toilet [36]. Thus, both somatic and autonomic nervous systems play a role in bladder control and health. Damage to the prefrontal cortex, such as with strokes or head trauma, can lead to urgency urinary incontinence because this part of the brain controls detrusor contraction. [36]

Impaired Bladder Filling

Both over- and under-activity of the detrusor muscle may lead to urgency and/or urinary urgency incontinence. The bladder capacity is approximately half a liter but impaired bladder relaxation may lead to limited urine storage. Groups of detrusor muscles are aligned heterogeneously and surrounded by connective tissue. During bladder filling, these smooth muscles must relax and if capacity is impaired, then pressure is heightened at lower volumes. This heightened pressure leads to urinary urgency and even incontinence. When the detrusor muscle contracts, the inner urethral sphincter must relax in order for the bladder to empty. Impairment of detrusor muscle relaxation may occur with hypertrophy of detrusor smooth muscle cells. Hypertrophy and hyperplasia of detrusor smooth muscle cells occur with any factor that increases bladder wall stress such as benign prostatic hyperplasia, or with bladder wall denervation in settings of spinal cord injury or diabetes. Detrusor hypertrophy can be reversible which is why treatment of benign prostatic hyperplasia can lead to gradual improvement of LUTS including urgency.

Diagnosis

Clinicians can best help patients by querying presence of LUTS among patients at high risk, which includes individuals with CKD. A detailed history of how LUTS started and progressed and associated co-morbidities such as diabetes or neurologic disorders will help determine need for referral to urology and urodynamic testing. Table 6.1 provides questions that can be used to query stress and urgency incontinence and nocturia. Questions on LUTS can be obtained from the International Consultation on Incontinence Questionnaire (ICIQ) [37]. These sex-specific modules are available in multiple languages and can be obtained without cost from the internet (www.iciq.net). The questionnaires have been previously validated and the short form module can be completed in 4 min. Each question is followed by a question on bother to determine if the patient is bothered by the symptom. Urodynamic testing can then be performed to determine post-void residual where patient is not completely emptying bladder, a common issue in diabetes. Generally, referral to Urology is indicated if LUTS are severe enough to impair CKD management and/or quality of life or if assistance with treatment is needed.

Table 6.1 Questions to diagnose overactive bladder, incontinence and nocturia. Questions obtained from the International Consultation on Incontinence Questionnaire (ICIQ). Questionnaire modules in multiple languages may be obtained from www.iciq.net

Urinary urgency	Do you have a sudden need to rush to the toilet to urinate?
Urgency incontinence	Does urine leak before you can get to the toilet?
Stress incontinence	Does urine leak when you cough or sneeze?
Nocturia	During the night, how many times do you have to get up to urinate, on average?
Bother	How much does this bother you? 0 (no bother) to 10 (a great deal). Bother question may be used for any LUTS question.

Management

Patients should be informed that LUTS is usually not a condition that can be cured but rather managed and mitigated. Treatment of LUTS should start with behavior management. Studies have shown that improvement in LUTS is optimized with behavior management with or without surgical or other interventions than with medications alone [24, 38]. Behavior management should include attention to dietary practices that may worsen LUTS and physical activity, especially exercises that strengthen the pelvic floor. Patients can be referred to physical therapy to strengthen and stretch the pelvic girdle [39–41]. Stress incontinence may be treated with Kegel exercises to strengthen the pelvic floor muscles [42]. Many older adults have mixed incontinence so strengthening the pelvic muscles may benefit the majority of patients with LUTS. Dietary factors may also play a role. While evidence supporting avoidance of certain foods that may irritate the bladder (acidic or spicy foods) remains limited [43], caffeine and alcohol do consistently increase urine output and may exacerbate LUTS.

Box 6.1 provides a list of factors that can be addressed by the patient to prevent or mitigate LUTS. Foods high in fiber may help with LUTS as constipation can exacerbate LUTS due to heightened pressure on the bladder from a distended colon and due to the convergence of neurons in the colon and bladder. With constipation, neurons that innervate the colon stimulate contraction and this can also heighten activity of detrusor smooth muscle [44]. Avoiding caffeine and alcohol helps to avoid higher urine output which can exacerbate LUTS.

In men with benign prostatic hyperplasia and LUTS, use of 5-alpha reductase enzyme inhibitors that convert testosterone to dihydrotestosterone can mitigate

Box 6.1 Non-medication Factors that can Exacerbate Lower Urinary Tract Symptoms (LUTS)

Factors that exacerbate LUTS	Reason
Constipation	Increases detrusor contractility
Caffeine	Increases urine output
Alcohol	Increases urine output
Carbonated beverages	Bladder irritant
High dose vitamin C	Bladder irritant
Foods with high acid content	Bladder irritant
Obesity-increases pressure on bladder	Increases pressure on bladder
Low physical activity	Reduces strength of pelvic muscles
Urinary tract infections	Bladder inflammation
Benign prostatic hyperplasia	Urinary outflow obstruction
Diabetes	Damages autonomic nerve innervation of bladder, reduces bladder contraction

prostate growth. Inhibition of prostate growth may be used to improve urinary flow and reduce urinary frequency, urgency incontinence and even nocturia. This medication class can also be used to treat male pattern baldness. Side effects include gynecomastia, erectile dysfunction, and decreased libido [45]. Alpha-1 adrenergic receptor antagonists reduce binding of adrenaline receptors on the inner urethral sphincter preventing muscle contraction and leading to increased urine flow. [46] Combination of alpha-1 adrenergic receptor antagonists with 5-alpha reductase inhibitors may be more effective than 1 drug class alone for incontinence and/or nocturia.

Medications for Overactive Bladder

Table 6.2 shows the commonly used medications for management of overactive bladder with or without incontinence. With the exception of mirabegron, these medications are muscarinic receptor antagonists which reduce detrusor contraction. Fesoteridine includes a quarternary ammonium compound to reduce the drug crossing into the blood-brain barrier and prevent anticholinergic effects, specifically central nervous system side effects like blurred vision, lightheadedness and headaches. Older individuals and individuals with creatinine clearance less than 30 mL/min are generally at heightened risk for side effects with anticholinergic medications and

Table 6.2 Drugs that may influence lower urinary tract symptoms

Alpha adrenergic antagonists [46]	Lowes bladder outlet resistance	Incontinence but may lessen urinary urgency
Alpha adrenergic agonists [66]	Contract bladder neck	Overflow urinary incontinence
Antipsychotics [67]	Lower bladder outlet resistance, or increase detrusor contraction	Urinary incontinence
Antidepressants [68, 69]	Depending on the drug-may increase urethral striatal muscle contraction	May improve stress incontinence but worsen urgency incontinence, depending on drug
Loop diuretics [4, 58, 70]	Increase urine output	Urinary urgency and incontinence, nocturia
Thiazide diuretics [58]	Nocturia	
Calcium channel blockers [58, 71]	Decrease detrusor smooth muscle contractility	Urinary retention and overflow incontinence, nocturia
Benzodiazepines [72]	Reduce detrusor smooth muscle contractility	Urinary retention and overflow incontinence
Angiotensin converting enzyme inhibitors and angiotensin receptor blockers [50]	Decreases detrusor overactivity and urethral sphincter tone	May improve urgency urinary incontinence but worsen stress incontinence
Estrogen [52–54, 56, 73]	Heightens detrusor contractility	Urinary incontinence, especially stress incontinence

dose should be reduced. Mirabegron is unique in that it is a beta-3 adrenergic receptor agonist and is only recommended as a second-line agent [47, 48]. While mirabegron does not usually lead to the anticholinergic symptoms of other medications for overactive bladder, it can increase blood pressure and is contraindicated in individuals with uncontrolled hypertension [49].

Medications that May Exacerbate LUTS

Multiple medications that are used to manage older adults with CKD may influence urinary symptoms. Use of angiotensin-converting enzyme inhibitors (ACEi) and angiotensin receptor blockers (ARB) was associated with lower prevalence of urgency urinary incontinence among men in a cross-sectional analysis of the U.S. adult non-institutionalized population [50]. No association was noted between ACEi/ARB use and urinary incontinence in women. This study did not find an association of any other antihypertensive medication use with self-reported stress or urgency incontinence in men or women [50]. A population-based observational study of over 5000 adults age 30–79 years living in Boston, Massachusetts found a significantly higher prevalence of self-reported LUTS among women using calcium channel blockers alone. This association was not noted in men. The urinary symptoms associated with calcium channel blocker use included nocturia, urgency and incontinence (Table 6.3).

Calcium channel blockers may block the L-type calcium channel receptors found in the smooth muscles of the bladder. Negative effects of calcium channel blockers on detrusor muscle contractility may require the presence of estrogen which plays a role in the regulation of L-type calcium channels in the urinary bladder [51]. The M3 receptors in the detrusor smooth muscle are G-protein coupled receptors that require opening of calcium channels and interaction with calmodulin to activate myosin light chain kinase and muscle contraction. The interaction of estrogen and L-type calcium channels explains why estrogen use in menopausal women increases risk of incontinence [52–54]. It should be noted that vaginal estrogen decreases vaginal dryness and urinary frequency and urgency in menopausal women [55]. Vaginal estrogen may also reduce incidence of recurrent urinary tract infections. However, oral estrogen with or without progestin is associated with a heightened risk of urinary incontinence, especially stress incontinence, thought due to heightened bladder contractility. [53, 54, 56]

Diuretics, both thiazide and loop diuretics, have been associated with increased risk and severity of LUTS in both men and women. Loop diuretics appear to show stronger associations with urinary incontinence and nocturia while thiazide diuretics are consistently associated with increased prevalence of urinary urgency and frequency [4, 57, 58]. Other medications such as clonidine and methyldopa can mimic norepinephrine and lead to contraction of muscles lining the inner urethral sphincter and prevent micturition. Alpha-adrenergic antagonist such as prazosin, doxazosin and terazosin block receptors that led to internal urethral sphincter muscle contraction and reduce resistance to urine flow. While these medications may improve LUTS in an individual with bladder outlet obstruction such as benign

Table 6.3 Drugs to treat overactive bladder

Drug	Mechanism of Action	Potential side effects	Considerations for use in CKD
Tolterodine (Detrol) [74–76]	Cholinergic muscarinic antagonist that competitively binds to M3 receptors	Dry mouth, dry eyes, constipation, dizziness, tiredness, blurred vision	Reduce dose with decreased glomerular filtration rate or liver disease and elderly
Oxybutynin (Ditropan XL) (Oxytrol) (Gelnique) [77]	Anticholinergic metabolite N-desethyloxybutynin competitively inhibits postganglionic muscarinic receptors	Dry mouth, dry eyes, constipation, dizziness, tiredness, blurred vision	Hepatically cleared but reduce dose recommended with decreased glomerular filtration rate and in older or frail adults
Trospium [77]	Cholinergic muscarinic antagonist	Dry mouth, indigestion, constipation but no CNS side effects	Reduce dose with creatinine clearance <30 mL/min and/or age 75+ years; side effects may be worse in patients with CKD
Solifenacin (Vesicare) [76, 77]	Cholinergic muscarinic antagonist	Dry mouth, dry skin, tiredness, headache, confusion	Reduce dose with creatinine clearance <30 mL/min and side effects may be worse in CKD
(Fesoterodine (Toviaz) [78, 79]	Cholinergic muscarinic receptor antagonist with quarternary ammonium group to prevent passage across blood brain barrier	Dry mouth, dry eyes, decreased sweating, blurred vision, headache	Do not exceed 4 mg daily if creatinine clearance <30 mL/min; avoid in children with creatinine clearance <30 mL/min
Mirabegron (Myrbetriq) [49, 80]	Beta-3 adrenergic receptor agonist	Increases blood pressure and urinary retention, constipation, dysuria	Should be used as second line therapy and may worsen blood pressure control

prostatic hyperplasia, alpha-adrenergic antagonists could increase urinary incontinence in individuals without bladder outlet obstruction. Use of alpha-adrenergic antagonists in women has been associated with a marked increase in urinary incontinence [52, 59].

Sodium-Glucose Cotransporter 2 Inhibitors

Sodium-glucose cotransporter 2 inhibitors (SGLT2i) increase urinary output and may exacerbate or initiate LUTS, especially nocturia. During the first week of treatment, urine volume and free water increase [60]. In a small study of men with type

2 diabetes initiated on SGLT2i, almost all men reported nocturia. Clinical trials have reported increased urination and nocturia which was reported by 5% treated with canagliflozin vs. 0.7% with placebo. All other SGLT2i are also associated with higher reported rates of increased urination versus placebo [61].

The SGLT2i drug class increases glucosuria which can lead to groin infections. While meta-analysis of clinical trials does not show significant differences in urinary tract infections between SGLT2i use vs. controls, genital infections are increased by over three-fold with SGLT2i use in persons with type 2 diabetes mellitus [62]. Only 1 genital infection was reported in the empagliflozin and placebo groups in the clinical trial of empagliflozin for adults with chronic kidney disease [63]. It should be noted that trial participants are generally healthier than the general clinic population and the distribution of side effects from medications may differ somewhat from clinical trials. Urinary incontinence is associated with dermatitis due to chronic moisture and chemical irritants that can be from the pads or briefs and shear mechanical stress on the skin [64, 65]. Given that SGLT2i increases glucosuria which can accelerate the growth of bacteria and yeast on the skin, this drug class will likely compound the increased risk of skin infections in patients with severe incontinence. Patients with urinary incontinence, especially if severe, should be informed of such risks in order to make an informed decision on whether to start SGLT2i.

Returning to the patient's case, the 85-year-old patient had urgency urinary incontinence which was not treated. Due to the severity of his incontinence, the patient was referred to a Urologist. Urodynamic testing on the patient confirmed presence of urgency urinary incontinence, which was attributed to diabetes causing autonomic nerve damage to bladder combined with benign prostatic hyperplasia. The patient was initiated on finasteride and doxazosin. After 2 months, his urinary urgency and incontinence decreased in severity, but he continued to wear adult briefs. The patient continued to decline SGLT2i due to concerns about groin infection.

References

1. Daugirdas SP, Markossian T, Mueller ER, Durazo-Arvizu R, Cao G, Kramer H. Urinary incontinence and chronic conditions in the US population age 50 years and older. Int Urogynecol J. 2020;31:1013–20. https://doi.org/10.1007/s00192-019-04137-y.
2. Dooley Y, Kenton K, Cao G, Luke A, Durazo-Arvizu R, Kramer H, Brubaker L. Urinary incontinence prevalence: results from the National Health and nutrition examination survey. J Urol. 2008;179:656–61. https://doi.org/10.1016/j.juro.2007.09.081.
3. Markland AD, Vaughan CP, Johnson TM 2nd, Goode PS, Redden DT, Burgio KL. Prevalence of nocturia in United States men: results from the National Health and nutrition examination survey. J Urol. 2011;185:998–1002. https://doi.org/10.1016/j.juro.2010.10.083.
4. Patel M, Vellanki K, Leehey DJ, Bansal VK, Brubaker L, Flanigan R, Koval J, Wadhwa A, Balasubramanian N, Sandhu J, et al. Urinary incontinence and diuretic avoidance among adults with chronic kidney disease. Int Urol Nephrol. 2016;48:1321–6. https://doi.org/10.1007/s11255-016-1304-1.

5. Akbar A, Liu K, Michos ED, Brubaker L, Markossian T, Bancks MP, Kramer H. Racial differences in urinary incontinence prevalence and associated bother: the multi-ethnic study of atherosclerosis. Am J Obstet Gynecol. 2021;224(80):e81–80e89. https://doi.org/10.1016/j.ajog.2020.07.031.

6. Akbar A, Liu K, Michos ED, Brubaker L, Markossian T, Bancks MP, Kramer H. Racial differences in urinary incontinence prevalence, overactive bladder and associated bother among men: the multi-ethnic study of atherosclerosis. J Urol. 2021;205:524–31. https://doi.org/10.1097/JU.0000000000001353.

7. Bansal R, Agarwal MM, Modi M, Mandal AK, Singh SK. Urodynamic profile of diabetic patients with lower urinary tract symptoms: association of diabetic cystopathy with autonomic and peripheral neuropathy. Urology. 2011;77:699–705. https://doi.org/10.1016/j.urology.2010.04.062.

8. Yang Z, Dolber PC, Fraser MO. Diabetic urethropathy compounds the effects of diabetic cystopathy. J Urol. 2007;178:2213–9. https://doi.org/10.1016/j.juro.2007.06.042.

9. Scarneciu I, Lupu S, Bratu OG, Teodorescu A, Maxim LS, Brinza A, Laculiceanu AG, Rotaru RM, Lupu AM, Scarneciu CC. Overactive bladder: a review and update. Exp Ther Med. 2021;22:1444. https://doi.org/10.3892/etm.2021.10879.

10. Abrams P, Kelleher CJ, Kerr LA, Rogers RG. Overactive bladder significantly affects quality of life. Am J Manag Care. 2000;6:S580–90.

11. Hubeaux K, Deffieux X, Ismael SS, Raibaut P, Amarenco G. Autonomic nervous system activity during bladder filling assessed by heart rate variability analysis in women with idiopathic overactive bladder syndrome or stress urinary incontinence. J Urol. 2007;178:2483–7. https://doi.org/10.1016/j.juro.2007.08.036.

12. Liao WC, Jaw FS. A noninvasive evaluation of autonomic nervous system dysfunction in women with an overactive bladder. Int J Gynaecol Obstet. 2010;110:12–7. https://doi.org/10.1016/j.ijgo.2010.03.007.

13. Akbar A, Liu K, Michos ED, Bancks MP, Brubaker L, Markossian T, Durazo-Arvizu R, Kramer H. Association of overactive bladder with hypertension and blood pressure control: the multi-ethnic study of atherosclerosis (MESA). Am J Hypertens. 2022;35:22–30. https://doi.org/10.1093/ajh/hpaa186.

14. Muntner P, Shimbo D, Carey RM, Charleston JB, Gaillard T, Misra S, Myers MG, Ogedegbe G, Schwartz JE, Townsend RR, et al. Measurement of blood pressure in humans: a scientific statement from the American Heart Association. Hypertension. 2019;73:e35–66. https://doi.org/10.1161/HYP.0000000000000087.

15. Coyne KS, Wein A, Nicholson S, Kvasz M, Chen CI, Milsom I. Economic burden of urgency urinary incontinence in the United States: a systematic review. J Manag Care Pharm. 2014;20:130–40. https://doi.org/10.18553/jmcp.2014.20.2.130.

16. Danforth KN, Townsend MK, Lifford K, Curhan GC, Resnick NM, Grodstein F. Risk factors for urinary incontinence among middle-aged women. Am J Obstet Gynecol. 2006;194:339–45. https://doi.org/10.1016/j.ajog.2005.07.051.

17. Gacci M, Simonato A, Masieri L, Gore JL, Lanciotti M, Mantella A, Rossetti MA, Serni S, Varca V, Romagnoli A, et al. Urinary and sexual outcomes in long-term (5+ years) prostate cancer disease free survivors after radical prostatectomy. Health Qual Life Outcomes. 2009;7:94. https://doi.org/10.1186/1477-7525-7-94.

18. Litwin MS, Lubeck DP, Stoddard ML, Pasta DJ, Flanders SC, Henning JM. Quality of life before death for men with prostate cancer: results from the CaPSURE database. J Urol. 2001;165:871–5.

19. Coyne KS, Sexton CC, Bell JA, Thompson CL, Dmochowski R, Bavendam T, Chen CI, Quentin CJ. The prevalence of lower urinary tract symptoms (LUTS) and overactive bladder (OAB) by racial/ethnic group and age: results from OAB-POLL. Neurourol Urodyn. 2013;32:230–7. https://doi.org/10.1002/nau.22295.

20. Coyne KS, Zhou Z, Bhattacharyya SK, Thompson CL, Dhawan R, Versi E. The prevalence of nocturia and its effect on health-related quality of life and sleep in a community sample in the USA. BJU Int. 2003;92:948–54. https://doi.org/10.1111/j.1464-410x.2003.04527.x.

21. Asplund R. Mortality in the elderly in relation to nocturnal micturition. BJU Int. 1999;84:297–301. https://doi.org/10.1046/j.1464-410x.1999.00157.x.

22. Guilleminault C, Lin CM, Goncalves MA, Ramos E. A prospective study of nocturia and the quality of life of elderly patients with obstructive sleep apnea or sleep onset insomnia. J Psychosom Res. 2004;56:511–5. https://doi.org/10.1016/S0022-3999(04)00021-2.

23. Tikkinen KA, Tammela TL, Huhtala H, Auvinen A. Is nocturia equally common among men and women? A population based study in Finland. J Urol. 2006;175:596–600. https://doi.org/10.1016/S0022-5347(05)00245-4.

24. Ridgway A, Cotterill N, Dawson S, Drake MJ, Henderson EJ, Huntley AL, Rees J, Strong E, Dudley C, Udayaraj U. Nocturia and chronic kidney disease: systematic review and nominal group technique consensus on primary care assessment and treatment. Eur Urol Focus. 2022;8:18–25. https://doi.org/10.1016/j.euf.2021.12.010.

25. Wu MY, Wu YL, Hsu YH, Lin YF, Fan YC, Lin YC, Chang SJ. Risks of nocturia in patients with chronic kidney disease—do the metabolic syndrome and its components matter? J Urol. 2012;188:2269–73. https://doi.org/10.1016/j.juro.2012.08.008.

26. Firsov D, Bonny O. Circadian regulation of renal function. Kidney Int. 2010;78:640–5. https://doi.org/10.1038/ki.2010.227.

27. Weiss JP, Everaert K. Management of nocturia and nocturnal polyuria. Urology. 2019;133S:24–33. https://doi.org/10.1016/j.urology.2019.09.022.

28. Ouslander JG, Nasr SZ, Miller M, Withington W, Lee CS, Wiltshire-Clement M, Cruise P, Schnelle JF. Arginine vasopressin levels in nursing home residents with nighttime urinary incontinence. J Am Geriatr Soc. 1998;46:1274–9. https://doi.org/10.1111/j.1532-5415.1998.tb04545.x.

29. Kikuchi Y. Participation of atrial natriuretic peptide (hANP) levels and arginine vasopressin (AVP) in aged persons with nocturia. Nihon Hinyokika Gakkai Zasshi. 1995;86:1651–9. https://doi.org/10.5980/jpnjurol1989.86.1651.

30. Boongird S, Shah N, Nolin TD, Unruh ML. Nocturia and aging: diagnosis and treatment. Adv Chronic Kidney Dis. 2010;17:e27–40. https://doi.org/10.1053/j.ackd.2010.04.004.

31. Chen YF, Durand J, Claycomb WC. Hypoxia stimulates atrial natriuretic peptide gene expression in cultured atrial cardiocytes. Hypertension. 1997;29:75–82. https://doi.org/10.1161/01.hyp.29.1.75.

32. Park HK, Paick SH, Kim HG, Park DH, Cho JH, Hong SC, Choi WS. Nocturia improvement with surgical correction of sleep apnea. Int Neurourol J. 2016;20:329–34. https://doi.org/10.5213/inj.1632624.312.

33. Agarwal R, Light RP, Bills JE, Hummel LA. Nocturia, nocturnal activity, and nondipping. Hypertension. 2009;54:646–51. https://doi.org/10.1161/HYPERTENSIONAHA.109.135822.

34. Fu FG, Lavery HJ, Wu DL. Reducing nocturia in the elderly: a randomized placebo-controlled trial of staggered furosemide and desmopressin. Neurourol Urodyn. 2011;30:312–6. https://doi.org/10.1002/nau.20986.

35. Andersson KE, Arner A. Urinary bladder contraction and relaxation: physiology and pathophysiology. Physiol Rev. 2004;84:935–86. https://doi.org/10.1152/physrev.00038.2003.

36. Fowler CJ, Griffiths D, de Groat WC. The neural control of micturition. Nat Rev Neurosci. 2008;9:453–66. https://doi.org/10.1038/nrn2401.

37. Abrams PAK, Gardener N, Donovan J, Advisory ICIQ, Board. The international consultation on incontinence modular questionnaire. J Urol. 2006;175:1063–6.

38. Balk EM, Rofeberg VN, Adam GP, Kimmel HJ, Trikalinos TA, Jeppson PC. Pharmacologic and nonpharmacologic treatments for urinary incontinence in women: a systematic review and network meta-analysis of clinical outcomes. Ann Intern Med. 2019;170:465–79. https://doi.org/10.7326/M18-3227.

39. Parker WP, Griebling TL. Nonsurgical treatment of urinary incontinence in elderly women. Clin Geriatr Med. 2015;31:471–85. https://doi.org/10.1016/j.cger.2015.07.003.
40. Scott KM, Gosai E, Bradley MH, Walton S, Hynan LS, Lemack G, Roehrborn C. Individualized pelvic physical therapy for the treatment of post-prostatectomy stress urinary incontinence and pelvic pain. Int Urol Nephrol. 2020;52:655–9. https://doi.org/10.1007/s11255-019-02343-7.
41. Thomas LH, Coupe J, Cross LD, Tan AL, Watkins CL. Interventions for treating urinary incontinence after stroke in adults. Cochrane Database Syst Rev. 2019;2:CD004462. https://doi.org/10.1002/14651858.CD004462.pub4.
42. Park SHK, Kang C-B. Effect of Kegel exercises on the management of female stress incontinence: a systematic review of randomized controlled trials. Adv Nursing. 2014;2014:1.
43. Bradley CS, Erickson BA, Messersmith EE, Pelletier-Cameron A, Lai HH, Kreder KJ, Yang CC, Merion RM, Bavendam TG, Kirkali Z, et al. Evidence of the impact of diet, fluid intake, caffeine, alcohol and tobacco on lower urinary tract symptoms: a systematic review. J Urol. 2017;198:1010–20. https://doi.org/10.1016/j.juro.2017.04.097.
44. Iguchi N, Carrasco A Jr, Xie AX, Pineda RH, Malykhina AP, Wilcox DT. Functional constipation induces bladder overactivity associated with upregulations of Htr2 and Trpv2 pathways. Sci Rep. 2021;11:1149. https://doi.org/10.1038/s41598-020-80794-0.
45. Busetto GM, Del Giudice F, D'Agostino D, Romagnoli D, Minervini A, Rocco B, Antonelli A, Celia A, Schiavina R, Cindolo L, et al. Efficacy and safety of finasteride (5 alpha-reductase inhibitor) monotherapy in patients with benign prostatic hyperplasia: a critical review of the literature. Arch Ital Urol Androl. 2020;91:205–10. https://doi.org/10.4081/aiua.2019.4.205.
46. Lepor H. Alpha blockers for the treatment of benign prostatic hyperplasia. Rev Urol. 2007;9:181–90.
47. Lerner LB, McVary KT, Barry MJ, Bixler BR, Dahm P, Das AK, Gandhi MC, Kaplan SA, Kohler TS, Martin L, et al. Management of lower urinary tract symptoms attributed to benign prostatic hyperplasia: AUA guideline part I-initial work-up and medical management. J Urol. 2021;206:806–17. https://doi.org/10.1097/JU.0000000000002183.
48. Ginsberg DA, Boone TB, Cameron AP, Gousse A, Kaufman MR, Keays E, Kennelly MJ, Lemack GE, Rovner ES, Souter LH, et al. The AUA/SUFU guideline on adult neurogenic lower urinary tract dysfunction: diagnosis and evaluation. J Urol. 2021;206:1097–105. https://doi.org/10.1097/JU.0000000000002235.
49. Sacco E, Bientinesi R. Mirabegron: a review of recent data and its prospects in the management of overactive bladder. Ther Adv Urol. 2012;4:315–24. https://doi.org/10.1177/1756287212457114.
50. Elliott CS, Comiter CV. The effect of angiotensin inhibition on urinary incontinence: data from the National Health and nutrition examination survey (2001-2008). Neurourol Urodyn. 2014;33:1178–81. https://doi.org/10.1002/nau.22480.
51. Sarkar SN, Huang RQ, Logan SM, Yi KD, Dillon GH, Simpkins JW. Estrogens directly potentiate neuronal L-type Ca2+ channels. Proc Natl Acad Sci USA. 2008;105:15148–53. https://doi.org/10.1073/pnas.0802379105.
52. Ruby CM, Hanlon JT, Boudreau RM, Newman AB, Simonsick EM, Shorr RI, Bauer DC, Resnick NM, Health A, Body CS. The effect of medication use on urinary incontinence in community-dwelling elderly women. J Am Geriatr Soc. 2010;58:1715–20. https://doi.org/10.1111/j.1532-5415.2010.03006.x.
53. Grodstein F, Lifford K, Resnick NM, Curhan GC. Postmenopausal hormone therapy and risk of developing urinary incontinence. Obstet Gynecol. 2004;103:254–60. https://doi.org/10.1097/01.AOG.0000107290.33034.6f.
54. Hendrix SL, Cochrane BB, Nygaard IE, Handa VL, Barnabei VM, Iglesia C, Aragaki A, Naughton MJ, Wallace RB, McNeeley SG. Effects of estrogen with and without progestin on urinary incontinence. JAMA. 2005;293:935–48. https://doi.org/10.1001/jama.293.8.935.
55. Qi W, Li H, Wang C, Li H, Fan A, Han C, Xue F. The effect of pathophysiological changes in the vaginal milieu on the signs and symptoms of genitourinary syndrome of menopause (GSM). Menopause. 2020;28:102–8. https://doi.org/10.1097/GME.0000000000001644.

56. Townsend MK, Curhan GC, Resnick NM, Grodstein F. Postmenopausal hormone therapy and incident urinary incontinence in middle-aged women. Am J Obstet Gynecol. 2009;200(86):e81–5. https://doi.org/10.1016/j.ajog.2008.08.009.
57. Ekundayo OJ, Markland A, Lefante C, Sui X, Goode PS, Allman RM, Ali M, Wahle C, Thornton PL, Ahmed A. Association of diuretic use and overactive bladder syndrome in older adults: a propensity score analysis. Arch Gerontol Geriatr. 2009;49:64–8. https://doi.org/10.1016/j.archger.2008.05.002.
58. Hall SA, Chiu GR, Kaufman DW, Wittert GA, Link CL, McKinlay JB. Commonly used antihypertensives and lower urinary tract symptoms: results from the Boston area community Health (BACH) survey. BJU Int. 2012;109:1676–84. https://doi.org/10.1111/j.1464-410X.2011.10593.x.
59. Marshall HJB, D. Alpha-adrenergic blockade and urinary incontinence. J Hypertension. 1993;11:1152–3.
60. Hallow KM, Helmlinger G, Greasley PJ, McMurray JJV, Boulton DW. Why do SGLT2 inhibitors reduce heart failure hospitalization? A differential volume regulation hypothesis. Diabetes Obes Metab. 2018;20:479–87. https://doi.org/10.1111/dom.13126.
61. Krepostman NK, H. Lower urinary tract symptoms should be queried when initiating sodium glucose co-transporter 2 inhibitors. Kidney360. 2021;2:751–4.
62. Liu J, Li L, Li S, Jia P, Deng K, Chen W, Sun X. Effects of SGLT2 inhibitors on UTIs and genital infections in type 2 diabetes mellitus: a systematic review and meta-analysis. Sci Rep. 2017;7:2824. https://doi.org/10.1038/s41598-017-02733-w.
63. Herrington WG, Baigent C, Haynes R. Empagliflozin in patients with chronic kidney disease. Reply. N Engl J Med. 2023;388:2301–2. https://doi.org/10.1056/NEJMc2301923.
64. Banharak S, Panpanit L, Subindee S, Narongsanoi P, Sanun-Aur P, Kulwong W, Songtin P, Khemphimai W. Prevention and care for incontinence-associated dermatitis among older adults: a systematic review. J Multidiscip Healthc. 2021;14:2983–3004. https://doi.org/10.2147/JMDH.S329672.
65. Gray M, Beeckman D, Bliss DZ, Fader M, Logan S, Junkin J, Selekof J, Doughty D, Kurz P. Incontinence-associated dermatitis: a comprehensive review and update. J Wound Ostomy Continence Nurs. 2012;39:61–74. https://doi.org/10.1097/WON.0b013e31823fe246.
66. Schwinn DA, Roehrborn CG. Alpha1-adrenoceptor subtypes and lower urinary tract symptoms. Int J Urol. 2008;15:193–9. https://doi.org/10.1111/j.1442-2042.2007.01956.x.
67. Ambrosini PJ. A pharmacological paradigm for urinary incontinence and enuresis. J Clin Psychopharmacol. 1984;4:247–53.
68. Wuerstle MC, Van Den Eeden SK, Poon KT, Quinn VP, Hollingsworth JM, Loo RK, Jacobsen SJ. Urologic diseases in America P. Contribution of common medications to lower urinary tract symptoms in men. Arch Intern Med. 2011;171:1680–2. https://doi.org/10.1001/archinternmed.2011.475.
69. Bae JH, Moon DG, Lee JG. The effects of a selective noradrenaline reuptake inhibitor on the urethra: an in vitro and in vivo study. BJU Int. 2001;88:771–5. https://doi.org/10.1046/j.1464-4096.2001.02389.x.
70. Asplund R. Pharmacotherapy for nocturia in the elderly patient. Drugs Aging. 2007;24:325–43. https://doi.org/10.2165/00002512-200724040-00005.
71. Peron EP, Zheng Y, Perera S, Newman AB, Resnick NM, Shorr RI, Bauer DC, Simonsick EM, Gray SL, Hanlon JT, et al. Antihypertensive drug class use and differential risk of urinary incontinence in community-dwelling older women. J Gerontol A Biol Sci Med Sci. 2012;67:1373–8. https://doi.org/10.1093/gerona/gls177.
72. Landi F, Cesari M, Russo A, Onder G, Sgadari A, Bernabei R, Silvernet HCSG. Benzodiazepines and the risk of urinary incontinence in frail older persons living in the community. Clin Pharmacol Ther. 2002;72:729–34. https://doi.org/10.1067/mcp.2002.129318.
73. Shamliyan TA, Kane RL, Wyman J, Wilt TJ. Systematic review: randomized, controlled trials of nonsurgical treatments for urinary incontinence in women. Ann Intern Med. 2008;148:459–73. https://doi.org/10.7326/0003-4819-148-6-200803180-00211.

74. Wefer J, Truss MC, Jonas U. Tolterodine: an overview. World J Urol. 2001;19:312–8. https://doi.org/10.1007/s003450100224.
75. Zinner NR, Mattiasson A, Stanton SL. Efficacy, safety, and tolerability of extended-release once-daily tolterodine treatment for overactive bladder in older versus younger patients. J Am Geriatr Soc. 2002;50:799–807. https://doi.org/10.1046/j.1532-5415.2002.50203.x.
76. Leone Roberti Maggiore U, Salvatore S, Alessandri F, Remorgida V, Origoni M, Candiani M, Venturini PL, Ferrero S. Pharmacokinetics and toxicity of antimuscarinic drugs for overactive bladder treatment in females. Expert Opin Drug Metab Toxicol. 2012;8:1387–408. https://doi.org/10.1517/17425255.2012.714365.
77. Lam S, Hilas O. Pharmacologic management of overactive bladder. Clin Interv Aging. 2007;2:337–45.
78. Malhotra B, Guan Z, Wood N, Gandelman K. Pharmacokinetic profile of fesoterodine. Int J Clin Pharmacol Ther. 2008;46:556–63. https://doi.org/10.5414/cpp46556.
79. Khullar V, Rovner ES, Dmochowski R, Nitti V, Wang J, Guan Z. Fesoterodine dose response in subjects with overactive bladder syndrome. Urology. 2008;71:839–43. https://doi.org/10.1016/j.urology.2007.12.017.
80. Corcos J, Przydacz M, Campeau L, Gray G, Hickling D, Honeine C, Radomski SB, Stothers L, Wagg A, Lond F. CUA guideline on adult overactive bladder. Can Urol Assoc J. 2017;11:E142–73. https://doi.org/10.5489/cuaj.4586.

Chapter 7
Hypertension in the Elderly

Sumaiya Ahmed and Swapnil Hiremath

Clinical Case Scenarios

Patient 1: A 78-year-old man, a retired federal bureaucrat with stage 3 chronic kidney disease, is seen in the clinic for follow-up. His past medical history includes coronary artery disease, peripheral arterial disease, and colon cancer. He is an ex-smoker. His sitting blood pressure in the clinic is 131/62 mmHg, and his standing blood pressure is 109/58 mmHg. His home medications include aspirin, atorvastatin, perindopril, hydrochlorothiazide, and amlodipine. Unlike previous visits, he is now using a 4-wheel walker, as he feels unsteady. His wife is accompanying him and volunteers that he is occasionally forgetful, though he has not been evaluated formally for cognitive impairment. Though they live independently, they are contemplating a move to an assisted living setting. You are faced with a decisional dilemma of escalating blood pressure therapy as it is not at target according to the latest guidelines, or considering lowering medications given your concern for hypotension-related adverse events.

Patient 2: An 82-year-old woman, a retired teacher with stage 3 chronic kidney disease is seen in the clinic for follow-up. She has a past medical history of atrial fibrillation, previous transient ischemic strokes, hypertension, and coronary artery disease. She is widowed and lives independently and does all her activities of daily

S. Ahmed
Division of Nephrology, Department of Medicine, The Ottawa Hospital and the University of Ottawa, Ottawa, ON, Canada
e-mail: sumaahmed@toh.ca

S. Hiremath (✉)
Division of Nephrology, Department of Medicine, The Ottawa Hospital and the University of Ottawa, Ottawa, ON, Canada

Clinical Epidemiology Program, Ottawa Hospital Research Institute, Ottawa, ON, Canada
e-mail: shiremath@toh.ca

© The Author(s), under exclusive license to Springer Nature Switzerland AG 2024
H. Kramer et al. (eds.), *Kidney Disease in the Elderly*,
https://doi.org/10.1007/978-3-031-68460-9_7

living on her own. She likes to do the Sunday crossword and enjoys curling in the winter. Her sitting blood pressure is 134/68 mmHg, and her standing blood pressure is 132/65 mmHg. She is on chlorthalidone and amlodipine for blood pressure control. Your clinical dilemma is to escalate blood pressure therapy based on the guideline targets or leave things be, based on her age and lack of symptoms.

Introduction

The treatment of hypertension (HTN) has been controversial for almost a century. The asymptomatic nature of the condition and the adverse effects with blood pressure (BP) lowering therapies were considered initial barriers. Epidemiological and trial data have made the benefits of BP lowering very clear. The advent of safe and effective pharmacotherapy has made the harms of BP lowering very low. However, in the elderly population, these concerns do arise even now. The absolute risks of harm from BP lowering are much higher than in the younger population, and the benefits are not as clear. In this chapter, we will discuss the trial evidence covering the benefits and harms of BP lowering and provide some practical suggestions for clinical practice.

Pathophysiology of Hypertension in the Elderly

The pathophysiology of HTN in the elderly can be explained by a combination of arterial stiffness, mechanical hemodynamic changes, neurohormonal and autonomic dysfunction, and aging kidneys [1]. Arterial stiffness occurs with age, and it is defined as the decrease in capacitance and elasticity, thereby reducing the ability to accommodate volume changes during the cardiac cycle [1]. As such, both systolic BP (sBP) and diastolic BP (dBP) increase with age; however, after the age of 60 years, there is a higher occurrence of central arterial stiffness [1]. Heightened arterial stiffness results in a rise in sBP while the dBP declines, thereby causing isolated systolic HTN and widened pulse pressure [1]. Hemodynamic mechanical changes also increase pulse pressure, as well as pulse-wave velocity, as it further decreases aortic elasticity and loss of recoil during diastole [1]. Central sBP increases as well due to the change in arterial structure which subsequently increases pressure waves in the ascending aorta [1]. Furthermore, neuro-hormonal changes include an elevation in endothelin-1 and reduction in bioavailability of nitric oxide which occurs as endothelial dysfunction develops and affects arterial dilation [1]. Lastly, aging is related to the increase sensitivity to salt in the kidneys because of nephron loss and a decrease in activity of the sodium/potassium and calcium adenosine triphosphate pumps, which causes vasoconstriction and vascular resistance [1].

Epidemiology

High BP is a well-known modifiable risk factor for cardiovascular disease (CVD) [2, 3] and the high prevalence of HTN has made it the largest contributor to the global burden of disease, affecting an estimated 1.39 billion people worldwide and leading to 10.4 million premature deaths each year [4]. As with many conditions, the prevalence of HTN and its severity increases with age [2]. For instance, the Framingham Heart Study demonstrated that more than 90% of participants with a normal BP at the age of 55 will eventually develop HTN [1, 5]. By the age of 60 years, 60% of the population will have developed HTN, and eventually 65% of men and 75% of women will develop HTN by age of 70 years [1].

Several large studies have demonstrated that elevated BP in elderly is associated with major complications such as increased risk of ischemic and hemorrhagic strokes, vascular dementia, Alzheimer's disease, coronary artery disease, cardiovascular (CV) related complications, atrial fibrillation, chronic kidney disease, and retinal diseases [1, 5–7]. In addition, observational studies have shown an association between elevated BP in middle age and cognitive impairment [5]. As such, treatment of elevated BP in the elderly is crucial and many trials over the last two decades have demonstrated the benefit.

Clinical Trial Evidence

Management of HTN in the elderly has been an area of uncertainty as the benefits were unclear and risks associated with treatment are associated with important adverse effects in this population. Many trials have been conducted over the years on management of HTN in the elderly to clarify the potential benefits (see Table 7.1 for details, and Fig. 7.1), and the target BP for treatment has slowly dropped from a sBP of 160 to an sBP of 120 mmHg. One of the first HTN trials specifically in the elderly was the Systolic HTN in the Elderly Program (SHEP) published in 2000 where 4736 participants ≥60 years with isolated systolic HTN were recruited with a target of a decrease in sBP of ≥20 mmHg from baseline to an sBP < 160 mmHg [6]. Chlorthalidone and either atenolol or reserpine were used as treatments and 65% of participants did achieve the targeted BP. The SHEP trial demonstrated that BP lowering reduced incidence of both ischemic (Relative Risk, RR: 0.63 (95% confidence interval [CI], 0.48–0.82) and hemorrhagic strokes (RR: 0.46; 95% CI, 0.21–1.02) [6]. The SHEP trial was later followed by the Hypertension in the Very Elderly Trial (HYVET) trial, which also demonstrated a reduction in stroke rate in the very elderly, defined as those >80 years, with BP lowering [8]. HYVET recruited 3845 participants with isolated systolic HTN and targeted BP reduction to less than 150/80 mmHg. Indapamide, and either perindopril or placebo, were used as the BP lowering agents and the average BP achieved was 144/78 mmHg in the treatment group and 159/84 mmHg in the control group. The study demonstrated that

Table 7.1 Summary of important trials on management of hypertension in the elderly

Trials	SHEP (2000) [6]	HYVET (2008) [8]	JATOS (2008) [9]	VALISH (2010) [10]	SPRINT Elderly (2016) [11]	STEP (2021) [12]
Participants	4736	3845	4418	3079	2636	8511
Duration, years	4.5	2.1	2	3.1	3.1	3.34
Study population	$\geq$ 60 years with isolated systolic hypertension	$\geq$ 80 years with sustained hypertension	65–85 years with essential hypertension	70–84 years with isolated systolic hypertension	$\geq$ 75 years with hypertension and high cardiovascular risk	60–80 years of age with hypertension
Blood pressure targets	Treatment: Decrease in baseline sBP of $\geq$ 20 mmHg	Treatment: < 150/80 mmHg Control: < 160/90	Treatment: < 140 mmHg Control: < 140–159 mmHg	Treatment: < 140 mmHg control: < 140–149 mmHg	Treatment: < 120 mmHg Control: < 140 mmHg	Treatment: 110–130 mmHg Control: 130–150 mmHg
Treatment arms	Protocol-based with chlorthalidone and either atenolol or reserpine as needed or placebo	Protocol-based with indapamide or placebo with either perindopril or placebo as needed	Efonidipine with an add-on agent if needed.	Valsartan with an add-on agent if needed.	Protocol based: Chlorthalidone among preferred agents	Protocol based with olmesartan, amlodipine, and hydrochlorothiazide
Achieved mean blood pressure, (mmHg)	65% of participants had a decrease of sBP of $\geq$ 20 mmHg from baseline to < 160	Treatment: 144/78 Control: 159/84	Treatment: 136/75 control: 146/78	Treatment: 137/75 control: 143/77	Treatment: 123/62 control: 135/67	Treatment: 127/76 Control: 136/79
Primary outcome	Ischemic stroke: RR: 0.63 (95% CI, 0.48–0.82) Hemorrhagic stroke: RR: 0.46 (95% CI, 0.21–1.02)	Stroke HR: 0.61 (95% CI, 0.38–0.99)	MACE and ESKD Rate per 1000 PYs: 22.6 vs 22.7, $p = 0.99$	MACE and ESKD HR: 0.89 (95% CI, 0.60–1.31)	MACE HR: 0.66 (95% CI 0.51–0.85)	MACE HR: 0.74 (95% CI 0.60–0.92)

Trials	SHEP (2000) [6]	HYVET (2008) [8]	JATOS (2008) [9]	VALISH (2010) [10]	SPRINT Elderly (2016) [11]	STEP (2021) [12]
Mortality	CV death HR 0.80 (95% CI 0.60–1.05) All cause death HR 0.87 (95% CI 0.73–1.05)	CV death HR 0.77 (0.60–1.01) All cause death HR 0.79 (95% CI 0.65–0.95)	All cause death 54 in treatment vs 42 in control group ($p = 0.22$)	CV death HR 0.97 (95% CI 0.42–2.25) All cause death HR 0.78 (0.46–1.33)	CV death HR 0.60 (0.33–1.09) All cause death HR, 0.67 (95% CI, 0.49–0.91)	CV death HR 0.72 (95% CI, 0.39 to 1.32) All cause death HR 1.11 (0.78–1.56)

SHEP Systolic Hypertension in the Elderly Program, *HYVET* Hypertension in the Very Elderly Trial, *JATOS* Japanese Trial to Assess Optimal Systolic Blood Pressure in Elderly Hypertensive patients, *VALISH* Valsartan in Elderly Isolated Systolic Hypertension, *SPRINT* Systolic Blood Pressure Intervention Trial, *STEP* Strategy of Blood Pressure Intervention in the Elderly Hypertensive Patients, *sBP* Systolic Blood Pressure, *RR* Relative Risk, *CI* Confidence Interval, *HR* Hazard Ratio, *MACE* Major Adverse Cardiovascular Events, *ESKD* End-stage Kidney Disease, *PY* Person-years, *CV* Cardiovascular

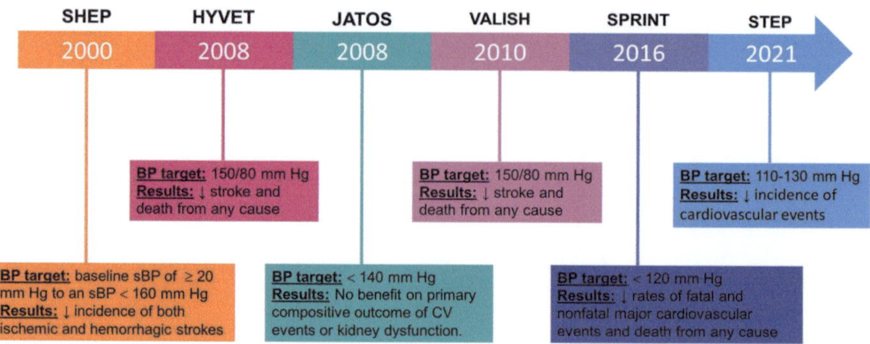

Fig. 7.1 Graphical summary of the landmark trials in hypertension management in the elderly

indapamide with or without an angiotensin converting enzyme-inhibitor was associated with a reduction in death from stroke (HR: 0.61, 95% CI, 0.38–0.99). This trial was stopped early (median follow-up, 1.8 years) because the second planned interim analysis showed a significant reduction in the incidence of strokes, as well as total mortality in the intervention arm compared to the control arm. Subsequently, two Japanese trials were conducted: Japanese Trial to Assess Optimal Systolic Blood Pressure in Elderly Hypertensive Patients (JATOS)[9] (Group, 2008) and Valsartan in Elderly Isolated Systolic Hypertension (VALISH) [10] (Ogihara T, 2004). JATOS recruited 4418 adults age 65–85 years with essential HTN with the intervention aimed to lower sBP to less than <140 mmHg. Both treatment and control arm had similar baseline BP; 171.6/89.1 mmHg and 171.5/89.1 mmHg respectfully. Efonidipine was the add-on agent if needed and average BP achieved was 135.9/74.8 mmHg in the treatment arm. Average BP achieved in the control arm was 145.6/78.1 mmHg, thus a difference of about 10/3 mmHg between the two arms. The trial reported no benefit on the primary composite outcome of CV events or kidney dysfunction with BP lowering vs. control arm and concluded that complex clinical features associated with aging may have contributed to the lack of difference in effect between the two treatments. VALISH recruited 3079 participants that were 70–84 years of age with isolated systolic HTN and target sBP < 140 mmHg in the treatment group. Baseline BP in both groups were comparable; 169.5/81.7 mmHg and 169.6/81.2 mmHg respectively. Valsartan was the add-on agent if needed and average achieved BP in the treatment group was 136.6/74.8 mmHg, while average BP in the control group was 142.0/76.5 mmHg. The difference in BP between both groups was 5.4/1.7 mmHg. The study also reported no benefit on primary composite outcome of CV events or kidney dysfunction (HR: 0.89, 95% CI, 0.60–1.31; $p = 0.38$) with blood pressure lowering. The systolic blood pressure intervention trial (SPRINT) conducted in 2015 evaluated the appropriate target BP for non-diabetic individuals. The trial recruited 9361 persons with an sBP of 130 mmHg or higher and an increased cardiovascular risk, but without diabetes, to an sBP target of less than 120 mmHg (intensive treatment) or a target of less than 140 mmHg (standard treatment). SPRINT reported a lower rate of fatal and nonfatal major cardiovascular death from any cause, although significantly higher rates of some adverse events were observed in the treatment arm [13]. The study had a prespecified subgroup of elderly (defined as those >75 years) which was reported separately [11]. 2636 participants ≥75 years with HTN and increased risk of CVD (either on basis of age ≥ 75 alone, or history of clinical or subclinical CVD, chronic kidney disease, a 10-year or Framingham risk score above 15%) were included in this subgroup analysis. BP target was <120 mmHg in the intensive treatment group and < 140 mmHg in the standard treatment group. A protocolized algorithm, including long-acting drugs and in particular chlorthalidone, was utilized to achieve BP targets. Average achieved BP was 123.4/62 mmHg in the treatment group. The study reported that the intensive treatment group resulted in significantly lower rates of fatal and nonfatal major CV events and death from any cause (RR: 0.66, 95% CI 0.51–0.85). Lastly, the most recent trial was the Strategy of Blood Pressure Intervention in Elderly Hypertensive Patients (STEP) in which 8511 participants were recruited who were 60–80 years of age with HTN [12]. Target BP was 110–130 mmHg and a protocol-based algorithm was used to control the BP which included olmesartan, amlodipine, and hydrochlorothiazide as needed. The achieved BP was 126.7/76.4 mmHg in the treatment group, and 135.9/79.2 mmHg in the control group. The trial reported that the intensive treatment group resulted in a lower incidence of CV events than standard treatment with a target of 130 to less than 150 mmHg (RR: 0.74, 95% CI 0.60–0.92). Similar to previous trials, STEP excluded patients with cognitive impairment and did not include their baseline functional status. Like the two Japanese trials (JATOS and VALISH) STEP trial only included East Asians and was not ethnically diverse, which limits the generalizability of their findings to other groups. Thus, overall, all but two trials report a benefit in lowering BP in the elderly population, and all but one trial also report a decrease in CV or all cause death with lowering of BP. The data are summarized in Table 7.1.

Guidelines

Despite the trial evidence discussed above, the HTN guidelines do differ in the guidance given, over the age cut-off for elderly, the BP at which BP lowering should begin, and the target BP (see Table 7.2). At the most liberal end is the American College of Physicians [19] which recommends a target sBP < 150 for the elderly, defined as those ≥60 years of age, and sBP < 140 only for those who are also at high CV risk. At the other end are the Australian [20] and Canadian [14] guidelines which both define the elderly as ≥75 years of age and recommend a target sBP of <120. Both these follow the definitions and targets from the SPRINT trial. The American College of Cardiology/American Heart Association (AHA/ACC) [2] guidelines which were published in 2017 had a blanket target of 130/80 for everyone, including the elderly, defined as ≥65 years. Despite the SPRINT trial findings, the AHA/ACC workgroup chose 130 rather than 120 given the concern that the achieved sBP in SPRINT in the intervention group was 123 and that the method of

Table 7.2 Summary of published guidelines for the management of hypertension in the elderly

Guidelines	HTN Canada 2020 [14]	ISH 2020 [15]	VA/DoD 2020 [16]	Japanese 2019 [17]	ESC/ESH 2018 [18]	ACP 2017 [19]	AHA/ACC 2017 [2]	Australia 2016 [20]
Definition of older patients	≥ 75 years	Not defined	≥ 60 years	≥ 65 years	Elderly 65–79 years Very old ≥ 80 years	≥ 60 years	≥ 65 years	≥ 75 years
Definition of hypertension (to initiate treatment) (mmHg)	sBP ≥ 130	≥ 140/90	sBP ≥ 150	≥ 140/90	Elderly: ≥ 140/90 Very old: ≥ 160/90	sBP ≥ 150	≥ 130/80	sBP ≥ 120
Blood pressure target (mmHg)	sBP < 120	< 140/80	sBP < 150 for most sBP < 140 if diabetes	65–74 years: < 130/80 ≥ 75 years: < 140/80	sBP 130–139 dBP 70–79	sBP < 150 for most sBP < 140 if high cardiovascular risk or history of stroke/TIA	< 130/80	sBP < 120

HTN Canada Hypertension Canada, *ISH* International Society of Hypertension, *Va/DoD* Veterans Affairs and the Department of Defense, *ESC/ESH* European Society of Cardiology, European Society of Hypertension, *ACP* American College of Physicians, *AHA/ACC* American Heart Association/American College of Cardiology, *sBP* Systolic Blood Pressure, *dBP* Diastolic Blood Pressure measuring BP in SPRINT, with an automated office BP (AOBP) monitor was not widely practiced. AOBP assesses BP after 5 min of resting and provides fully automated readings over a 5-min period while the patient is quietly resting alone. The AOBP method more closely matches the mean daytime BP than the numbers obtained with a casual office BP. This method also minimizes white coat HTN and can lead to sBP measurements about 7–12 mmHg lower than a single automated/oscillometric BP measurement, which is most commonly used [21]. For similar reasons related to BP measurement and other concerns with SPRINT, the European [18] and the International Societies [15] also chose a more liberal target of <140/80 for the elderly. Notably, the European guidelines [18] also have a floor of 130/70 for the BP target, recommending BP not be lowered below this, which would be difficult in practice given the high prevalence of isolated systolic HTN (coupled with low diastolic BP) in the elderly. Similarly, the Department of Veterans Affairs and the Department of Defense guidelines (VA/DoD) recommend treating to an sBP < 150 for most with added benefit of lowering sBP further for those between 130 and 150 for patients ≥60 years [16]. Lastly, the Japanese guidelines [17], in keeping with the two Japanese trials, also suggest somewhat liberal targets at two different age cut-offs: < 130/80 for those 65–74 years age, and < 140/80 for those ≥75 years age.

This veritable smorgasbord of guidelines does create some confusion for the practitioner. If we review some of the eligibility and the adverse effects from the same trials, we can understand how different societies and workgroups came to divergent guidance based on the same set of evidence.

Pitfalls in Lowering BP in Elderly

Lowering BP does lower the risk of several cardiovascular outcomes, but also comes with certain baggage. There is an increase in hypotension-related adverse effects, which are particularly important in certain participants, such as the elderly. Common adverse effects of lowering BP are postural orthostasis and/or post-prandial hypotension, dizziness, falls, risk of kidney failure, electrolyte imbalances, and polypharmacy, all of which are more clinically relevant in the elderly population [5]. However, when it comes to the RCT evidence, the overall safety outcomes reported are mostly similar in both groups with a few notable exceptions (see Table 7.3). The two Japanese trials which did not report a significant benefit with BP lowering [9, 10] (JATOS and VALISH) also did not report more adverse events with BP lowering. This is also in keeping with the small, achieved difference in BP (< 10 mmHg in sBP between arms) in these two trials. The other trials did report more hypotension-related adverse events in the lower BP arm, and other adverse events possibly related to the drugs used (e.g., electrolyte disorders from thiazides, ankle swelling from calcium channel blocker). However, notably despite an increase in hypotension, there was no increase in fractures in the most recent trials (STEP and SPRINT) [11,

Table 7.3 Select exclusion criteria and adverse effects in trials of hypertension in the elderly

Trials	Select relevant exclusion criteria	Select adverse effects in lower BP arm
SHEP (2000) [6]	Other serious illnesses (cancer, alcoholic liver disease, established renal dysfunction, with competing risk for the SHEP primary end point or the presence of medical management problems)	Falls (2.5% higher) Nocturia (2.0% higher) Unusual joint pain (3.6% higher) Severe headaches (1.1% lower)
HYVET (2008) [8]	Condition expected to severely limit survival, e.g. terminal illness. Clinical diagnosis of dementia Resident in a nursing home Unable to stand up or walk Standing sBP < 140 mmHg	Serious adverse events 448 in the placebo group and 358 in the active-treatment group ($P = 0.001$). Only five of these events (three in the placebo group and two in the active-treatment group) were classified by the investigators as possibly having been due to the trial medication
JATOS (2008) [9]	Recent stroke or acute coronary syndrome Congestive heart failure of NYHA class II or higher Malignant disease or collagen disease	Adverse events overall similar ($p = 0.99$) Treatment discontinuation due to adverse events also similar ($p = 0.99$)
VALISH (2010) [10]	Recent stroke or acute coronary syndrome Severe heart failure ($\geq$NYHA functional classification III) Severe aortic stenosis or valvular disease Other patients who are judged to be inappropriate for The study by the investigator	Overall similar 18.2% vs 17.9% ($p = 0.85$) Those related to valsartan (5.6% versus 4.4%; $p = 0.13$)
SPRINT Elderly (2016) [11]	Recent stroke or acute coronary syndrome One-minute standing SBP <110 mmHg Symptomatic heart failure within the past 6 months or left ventricular ejection fraction <35% A medical condition likely to limit survival to <3 years or a malignancy other than non-melanoma skin cancer within the last 2 years Institutionalized or wheelchair bound	Overall serious adverse events HR, 0.99 (95% CI, 0.89–1.11) Syncope: 3.0% vs 2.4%, HR, 1.23 (95% CI, 0.76–2.00) Electrolyte abnormalities (4.0% vs 2.7%; HR, 1.51 (95% CI, 0.99–2.33) Acute kidney injury or renal failure (5.5% vs 4.0%; HR, 1.41 (95% CI, 0.98–2.04)
STEP (2021) [12]	Recent stroke or acute coronary syndrome New York heart association class III-IV Severe liver or kidney disease Cognitive impairment	Hypotension, RR 1.31 (95% CI 1.02–1.68) Fracture RR 0.79 (95% CI 0.40–1.56) 30% reduction in GFR RR 0.90 (95% CI 0.63–1.30)

SHEP Systolic Hypertension in the Elderly Program, *HYVET* Hypertension in the Very Elderly Trial, *sBP* Systolic Blood Pressure, *NYHA* New York Heart Association, *JATOS* Japanese Trial to Assess Optimal Systolic Blood Pressure in Elderly Hypertensive patients, *VALISH* Valsartan in Elderly Isolated Systolic Hypertension, *SPRINT* Systolic Blood Pressure Intervention Trial, *HR* Hazard Ratio, *CI* Confidence Interval, *STEP* Strategy of Blood Pressure Intervention in the Elderly Hypertensive Patients, *RR* Relative Risk, *GFR* Glomerular Filtration Rate

12]. These aspects make sense in the assessment of the totality of the trial methods including the eligibility criteria (see Table 7.3).

Perusing the exclusion criteria of the trials does allow one to understand why the adverse effects with BP lowering are lower than what one would expect to see in real life. These trials were designed to exclude individuals at high risk for adverse events with BP lowering. Apart from usual exclusions (such as a recent stroke or acute coronary syndrome), these trials also excluded individuals in a nursing home (HYVET, SPRINT) [8, 11], those with a standing BP below a certain threshold (sBP < 110 in SPRINT, sBP < 140 in HYVET), and those with cognitive impairment or dementia (HYVET, STEP) [8, 12]. These exclusions are important to keep in mind while making BP-lowering decisions in the elderly.

Outcomes and Shared Decision-Making

From the previous discussion of the benefits and adverse events, it is important to consider patient safety, quality of life, life expectancy, time-to-benefit from therapy when treating BP in these patients. Patient selection for intensive BP lowering is important to avoid adverse events. However, age and frailty are not synonymous and older patients are often at high CV risk and deserving of receiving the benefit of BP lowering. It is crucial to have a shared decision-making process where patients are involved in whether benefits associated with treating BP outweigh the risks. Valuing stroke prevention may be important for some while avoiding hypotensive falls and pill burden might be more important for others.

HTN management is not straightforward, and many patients may not appreciate the complexity behind it. They may be hesitant with respect to adherence to treatment despite benefits that have been supported by clinical trials [5]. In addition to initial acceptance of treatment, the long-term treatment plan is complex with follow-up appointments, adjustments in drug administration, and potential side effects. Few studies have been conducted on patient drug adherence in older age and the long-term adherence and management does not get simpler [5]. As such, involving patients in the decision-making process can assist with patient adherence. It may also be safer for patients as they will understand the benefits and risks associated with treatment. On the other hand, Benneton et al. [5] also discuss that physicians may not be convinced of the benefits of treating elderly patients with HTN as most previous studies have been observational and trials are conducted in a controlled setting where most participants are adherent to treatment plan and stringent follow up [5].

As such, a shared decision-making model between the patient and healthcare provider will help with patient's understanding of the advantages and disadvantages associated with treatment, as well as patient adherence. The shared decision-making process is often seen as more complicated however it is highly relevant in elderly patients with multi-comorbidities. The latter allows healthcare providers to focus on the goals and wishes of the patient and cater the treatment plan based on that.

Drug Classes and Deprescribing

Drugs of the first line, in particular angiotensin converting enzyme inhibitors (ACEi) and thiazide-like diuretics (indapamide or chlorthalidone) were commonly used in the trials that demonstrated benefit. It is important to be alert and also avoid the prescribing cascade which is adding a drug to counteract another drug's side effects. For example, adding a diuretic to counteract the side effect of development of peripheral edema with a calcium channel blocker—which is due to vasodilation and better treated by using a low dose in combination with an ACEi or an angiotensin receptor blocker. Drug classes that should be avoided in the elderly include alpha-adrenergic antagonists, in particular, that are associated with hypotension-related adverse events [22].

Aging is associated with multiple morbid conditions and multiple medications for each condition leading to polypharmacy. The latter is associated with significant adverse events and higher hospitalization rate [23]. Shepperd et al. discuss the importance of deprescribing which is defined as eliminating an inappropriate or unnecessary medication, supervised by a licensed healthcare professional in order to decrease the burden of medication and prevent adverse effects. CVs are considered good targets for deprescribing since they are started for preventive measures rather than treating an acute illness or symptom. A recent Cochrane review found no evidence of association between withdrawing anti-HTN medication in the elderly and mortality, myocardial infarction, stroke or hospitalisation [24]. BP did increase by 10/4 mmHg in the six trials included, however, follow-up was short which prevented firm conclusions on risks with deprescription. The Optimising Treatment for Mild Systolic Hypertension in the Elderly (OPTIMISE) trial examined the short-term safety and efficacy of anti-HTN deprescribing [25]. Recruited participants were aged 80 years or older, with sBP at baseline <150 mmHg and prescribed two or more antihypertensive treatments for at least 12 months prior to enrollment. Patients with a history of heart failure, myocardial infarction/stroke in the last 12 months, secondary HTN or lack of capacity to consent were excluded from the study. Participants were randomized to either medication reduction or standard care. An algorithm was provided to physicians on the choice of drug for withdrawal. A total of 569 participants were randomized, 560 of whom were multimorbid and mean age was 85 years. The trial lasted for 12 weeks. The findings demonstrated that medication reduction was associated with an important increase in BP (3/2 mmHg) but no differences in quality of life, frailty, side effects or serious adverse events. However, the study was not powered to detect differences in clinical outcomes such as adverse CV events or death. Further research is needed to establish long-term outcomes in deprescribing anti-HTN medications in asymptomatic individuals as it remains unclear on the potential long-term effects. However, the trajectory of BP in the years prior to death has been known to be one of decline [26]. The changes in sBP from peak values ranged from −8.5 mmHg (95% CI, −9.4 to −7.7) for those dying aged 60 to 69 years to −22.0 mmHg (95% CI, −22.6 to −21.4) for those dying at 90 years or older; overall, 64.0% of individuals had SBP changes of greater than −10 mmHg. Thus, in this scenario of declining BP, or in presence of hypotension symptoms, deprescribing BP medications may be the appropriate action.

Unanswered Questions

As mentioned previously, dBP will typically be lower than sBP in older adults due to central arterial stiffness. dBP below 60 or 65 mmHg in patients with isolated systolic HTN and known coronary artery disease has been associated with higher risk of stroke and CV events [27]. Though the SPRINT data does suggest benefit of intensive BP lowering across tertiles of dBP, the safety of intensive sBP lowering in the setting of very low dBP (< 60) in the elderly would benefit from more data [28]. As mentioned above, though deprescribing reduces the pill burden, the longer-term safety remains uncertain. Lastly, newer BP-lowering agents and device therapy are now making it into the clinical realm. The elderly population often gets excluded in phase 3 trials, and their efficacy/safety would remain to be established.

Conclusion

John H. Hay is quoted as saying, "The greatest danger to a man with high blood pressure lies in its discovery because then some fool is certain to try and reduce it" [29]. HTN management in the elderly is complex and an individualized approach is mandatory. The latter allows the values and goals of the patient to be considered, as well as their overall health status to provide proper care [30].

Discussion of Clinical Case Scenarios

Though patient 1 has an sBP not at target and pre-existing vascular disease with high risk of adverse CV outcomes, he also has several concerning features suggesting high risk of adverse outcomes with BP lowering. He has a significant orthostatic drop in BP with a sBP < 110 mmHg, and though not explicit, there is a concern of early cognitive impairment and falls—such that they are moving to an assisted living facility. Such a patient would not have been enrolled in the trials demonstrating benefit (SPRINT, STEP) and one should be cautious about extrapolating those data for this patient. Indeed, one could even consider deprescribing or reducing some of his BP-lowering medications given the concern for falls and orthostatic hypotension.

The second patient is older, but she is independent and active. She has no major red flags of concern and has no orthostatic drop. Despite the age, her risk profile suggests a high risk of future CV outcomes, and it would be reasonable to discuss the benefits of intensive BP lowering (< 130, or even <120) as appropriate and escalate BP-lowering therapy.

References

1. Oliveros E, Patel H, Kyung S, Fugar S, Goldberg A, Madan N, Williams KA. Hypertension in older adults: assessment, management, and challenges. Clin Cardiol. 2020;43(2):99–107. https://doi.org/10.1002/clc.23303.
2. Kulkarni A, Mehta A, Yang E, Parapid B. Older adults and hypertension: beyond the 2017 guideline for prevention, detection, evaluation, and management of high blood pressure in adults. Am Heart Assoc. 2008;58(10):1117–29.
3. Blood Pressure Lowering Treatment Trialists' Collaboration. Age-stratified and blood-pressure-stratified effects of blood-pressure-lowering pharmacotherapy for the prevention of cardiovascular disease and death: an individual participant-level data meta-analysis. Lancet (London, England). 2021;398(10305):1053–64. https://doi.org/10.1016/S0140-6736(21)01921-8.
4. Philip R, Beaney T, Appelbaum N, Gonzalvez CR, Koldeweij C, Golestaneh AK, Poulter N, Clarke JM. Variation in hypertension clinical practice guidelines: a global comparison. BMC Med. 2021;19(1):117. https://doi.org/10.1186/s12916-021-01963-0.
5. Benetos A, Petrovic M, Strandberg T. Hypertension management in older and Frail older patients. Circ Res. 2019;124(7):1045–60. https://doi.org/10.1161/CIRCRESAHA.118.313236.
6. Perry HM Jr, Davis BR, Price TR, Applegate WB, Fields WS, Guralnik JM, Kuller L, Pressel S, Stamler J, Probstfield JL. Effect of treating isolated systolic hypertension on the risk of developing various types and subtypes of stroke: the systolic hypertension in the elderly program (SHEP). JAMA. 2000;284(4):465–71. https://doi.org/10.1001/jama.284.4.465.
7. Bulpitt CJ, Beckett NS, Cooke J, Dumitrascu DL, Gil-Extremera B, Nachev C, Nunes M, Peters R, Staessen JA, Thijs L, Hypertension in the Very Elderly Trial Working Group. Results of the pilot study for the hypertension in the very elderly trial. J Hypertens. 2003;21(12):2409–17. https://doi.org/10.1097/00004872-200312000-00030.
8. Beckett NS, Peters R, Fletcher AE, Staessen JA, Liu L, Dumitrascu D, Stoyanovsky V, Antikainen RL, Nikitin Y, Anderson C, Belhani A, Forette F, Rajkumar C, Thijs L, Banya W, Bulpitt CJ, HYVET Study Group. Treatment of hypertension in patients 80 years of age or older. N Engl J Med. 2008;358(18):1887–98. https://doi.org/10.1056/NEJMoa0801369.
9. JATOS Study Group. Principal results of the Japanese trial to assess optimal systolic blood pressure in elderly hypertensive patients (JATOS). Hypertension Res. 2008;31(12):2115–27. https://doi.org/10.1291/hypres.31.2115.
10. Ogihara T, Saruta T, Matsuoka H, Shimamoto K, Fujita T, Shimada K, Imai Y, Nishigaki M. Valsartan in elderly isolated systolic hypertension (VALISH) study: rationale and design. Hypertension Res. 2004;27(9):657–61. https://doi.org/10.1291/hypres.27.657.
11. Williamson JD, Supiano MA, Applegate WB, Berlowitz DR, Campbell RC, Chertow GM, Fine LJ, Haley WE, Hawfield AT, Ix JH, Kitzman DW, Kostis JB, Krousel-Wood MA, Launer LJ, Oparil S, Rodriguez CJ, Roumie CL, Shorr RI, Sink KM, Wadley VG, SPRINT Research Group. Intensive vs standard blood pressure control and cardiovascular disease outcomes in adults aged ≥75 years: a randomized clinical trial. JAMA. 2016;315(24):2673–82. https://doi.org/10.1001/jama.2016.7050.
12. Zhang W, Zhang S, Deng Y, Wu S, Ren J, Sun G, Yang J, Jiang Y, Xu X, Wang TD, Chen Y, Li Y, Yao L, Li D, Wang L, Shen X, Yin X, Liu W, Zhou X, Zhu B, STEP Study Group. Trial of intensive blood-pressure control in older patients with hypertension. N Engl J Med. 2021;385(14):1268–79. https://doi.org/10.1056/NEJMoa2111437.
13. SPRINT Research Group, Wright JT Jr, Williamson JD, Whelton PK, Snyder JK, Sink KM, Rocco MV, Reboussin DM, Rahman M, Oparil S, Lewis CE, Kimmel PL, Johnson KC, Goff DC Jr, Fine LJ, Cutler JA, Cushman WC, Cheung AK, Ambrosius WT. A randomized trial of intensive versus standard blood-pressure control. N Engl J Med. 2015;373(22):2103–16. https://doi.org/10.1056/NEJMoa1511939.
14. Rabi DM, McBrien KA, Sapir-Pichhadze R, Nakhla M, Ahmed SB, Dumanski SM, Butalia S, Leung AA, Harris KC, Cloutier L, Zarnke KB, Ruzicka M, Hiremath S, Feldman RD, Tobe SW, Campbell TS, Bacon SL, Nerenberg KA, Dresser GK, Fournier A, Daskalopoulou

SS. Hypertension Canada's 2020 comprehensive guidelines for the prevention, diagnosis, risk assessment, and treatment of hypertension in adults and children. Can J Cardiol. 2020;36(5):596–624. https://doi.org/10.1016/j.cjca.2020.02.086.

15. Unger T, Borghi C, Charchar F, Khan NA, Poulter NR, Prabhakaran D, Ramirez A, Schlaich M, Stergiou GS, Tomaszewski M, Wainford RD, Williams B, Schutte AE. 2020 International Society of Hypertension global hypertension practice guidelines. J Hypertens. 2020;38(6):982–1004. https://doi.org/10.1097/HJH.0000000000002453.

16. Tschanz CMP, Cushman WC, Harrell CTE, Berlowitz DR, Sall JL. Synopsis of the 2020 U.S. Department of Veterans Affairs/U.S. Department of Defense clinical practice guideline: the diagnosis and Management of Hypertension in the primary care setting. Ann Intern Med. 2020;173(11):904–13. https://doi.org/10.7326/M20-3798.

17. Umemura S, Arima H, Arima S, Asayama K, Dohi Y, Hirooka Y, Horio T, Hoshide S, Ikeda S, Ishimitsu T, Ito M, Ito S, Iwashima Y, Kai H, Kamide K, Kanno Y, Kashihara N, Kawano Y, Kikuchi T, Kitamura K, Hirawa N. The Japanese Society of Hypertension Guidelines for the Management of Hypertension (JSH 2019). Hypertension Res. 2019;42(9):1235–481. https://doi.org/10.1038/s41440-019-0284-9.

18. Benetos A, Bulpitt CJ, Petrovic M, Ungar A, Agabiti Rosei E, Cherubini A, Redon J, Grodzicki T, Dominiczak A, Strandberg T, Mancia G. An expert opinion from the European Society of Hypertension-European Union Geriatric Medicine Society Working Group on the Management of Hypertension in very old, frail subjects. Hypertension (Dallas, Tex. : 1979). 2016;67(5):820–5. https://doi.org/10.1161/HYPERTENSIONAHA.115.07020.

19. Qaseem A, Wilt TJ, Rich R, Humphrey LL, Frost J, Forciea MA, Clinical Guidelines Committee of the American College of Physicians, The Commission on Health of the Public, Science of the American Academy of Family Physicians, Fitterman N, Barry MJ, Horwitch CA, Iorio A, McLean RM. Pharmacologic treatment of hypertension in adults aged 60 years or older to higher versus lower blood pressure targets: a clinical practice guideline from the American College of Physicians and the American Academy of family physicians. Ann Intern Med. 2017;166(6):430–7. https://doi.org/10.7326/M16-1785.

20. Gabb GM, Mangoni AA, Arnolda L. Guideline for the diagnosis and management of hypertension in adults −2016. Med J Aust. 2017;206(3):141. https://doi.org/10.5694/mja16.01132.

21. Bakris GL. The implications of blood pressure measurement methods on treatment targets for blood pressure. Circulation. 2016;134(13):904–5. https://doi.org/10.1161/CIRCULATIONAHA.116.022536.

22. Hiremath S, Ruzicka M, Petrich W, McCallum MK, Hundemer GL, Tanuseputro P, Manuel D, Burns K, Edwards C, Bugeja A, Magner P, McCormick B, Garg AX, Rhodes E, Sood MM. Alpha-blocker use and the risk of hypotension and hypotension-related clinical events in women of advanced age. Hypertension (Dallas, Tex. : 1979). 2019;74(3):645–51. https://doi.org/10.1161/HYPERTENSIONAHA.119.13289.

23. Sheppard JP, Payne RA. Deprescribing antihypertensives in patients with multimorbidity. Prescriber. 2020;31:16–9. https://doi.org/10.1002/psb.1870.

24. Reeve E, Jordan V, Thompson W, Sawan M, Todd A, Gammie TM, Hopper I, Hilmer SN, Gnjidic D. Withdrawal of antihypertensive drugs in older people. Cochrane Database Syst Rev. 2020;6(6):CD012572. https://doi.org/10.1002/14651858.CD012572.pub2.

25. Sheppard JP, Burt J, Lown M, Temple E, Benson J, Ford GA, Heneghan C, Hobbs FDR, Jowett S, Little P, Mant J, Mollison J, Nickless A, Ogburn E, Payne R, Williams M, Yu LM, McManus RJ. Optimising treatment for mild systolic hypertension in the elderly (OPTiMISE): protocol for a randomised controlled non-inferiority trial. BMJ Open. 2018;8(9):e022930. https://doi.org/10.1136/bmjopen-2018-022930.

26. Delgado J, Bowman K, Ble A, Masoli J, Han Y, Henley W, Welsh S, Kuchel GA, Ferrucci L, Melzer D. Blood pressure trajectories in the 20 years before death. JAMA Intern Med. 2018;178(1):93–9. https://doi.org/10.1001/jamainternmed.2017.7023.

27. Laubscher T, Regier L, Stone S. Hypertension in the elderly: new blood pressure targets and prescribing tips. Can Fam Physician. 2014;60(5):453–6.

28. Beddhu S, Chertow GM, Cheung AK, Cushman WC, Rahman M, Greene T, Wei G, Campbell RC, Conroy M, Freedman BI, Haley W, Horwitz E, Kitzman D, Lash J, Papademetriou V, Pisoni R, Riessen E, Rosendorff C, Watnick SG, Whittle J, SPRINT Research Group. Influence of baseline diastolic blood pressure on effects of intensive compared with standard blood pressure control. Circulation. 2018;137(2):134–43. https://doi.org/10.1161/CIRCULATIONAHA.117.030848.
29. Elias MF, Goodell AL. Setting the record straight for two heroes in hypertension: John J Hay and Paul Dudley White. J Clin Hypertension (Greenwich, Conn). 2019;21(9):1429–31. https://doi.org/10.1111/jch.13650.
30. Giffin A, Madden KM, Hogan DB. Blood pressure targets for older patients-do advanced age and frailty really not matter? Can Geriatr J. 2020;23(2):205–9. https://doi.org/10.5770/cgj.23.429.

Chapter 8
Diabetic Nephropathy in Advanced Age Patients

Christos P. Argyropoulos and Maria-Eleni Roumelioti

Introduction

Case Vignette Introduction

Ms X is an 80-year-old woman who is scheduled to see you for a new appointment to investigate her "kidney disease". She has had diabetes type 2 requiring medications for 20 years, but her primary care physician has told her she had had "pre-diabetes" for another 10 years prior to that. Her diabetes was complicated by the development of neuropathy, but not retinopathy. A review of her lab records sent over by the endocrinologist shows that she has kept her hemoglobin A1c to between 7–7.8%, with most measurements over 7.5%. Her most recent estimated glomerular filtration rate is 40 mL/min/1.73 m², and her LDL is 70 mg/dL. While she is currently living independently, she is having increasing difficulty performing the activities of daily leaving, while taking care of her husband with progressive cognitive decline. She has many questions about the diagnosis of her kidney disease ("I feel fine") and the approach to management. We will use her case to illustrate the nuances of taking care of kidney disease in a patient with an advanced age and diabetes type 2.

Diabetes mellitus (DM) and chronic kidney disease (CKD) represent major health issues and are highly prevalent in older adults. One should not overlook the fact that the process of aging and the long-term complications of DM affect multiple organs including the kidneys. Historically known as diabetic nephropathy (DN), CKD in patients with DM is often abbreviated as diabetic kidney disease (DKD) and is the major cause of CKD and end-stage kidney disease (ESKD) in those over 60 years old [1]. However, diabetic kidney disease infers the absence of other etiologies and in adults with advanced age, other factors could be operative such as

C. P. Argyropoulos (✉) · M.-E. Roumelioti
Internal Medicine, University of New Mexico Hospitals, Albuquerque, NM, USA
e-mail: cargyropoulos@salud.unm.edu

H. Kramer et al. (eds.), *Kidney Disease in the Elderly*, https://doi.org/10.1007/978-3-031-68460-9_8

previous AKI episodes, medications, cholesterol emboli, and other glomerular disease. Most patients with diabetes and CKD are never biopsied but a third of new ESKD cases in those over 75 years old are attributed to diabetes.

The growing population of older patients with diabetes and CKD poses many great challenges. General diagnostic criteria and treatment options, although widely available, need to be applied with caution. Multidisciplinary medical management due to co-existing comorbidities is also required and these patients may eventually enter assisted living or a nursing home. Adults with advanced age, diabetes and CKD often have psychiatric disorders, audiovisual impairments, plus neuropathy that impairs proprioception and balance. In addition, diabetic-caused vascular disease increases the risk of cognitive impairment and in this vulnerable population challenges adherence to complex medical regimens [2].

CKD care for older patients with diabetes has to recognize the wider challenges faced by a globally reduced workforce in the field. Though guidelines have incorporated fixed, non-age dependent criteria for referral to nephrology, strict adherence to such criteria may lead to referral of lower-risk advanced age patients who may not derive benefit as compared to younger individuals [3], while the likelihood of regression, i.e., a spontaneous improvement in kidney filtration, often exceeds the likelihood of progression [4]. CKD in the setting of diabetes is often a non-proteinuric form of kidney disease [5–8] and the presence of proteinuria or CKD in an older patient with diabetes doe not necessarily reflect diabetic kidney disease. This creates challenges in translating interventions which are often tested in populations with some degree of proteinuria to those patients with (near-) normoalbuminuria. Nevertheless, recent therapeutic improvements in the field of DKD apply equally to advanced age and younger patients and can be deployed either in primary or as pillars of therapy in a multidisciplinary management program for diabetes.

Definition, Epidemiology, and Health Resource Utilization

The typical form of DKD, and the disease most often associated with the historical term DN, is a syndrome characterized by the presence of pathological quantities of urine albumin excretion (>500 mg/24 h in at least three consecutive samples), diabetic glomerular lesions, and loss of GFR in patients with pre-existing diabetes [9]. Diabetic kidney disease is a major micro-vascular and macro-vascular complication of both type I and type II.

Over the past 30 years the incidence and prevalence of diabetes, especially type 2 DM, as an attributed cause of ESKD has increased [5] and has become a global pandemic. This is largely a result of the increasing prevalence of DM per se. In a National Health and Nutrition Examination Survey (NHANES analysis: 2003–2004 until 2013–2014) the estimated frequency of DM increased by nine million, affecting 30.2 (13%) million US adults [5]. The 2020 National Diabetes Statistics report that incorporated data from 2013–2018 suggests very little improvement [10]. Among the advanced age patients, the historically reported incidence of diagnosed

DM is 10–18%, but this appears to be increasing. Notably, between 1994 and 2004, the prevalence of DM in the age group over 65 in the United States increased by 62%. In the United States' National Diabetes Statistics Report [10], the prevalence of diagnosed and total diabetes was 21.4% and 26.8% respectively, in those over 65. The International Diabetes Federation Atlas [11] projects similar patterns world-wide and an increasing trend of DM up to 2045.

The higher rates of DM threaten the improvement in the *incidence rates* of CKD which has been observed in recent years [12]. For example, the prevalence of CKD among the advanced age patients decreased from 43.2% to 36.8% for time periods 2003–2006 and 2015–2018 respectively, while the prevalence of CKD with diabetes decreased from 41.5% to 36.3% during the same period. Using estimates from NHANES [5], approximately 26.2% of US adults with diabetes would meet the criteria for CKD using either a criterion of reduced estimated glomerular filtration rate (eGFR), or increased albuminuria, and nearly 56% of these individuals with CKD would have albuminuria. The unadjusted prevalence of albuminuria in those older than 65-year-old was nearly 35% higher than in those younger than 65 (32.3% vs 23.9%). Similar findings are noted in non-US populations [13]. Projections derived prior to the COVID-19 pandemic, that factored in the various temporal trends, however, predict a stabilization of the incidence, but rising prevalence in the ESKD from 2015 to 2030 [14]. It is important to realize that subgroups continue to experience higher rates of ESKD due to DM; these groups include African Americans, Hispanic Americans and American Indians [5], and these changes highlight the disparities in the provision of diabetes and kidney care in the United States.

The overall cost of care for patients with diabetes and CKD is substantial. The USRDS 2021 report tabulated US Medicare costs for individuals older than 65. Excluding ESKD costs, total Medicare expenditures were 23.9% for patients with DM, 13.6% among those with CKD and nearly half of the CKD related costs (6.8% out of 13.6%) were generated for advanced age patients with CKD and DM. Not adjusted for inflation, the per-person spending for older patients with CKD and DM was $54,489 for CKD stage 4 and $47,168 for stage 3, which were substantially higher than the corresponding figures for older individuals with CKD but without DM ($43,640 for stage 4–5 and $30,743 for stage 3). The three larger categories of costs included inpatients costs (24.8% of total), physician/supplier (17.2%), and medications (10.7%).

Pathophysiology, Pathology, and Natural History

Case Vignette Continued

Ms X is really puzzled about her referral for evaluation of kidney disease. She says that her diabetes provider has always congratulated on her meticulous control of her glycemia for years and is puzzled that her kidney function is now below normal. She questions you specifically to rule out the possibility that her "slowing" kidney function is not due to diabetes, but part of her normal aging. Or could it even be due to both factors?

The aging process in the kidney starts to occur at the end of third decade of life and.aging abnormalities in the kidney include vascular changes, fibrosis due to global sclerosis and collagen accumulation, increased mesangial and endothelial cell numbers, mesangial matrix expansion, basement membrane thickening, podocyte depletion, interstitial fibrosis and tubular atrophy [15]. Nephron loss occurs with advancing age [16], but this loss is not associated with increase in single nephron GFR and hyperfiltration [17, 18]. DM may accelerate biologic aging at both the cellular and the organ level, by leading to hyperfiltration, an increase in the single nephron GFR and an accelerated loss of kidney function. Hence, DKD in the advanced age patients could be thought as yet another demonstration of the "Brenner hypothesis", i.e. that hyperfiltration drives the progression of kidney disease [19, 20] in a limited (due to aging) kidney functional reserve. Hyperglycemia and the subsequent oxidant stress may hinder the limited auto-repair capability of the aged kidney tissue and contribute to accelerated nephron loss in diabetes. Early genetic studies showed that there is an overlap of loci associated with albuminuria in aging mice and human patients with diabetes [21]. One significant and eight suggestive loci were found, while two of the nine mouse loci for age-related albuminuria were significantly associated with diabetic nephropathy. This suggests a common pathway of renal senescence and diabetic-related kidney disease.

In older patients with diabetes, pathologic changes are also the result of the accumulation of advanced glycation end products (AGEs) [22]. The expression of receptors for AGEs or RAGR (cell surface receptor of AGEs) is increased in both aging and DM. AGEs favor oxidation and inflammation [23, 24] and increase the likelihood of age-and diabetic-related CKD [25]. The complexity of the molecular mechanisms underlying the progression of DKD in older patients [26] reveals a complex interplay between oxidative stress, inflammation and hyperglycemia have emerged.

Translational medicine efforts have continuously refined our understanding of DKD, and various prognostic markers have been tentatively identified as mapping to pathways associated with aging, inflammation, oxidative stress and ischemia-reperfusion in addition to the more traditional factors of glycemia and generation of AGE products [27]. Inflammation and tissue fibrosis in DKD may be the result of aberrant activation of the mineralocorticoid receptor. While most nephrologists associate aldosterone and other endogenous mineralocorticoids with electrolyte transport in the distal nephron, the first studies with these hormonal agonists showed that systemic administration of mineralocorticoids may promote damage in many vascular beds (including the kidney) and tissue fibrosis [28]. Mineralocorticoid receptor signaling links together tissue injury, oxidative stress, inflammation, arterial hypertension and fibrosis in both the cardiovascular system and the kidney [29–31]. While this rather complex pathophysiology has yet to translate to therapeutic advances [32], targeting hyperfiltration, with sodium glucose co-transporter two inhibitors, and the final common pathway of inflammation and fibrosis with non-steroidal mineralocorticoid receptor antagonists, can slow kidney disease progression.

Pathology

The 2010 Pathologic Classification of Diabetic Nephropathy [33] recognizes that DKD may affect all structures and compartments within the kidney: glomeruli, arterioles, mesangium, tubules and the interstitium. In particular, one may observe the following lesions:

(a) *Glomeruli:* (1) diffuse intracapillary glomerulosclerosis with mesangial widening, thickening of the capillary wall and glomerular basement membrane, capillary dilation and formation of microaneurysms, and eventually capillary narrowing and reduced glomerular circulation, (2) nodular intercapillary (Kimmelstiel and Wilson) glomerulosclerosis.
(b) *Arterioles:* subintimal hyaline deposits (exudative or insudative lesions) [34] in afferent and efferent arterioles (hyaline arteriosclerosis). Deposits may also present in capillary walls (fibrin caps) and Bowman capsules (capsular drops) [35]. Capsular drops are in general considered to be specific for DKD [36], and may also be observed in 5.3% of biopsies without diabetes [34]. Capsular drops are useful to distinguish between diabetic and non-diabetic causes of glomerulosclerosis [33].
(c) *Mesangium:* DKD is defined histologically by mesangial matrix expansion/ mesangiolysis and mesangial cell proliferation, and is estimated through the mesangial fractional volume (Vv[mes/glom]). Mesangial fractional volume correlates with GFR and the presence of albuminuria and hypertension [35].
(d) *Tubules and Interstitium:* tubular atrophy and basement membrane thickening, interstitial space expansion and eventually fibrosis [37].

Based on these observations, a staging system has been proposed based on the glomerular pathology, with a separate quantitative evaluation for interstitial and vascular lesions (Table 8.1 and Table 8.2). The glomerular stage is assigned on the basis of the most severe lesion observed in the kidney biopsy, e.g., a biopsy showing Kimmelstiel–Wilson nodules and global sclerosis in >50% of the glomeruli will be assigned a stage IV rather than III.

Some of the histologic lesions can be related to biological aging, while others may be related to age, chronic inflammation or vascular disease [38]. Older patients with type II diabetes may also have renal artery stenosis (RAS) leading to kidney ischemia [39] or intrarenal arterial hyalinosis lesions [40]. While hyalinosis of the efferent arteriole is relatively specific for DKD, afferent arteriolar hyalinosis may be observed in other conditions e.g., hypertensive nephropathy. In recent years there has been an increasing prevalence of patients with normoalbuminuric kidney disease in advanced age patients with diabetes, and this clinical phenotype may be associated with an interstitial, tubular atrophy or vascular form of kidney injury [41,

Table 8.1 Glomerular staging system for diabetic kidney disease

Class	Description	Defining feature
I	Mild or nonspecific LM changes and EM-proven GBM thickening	GBM > 395 nm in female and > 430 nm in male individuals 9 years of age and older
IIa	Mild mesangial expansion	Mild mesangial expansion in >25% of the observed mesangium
IIb	Severe mesangial expansion	Severe mesangial expansion in >25% of the observed mesangium
III	Nodular sclerosis (Kimmelstiel–Wilson lesion)	At least one convincing Kimmelstiel–Wilson lesion
IV	Advanced diabetic glomerulosclerosis	Global glomerular sclerosis in >50% of the glomeruli

EM electron microscopy, *LM* light microscopy, *GBM* glomerular basement membrane

Table 8.2 Interstitial and vascular lesions in diabetic kidney disease

Lesion	Criteria	Score
Interstitial lesions		
IFTA	No IFTA	0
	<25%	1
	25% to 50%	2
	>50%	3
Interstitial inflammation	Absent	0
	Infiltration in areas with IFTA	1
	Infiltration in areas without IFTA	2
Vascular lesions		
Arteriolar hyalinosis	Absent	0
	At least one area of arteriolar hyalinosis	1
	More than one area of arteriolar hyalinosis	2
Large vessels		Yes/no
Arteriosclerosis (score worst artery)	No intimal thickening	0
	Intimal thickening less than thickness of media	1
	Intimal thickening greater than thickness of media	2

IFTA interstitial fibrosis and tubular atrophy

42] than more typical glomerular lesions of diabetes. Notwithstanding these observations, serial biopsy studies have shown that among patients with DM and normo−/microalbuminuria, loss of kidney function is associated with mesangial expansion [43], underscoring the importance of the mesangium as an early initiator of DKD. More recent molecular phenotyping in the multicenter TRIDENT (Transformative Research in Diabetic Nephropathy) study [44] showed that glomerular lesions (glomerulosclerosis/mesangiolysis) and podocyte injury were the strongest predictors for the rate of decline in kidney function, but interstitial fibrosis was a very strong predictor of eGFR at the time of the kidney biopsy. Such data would point toward the glomerulus as the site of initiation of the typical DKD lesion with tubulointerstitial lesions being an outcome, rather than a cause of

DKD. However, the tubule itself may be an important site of action of therapies that reduce the rate of progression of DKD, as we will discuss below in the section about therapies.

Autopsy findings may shed some light into the natural history of the histopathologic changes of DKD in relation to the clinical manifestations [45]. Data analyzed from 168 patients with either type 1 or 2 diabetes found that histopathologic changes attributable to DKD were present in 106 patients, while in 20 out of those 106 patients, clinical manifestations associated with DKD had been absent during their lifetimes. Underdiagnosed DKD encompassed all classes except the sclerotic class. Microalbuminuria or macroalbuminuria was not associated with the presence of histologically proven DKD. Hence, *kidney lesions associated with diabetes may develop before the onset of clinical laboratory abnormalities.*

Natural History

Structural changes lead inevitably to functional changes. The natural history of DKD is easier to study on patients with type I DM since the onset of the disease can be specified most of the times. Unfortunately, the onset date for type II DM is difficult to establish because the diagnosis is often incidental. Almost 50% of these patients are unaware of their disease. The first important step is the accurate assessment of kidney function (eGFR) and assessment for kidney damage (urine albumin to creatinine ration, UACR) in older patients. With aging, kidney function shows a moderate reduction due to a proportionate blood flow reduction even without diabetes. Normal GFR when measured as inulin clearance is about 80 mL/min/1.73m^2 for the 75–79 years age group, and 65 mL/min/1.73m^2 for those 80–89 years old. The CKD determination of an older patient needs to consider the age appropriate loss of GFR due to nephron senescence [46]. The typical DKD lesion is thought to progress through 5 stages, with albuminuria and eGFR being the main determinants of kidney function for each stage.

Glomerular hyperfiltration and kidney hypertrophy initiate DKD (**Stage 1**). Age-unadjusted definitions of hyperfiltration propose a range of 125–175 mL/min/1.73m^2. Approximately one-third of patients with type I DM patients have a 20–40% higher eGFR than age-matched patients without diabetes. Glomerular hyperfiltration due to hyperglycemia may be controlled with intensive insulin-therapy but is also a sign of future clinical DKD [47]. As discussed previously, the hyperfiltration and increase in the single nephron GFR may be a key factor in the acceleration of the physiologic, age-related kidney senescence.

Early glomerular lesions (glomerular basement membrane thickening, mesangial matrix widening) occur as soon as 18–36 months after the initial diagnosis and become more prominent 3.5–5 years later [48]. These histologic changes define **Stage 2**. The UACR is normal in this stage and DKD is silent, since neither markers of impaired filtration (eGFR), nor markers of kidney damage (UACR) will be abnormal. However, intense exercise or poorly controlled hyperglycemia may unmask microalbuminuria.

Stage 3 is the stage of *microalbuminuria* (>30 mg/24 h or 20 μg/min and < 300 mg/24 h or 200 μg/min detected in two or more urine specimens over three or more months); the first laboratory evidence of DKD or else 'insipient DKD'. Hypertension may also be present in Stage 3. Microalbuminuria is not a consistent finding and may be exacerbated by fever, exercise, high salt consumption, hypertension, poorly controlled hyperglycemia, and congestive heart failure [49]. Screening is performed by measuring the UACR in a morning urine sample. Measurements of albumin levels are also performed in 24-h or short-term urine collections and are more accurate than the screening process. After 5–10 years of having type I DM approximately 25–40% of the patients show persistent microalbuminuria [50]. In both types of DM persistent microalbuminuria is an ominous sign of kidney damage, signifying progression to CKD and eventually to ESKD. Therefore, this finding has become an essential part of the treatment strategies of DKD [51].

Stage 4 is the stage of overt or clinical DKD. It is characterized by an increase in albuminuria (> 300 mg/24 h to nephrotic range), progressive decline of eGFR and worsening hypertension. Systolic and diastolic hypertension accelerate the rate of kidney function decline. Aggressive blood pressure control is essential at this point, otherwise eGFR declines at a linear rate (7.5–28 mL/min/year) [52, 53].

Stage 5 is the stage of ESKD. For approximately 30–40% of patients with type I DM the development of ESKD is inevitable after 20–40 years of suboptimal management of the disease. The interval between Stage 4 and 5 has increased in the most recent years due to the availability of more effective treatments for uncontrolled hyperglycemia and hypertension as we will discuss below in the treatment section of this chapter.

In summary, the classic presentation is the occurrence of albuminuria leading to a GFR decline/loss of kidney function over time. Microalbuminuria is the first clinical sign of DKD and precedes albuminuria. Albuminuria in the advanced age diabetic patients can be the result of other conditions, while atypical presentations of kidney disease in this population (without albuminuria) are often observed [54]. Other studies have suggested that normoalbuminuric DKD may be more likely in older, female patients, those who maintain higher insulin sensitivity or better diabetes control and those treated with inhibitors of the renin angiotensin system [5, 55–57]. Numerous studies (reviewed in [58, 59]) have defined risk factors that increase susceptibility to, initiate the disease process among those susceptible or accelerate the progression of kidney disease once it has been initiated (Table 8.3).

The typical natural history of DKD, sees the development of ESKD within 25 years after the development of diabetes [2, 33, 58], yet many individuals will reach a (cardiovascular) end point or die prior to the anticipated need for dialysis. Such competing risks for total and cardiovascular mortality are particularly relevant for advanced age individuals with CKD, in whom the relative risk of death may be higher in those older than 75 years. In the subgroup of patients aged 75–84 with DM but without cardiovascular disease, the risk of death was 2.6 times higher than

Table 8.3 Risk factors of diabetic kidney disease

Demographics	Older age, male gender, race/ethnicity (Black, American Indian, Hispanic, Asian/Pacific Islanders
Hereditary	Family history of DKD, genetic kidney diseases
Systemic conditions	Hyperglycemia, microalbuminuria, hypertension, obesity, hyperlipidemia, hyperuricemia, arteriosclerosis, coronary artery disease, heart failure, renal arterial stenotic lesions, infections
Dietary habits	High protein intake, high salt intake
Nephrotoxins	NSAIDs, COX-2 inhibitors, radiocontrast agents
Lifestyle/other	Tobacco use, lack of exercise, alcohol consumption/acute kidney injury

kidney failure, but was 10 times higher in those who were older than 85 years old. Presence of cardiovascular disease magnified the relative risk of death over that of kidney failure, underscoring the need for management of the total cardiovascular and kidney risk in this patient population.

Diagnosis

Case Vignette Continued
Having discussed the risk factors for chronic kidney disease in diabetes, Ms X would like to explore a diagnostic path that secures the diagnosis of (diabetic) chronic kidney disease. She is worried that she will need a biopsy and is inquiring if one can possibly make the diagnosis, or at least exclude other conditions via non-invasive means.

Clinical Criteria

Screening for DKD in older adults follows the general population guidelines and includes measurement of eGFR and UACR upon diagnosis and (at least) annually thereafter. CKD can be diagnosed either on the basis of impaired eGFR, or the presence of albuminuria and this is the guideline-based approach. The Healthcare Effectiveness Data and Information Set (HEDIS) Kidney Health quality measure has formalized the importance of obtaining both measures for quality improvement and will track the percentage of adults who will receive an annual determination of both eGFR and urine albumin to creatinine ratio (UACR) in clinical practice [60]. Nevertheless, normal age-related loss of kidney function should also be considered when caring for an advanced age individual patient as a potential cause of a reduced eGFR value (but not albuminuria). Recognition of this phenomenon has led to proposals for an age-adapted definition of CKD [46], by adopting a threshold of <45 mL/min/1.73m^2 instead of the <60 mL/min/1.73m^2. However, such definitions are not endorsed in the guidelines, hence the fixed age-independent threshold of

60 mL/min/1.73m^2 will be assumed in this chapter. The possibility of a kidney lesion not related to diabetes should also be considered when investigating individual patients. The timing of the diagnosis of CKD relative to the development of DM may provide some clues. If the CKD pre-dated DM, then the likelihood of a non-diabetic lesion is particularly high [61]. However, the two conditions are often diagnosed simultaneously or within 5–10 years of each other, so this criterion cannot often be applied. To properly evaluate older diabetic patients with kidney disease we must consider the different and frequently overlapping histologic changes of DKD and "normal" aging, the increase in non-diabetic lesions (e.g., vasculitis or glomerulonephritis), the presence of kidney dysfunction without albuminuria, and last the increased incidence of renovascular disease (RAS) due to atherosclerosis and obstructive uropathy in male patients. The typical workup for an older patient with diabetes who first presents for evaluation of DKD should include a complete urinalysis with a microscopic exam, UACR, creatinine/eGFR, glucose, sodium, potassium, chloride, bicarbonate calcium, phosphorus, serum albumin and a complete blood count. A limited battery of serological tests for hepatitis B and C, antinuclear antibodies, rheumatoid factors, complement levels (C3/C4), serum and urine protein electrophoresis, a free light chain assay and a kidney ultrasound would allow to screen for most common non-DKD lesions. If a patient with diabetes has typical and advanced retinopathy [62–65], albuminuria and negative serologies, most clinicians would diagnose the patient with DKD and would not proceed to obtain a kidney biopsy. In the advanced age patient, vascular disease related to atherosclerosis, hypertension, and RAS-related ischemia [39, 66] may also be present, and thus attention should be paid to the clinical history and or imaging findings (pronounced kidney size asymmetry) to determine the likelihood of such conditions.

Kidney Biopsy Indications

The indications to perform a diagnostic kidney biopsy in a patient with diabetes are still controversial. Based on past studies and numerous debates the following list summarizes when to consider non-DKD and/or pursue a kidney biopsy [67–70]. The indications rest on the so-called atypical features for a DKD lesion, which are summarized below:

1. Absence of diabetic retinopathy.
2. Albuminuria developing less than 5 or more than 25 years since the onset of Type I DM.
3. Immunological markers or active urinary sediment.
4. Nephritic syndrome.
5. Hematuria.
6. Rapid decline in kidney function (eGFR, > 5 mL/min/1.73m^2/year).
7. Acute Kidney Injury.

8. Significant reduction in eGFR (>30%) after initiation of inhibitors of the renin angiotensin system.
9. Acute/sudden onset of macroalbuminuria or the nephrotic syndrome.

It is important to note that such criteria are post-hoc and are justified on the basis of histological findings of patients who underwent a kidney biopsy. Nonetheless, studies of patients with diabetes and CKD who underwent a kidney biopsy may be subject to selection bias regarding the moment in time at which the biopsy was performed [71–73]. A recent meta-analysis of 48 studies [69] examined the histologic findings of patients with diabetes who undergo kidney biopsies using clinical criteria. There was considerable variability in the detection rate of a non-DKD lesion in this pooled cohort of 4876 kidney biopsies: the prevalence of typical DKD, non-DKD and mixed forms ranged from 6.5 to 94%, 3 to 82.9% and 4 to 45.5% of the overall diagnoses, respectively. Among this diversity of studies, the outcome of a kidney biopsy can be predicted as reliably as flipping a coin: only 50% of biopsies ordered this way will demonstrate a typical DKD lesion, and the remaining 50% will show non-diabetic or mixed forms of pathology. Of interest, very few patients in this meta-analysis were older than 60 years old; thus the translation of these findings to the advanced age population is fraught with nuance. Kidney biopsies in patients with advanced age may be performed for different indications than the younger patients and the findings may be skewed toward diagnoses (such as rapidly progressive or membranous glomerulonephritis) that are more commonly seen in older adults. In the few studies that have specifically enrolled older individuals with or without diabetes and various kidney disease syndromes, the prevalence of a DKD diagnosis [74–76] was as variable (range 17–73%) as the studies in the younger individuals. Since the histologic diagnosis cannot be predicted from clinical criteria [77] and considering the lack of an age-related safety concern (bleeding rate of 2–3%) in kidney biopsies in various studies [78–80], it may be reasonable to apply the same criteria for ordering kidney biopsies in advanced age patients with diabetes and atypical features for DKD.

Treatment

Case Vignette Continued
Ms X, receives a comprehensive laboratory work up that included markers of immune-mediated kidney disease (antinuclear antibodies, anti-neutrophilic cytoplasmic antibodies, complement levels), hepatitis B and C serologies, serum free-light chain assays, serum and urine protein electrophoresis, which were non-revealing. A kidney ultrasound did not reveal any evidence for obstruction. Her urine albumin to creatinine ratio came back at 500 mg/g creatinine. She would like to discuss with you a comprehensive management plan that is not limited to medications. She is particularly worried about the development of hypoglycemia that may interfere with her ability to take care of her husband. She would like to avoid drastic

changes to her medication regimen, which includes metformin, a daily aspirin, a DPP4 inhibitor (linagliptin) and amlodipine.

The treatment of CKD and diabetes in the advanced age patients requires special attention because of the multiple concomitant medical problems and comorbidities associated with advanced age. Areas of intervention include the encouragement of a healthy lifestyle, glycemic and blood pressure control, followed by initiation and maintenance of guideline directed appropriate anti-proteinuric and anti-fibrotic therapies. We propose a model to organize care that should be delivered to older patients with DKD (Fig. 8.1).

Healthy lifestyle modifications should include smoking cessation and moderate exercise for at least 150 min/week, while types of exercise for these patients may include both aerobic and resistance training activities [81]. Special considerations of exercise programs in the older patient living with diabetes do apply, as there are contraindications for the practice of specific exercise modalities [82], and special attention should be based to the propensity to hypoglycemia and orthostatic hypotension in individuals who may be suffering from autonomic dysregulation. The Vivifrail multicomponent exercise program has been introduced to tailor the prescription of physical therapies that are individualized according to the older adult's functional capacity limitations [83].

Sodium restriction to less than 2 g a day is key for hypertension control, especially under conditions of a diet poor in fresh vegetables. In the latter case, increasing levels of sodium intake has been associated with increased incidence of diabetic retinal disease [84]. While a DASH diet should be encouraged for hypertension control, it may lead to hyperkalemic episodes in individuals with hyporeninemic hypoaldosteronism. Past studies on dietary protein restriction have failed to show a clear benefit in DKD [66, 85, 86]. Current ADA guidelines suggest limiting protein intake to 0.8–1.0 g/kg/day in those with DM and CKD. One should be aware that severe protein restriction may lead to malnutrition, especially in older diabetics with nephrotic range proteinuria or nephrotic syndrome.

Fig. 8.1 Comprehensive care model for advanced age patients with diabetic kidney disease

Areas of Intervention	Lifestyle Changes
Encourage a health life style Blood Pressure Control Glycemic Control Antiproteinuric therapies Antifibrotic therapies	Smoking Cessation Exercise 150 min/week Protein 0.8 g/kg/d Sodium < 2 g/day
Targets of Therapy BP < 120 mmHg A1c : < 7 % LDL-C based on ASCVD UACR as close to 30mg/g as possible	**Pillars of Therapy** **ACEi/ARB** for UACR> 30mg/g **SGLT2i** irrespective of proteinuria **Finerenone** for high CVD risk or proteinuria on ACEi/ARB **GLP1RA** for high CVD risk, suboptimal glycemic control, obesity

Hyperglycemia and hypertension are potentially modifiable, and constitute major intervention targets. The standard therapeutic goals of DKD are: (1) individualized blood glucose control, (2) blood pressure control (<120 mmHg, noting that the ratio of benefits to harm is less certain to those over 90 years old). The risks of tight glycemic control have been demonstrated in numerous studies [87–91] due to impaired physiologic responses to hypoglycemia and more severe hypoglycemia unawareness. The advanced age patients in general and those with CKD will require a highly individualized approach to glycemic control and the A1c target that considers age-related conditions, situational factors, comorbidities and life expectancy.

The European Diabetes Working Party for Older People in 2011 [92] published clinical guidelines for older individuals (defined as those ≥70 years of age) [93]. According to these guidelines, one may target an HbA1c goal of 7–7.5% and a fasting glucose target range of 6.5–7.5 mmol/L (117–135 mg/dL) in those without major comorbidities, but should allow higher goals, i.e., an HbA1c goal of 7.6–8.5% and a fasting glucose target range of 7.6–9.0 mmol/L (137–162 mg/dL) in frail individuals with comorbidities.

The American Diabetes Association (ADA) standards of care in diabetes [94] put forward a more expansive framework that simultaneously addresses glycemic targets, blood pressure and lipid management (Table 8.4). In that framework, coexisting chronic illnesses are defined as conditions that are serious enough to require medications or lifestyle management. Examples of such conditions include arthritis, cancer, heart failure, depression, emphysema, falls, hypertension, incontinence, Stage 3 or worse CKD, myocardial infarction, and stroke. End-stage chronic illness, such as stage 3–4 heart failure or oxygen-dependent lung disease, dialysis dependent ESKD, or uncontrolled metastatic malignancy should trigger a movement away from HbA1c goals, toward an approach that bases management on the avoidance of glycemia extremes. It should be noted that the blood pressure targets that the ADA proposes differ from those in the KDIGO guidelines. Patients and their health care providers should engage in shared decision-making to individualize targets based among other things on side effects of therapy that impair the quality of life of older diabetics.

Current evidence about the effects of statins in older individuals with diabetes is not as strong as in younger individuals. When used for primary and secondary prevention, benefits may be realized for those individuals whose life expectancy exceeds the time frames (2–6 years) of the clinical trials [95]. Alternatively, one may use the time to benefit for a therapy, which for statins was 2.5 years [96] and treat individuals who are likely to live longer than this time frame. Many advanced age individuals with CKD stage 3a-5 will thus benefit from statin therapy, and in fact the KDIGO clinical practice guidelines [92] about treatment of lipids in CKD recommends treatment with a statin or a statin/ezetimibe in patients older than 50 years old. These recommendations are largely based on the SHARP trial [97] that randomized 9270 participants with CKD (mean eGFR of 27 mL/min/1.73 m^2) to receive simvastatin 20 mg plus ezetimibe 10 mg daily or placebo, and followed them for 5 years. Statin plus ezetimibe therapy reduced the primary outcome of major atherosclerotic event (coronary death, myocardial infarction, need for

Table 8.4 Glycemic control target in advanced age

Patient characteristics health status	Rationale	HbA1C goal	Fasting or pre-prandial glucose	Bedtime glucose	Blood pressure	Lipids
Healthy Fewer than three coexisting chronic illnesses AND intact cognitive and functional status	Longer remaining life expectancy	<7.0–7.5% (53–58 mmol/Mol)	80–130 mg/dL (4.4–7.2 mmol/L)	80–180 mg/dL (4.4–10.0 mmol/L)	<140/90 mmHg	Statin unless contraindicated or not tolerated
Complex At least three coexisting chronic illnesses OR 2+ instrumental ADL impairments OR mild-to-moderate cognitive impairment	Intermediate remaining life expectancy, high treatment burden, hypoglycemia vulnerability, fall risk	<8.0% (64 mmol/Mol)	90–150 mg/dL (5.0–8.3 mmol/L)	100–180 mg/dL (5.6–10.0 mmol/L)	<140/90 mmHg	Statin unless contraindicated or not tolerated
Very complex Long-term care facility resident OR End-stage chronic illnesses OR moderate-to-severe cognitive impairment OR 2+ ADL impairments	Limited remaining life expectancy makes benefit uncertain	Avoid reliance on HbA1C; glucose control decisions should be based on avoiding hypoglycemia and symptomatic hyperglycemia	100–180 mg/dL (5.6–10.0 mmol/L)	110–200 mg/dL (6.1–11.1 mmol/L)	<150/90 mmHg	Consider likelihood of benefit with statin

revascularization, non-hemorrhagic stroke) by 17% (95% CI: 0.06–0.26), largely due to reductions in stroke and need for revascularization, without affecting the progression to dialysis.

For the pharmacological therapy of DKD in advanced age patients we propose that clinicians adopt a *pillar model* that considers four major drug classes: angiotensin converting enzyme inhibitors (ACEi) or angiotensin receptor blockers (ARBs), sodium-glucose co-transporter two inhibitors (SGLT2i) and GLP1 (glucagon-like peptide1) receptor agonists (either pure or in dual agonist of the gastric inhibitor peptide receptor). This pillar model is based on multiple randomized controlled trials (RCTs) that show that each of these agents in isolation, may have discrete beneficial effects on cardiovascular and kidney outcomes.

Case Vignette Continued
Based on the degree of albuminuria and an elevated blood pressure (155/85) Ms X is prescribed lisinopril 40 mg per day. She inquires about the laboratory follow-up to ensure she "is safe to take this new drug" and whether this is going to be the only medication she will have to take for her kidney disease.

Inhibitors of the Renin-Angiotensin System

These include ACEi or ARBs and are well established in clinical practice since the pivotal trials of irbesartan (Irbesartan Diabetic Nephropathy Trial, IDNT) [98] and losartan (Reduction of Endpoints in NIDDM with the Angiotensin II Antagonist Losartan, RENAAL) [19]. The results of these landmark trials have been instrumental in informing the design of subsequent RCTs by providing a standard of care therapy, a backbone to which investigational therapies are added on. IDNT and RENAAL not only suggested the optimal way to use these agents, i.e., to escalate the dose until the maximally tolerated one (in terms of side effects of hypotension, hyperkalemia or acute kidney injury) is individualized for each patient, but also suggested residual albuminuria as marker of increased cardiovascular and kidney disease risk [99, 100]. In fact, residual albuminuria on a maximum tolerated dose of an inhibitor of the renin angiotensin system had been a major inclusion criterion in the SGLT2i and finerenone trials. Despite their unequivocal benefit in DKD, inhibitors of the renin angiotensin system continue to be underutilized, even when absolutely indicated. In a recent analysis only 17% of patients with diabetes initiated these agents [101] within 12 months of diagnosis of CKD [102]; utilization appears to top out at ~60% of eligible patients with no racial disparities in utilization [103]. Even when initiated though, the use of these agents is suboptimal because of submaximal dosing; in a recent study only one-third of patients were maintained om a maximal dose, despite the absence of potential contraindications to dose escalation (systolic blood pressure < 120 mmHg, eGFR <15 mL/min per 1.73 m^2, serum potassium level greater than 5.0 mEq/L, or acute kidney injury within the prior year). The British Clinical Diabetologists and the UK kidney association have recently released guidelines about the management of ACEi and ARBs in patients with diabetes and CKD [104]. Of note the guideline does not explicitly consider older individuals and thus one is left to extrapolate these recommendations to such patients:

1. When prescribing ACEi or ARBs, kidney function and potassium level should be checked within 7–10 days after initiation.
2. A decrease in the eGFR up to 30% may be observed and is reversible.
3. More pronounced drops in kidney function, should prompt investigation for underlying causes such as RAS, sepsis, volume depletion or concomitant medications, e.g., NSAIDs.
4. If no alternative explanation for the deterioration in kidney function is found, then one may reduce the angiotensin system inhibitor to a previously tolerated dose, or stop them altogether.
5. While an elevation in the serum potassium over 5 mEq/L has traditionally been considered a contraindication for the initiation of inhibitors of the renin angiotensin system, the recently introduced potassium binders patiromer and sodium zirconium cyclosilicate may allow the optimization of dosing of these agents.
6. Combination therapy with ACEi, direct renin inhibitors and ARBs should not be undertaken due to multiple clinical trials demonstrating higher risks of side effects such as hypotension, hyperkalemia and acute kidney injury with these therapies [105], and no conclusive evidence of clinical benefit.
7. In advanced (stage 4 and 5) CKD the incidence of hyperkalemia and kidney injury may be substantial, but discontinuation [106] of the inhibitors of the renin angiotensin system was associated with higher death rates (hazard ration 1.39, 95% CI 1.20–1.60), numerically higher risk of progression to ESKD (HR 1.19, 95% CI: 0.86–1.65) and a lower risk for hyperkalemia HR, 0.65; 95% CI, 0.54–0.79). The STOP-ACEi [107, 108] RCT provided clinical evidence about the benefits vs. harm of stopping the inhibitors of the renin angiotensin system in advanced CKD. The study enrolled patients with advanced CKD (eGFR was ~18 mL/min/1.73 m^2 at baseline) and the primary outcome was the difference in eGFR between the arm of patients who were maintained on inhibitors of the renin angiotensin system and those who had these drugs discontinued. There was no difference in the primary outcome at 3 years between participants older than 65 years (− 0.32, 95% CI -2.72—2.09 mL/min/1.73 m^2) and those younger than 65 years (− 0.32, 95%CI -2.92—2.28 mL/min/1.73 m^2). ESKD occurred in 128 patients (62%) in the discontinuation group and in 115 patients (56%) in the continuation group (HR, 1.28; 95% CI, 0.99 to 1.65). There was a similar number of cardiovascular events (108 vs. 88) and deaths (20 vs. 22).

Case Vignette Continued

Ms X comes back to the office after 3 months. Her blood pressure is 125/73, her potassium level is 4.7 and her albuminuria decreased by 40%, but still measures 300 mg/g of creatinine in multiple measurements. Her eGFR is 38 mL/min/1.73 m^2. She is very certified about the reduction in blood pressure, and that her urine does not show "so high a kidney damage marker level", and she would like to explore *additional pharmaceutical options to reduce her risk for heart and kidney issues, risk that is related to her persistent albuminuria.*

Sodium-Glucose Co-Transporter Two Inhibitors (SGLT2i)

SGLT2i are orally administered inhibitors of the SGLT2 transporter. They are small molecules that act on the luminal side in the proximal tubule of the kidney. Originally, SGLT2i were introduced as modest antiglycemics [109] that reduced HbA1c by −0.81 to−1.02% in treatment naive patients and − 0.57 to −0.63% in those treated with metformin. When used to reduce HbA1c, the efficacy of these drugs rapidly declines as the eGFR drops [110, 111] below 60 mL/min/1.73 m^2, as their glucosuric effect depends on the total GFR. However, their effects on reducing the kidney hyperfiltration is expected to be maintained at low GFRs, as hyperfiltering nephrons will be present at all levels of kidney disease according to the Brenner's hypothesis.

The cardiorenal benefits of SGLT2i were first demonstrated on the cardiovascular safety trials for empagliflozin (EMPA-REG OUTCOME) [112, 113], canagliflozin (integrated CANVAS program consisting of two clinical trials, CANVAS and CANVAR-R) [114–116], dapagliflozin (DECLARE-TIMI-58) and ertugliflozin (VERTIS-CV). In these trials the use of the SGLT2i were associated with statistically and clinically meaningful reductions in Major Adverse Cardiovascular events (a composite of cardiovascular death, non-fatal myocardial infarction, or stroke) in the case of the empagliflozin and canagliflozin trials and non-inferior effects for dapagliflozin and ertugliflozin. In the same trials, beneficial effects were consistently seen for heart failure hospitalizations for all four commercially available SGLT2i and a composite kidney specific outcome that included progression to dialysis dependency/need for kidney transplantation and declines in eGFR when the definition of the secondary kidney outcomes was harmonized across the four trials [110]. SGLT2i have also been trialed in heart failure with reduced (dapagliflozin, DAPA-HF [117] and empaglifozin EMPEROR-REDUCED [118]) and preserved (dapagliflozin, DELIVER [119] and empagliflozin EMPEROR-PRESERVED [120]) ejection fraction. Dedicated kidney specific outcomes for SGLT2i include the CREDENCE trial (canagliflozin) [121], the DAPA-CKD (dapagliflozin) [122] and EMPA-KIDNEY (empagliflozin) [123]. The latter studies used SGLT2i on a background of maximum tolerated dose of an ACEi or an ARB, which is part of the standard of care for the management of DKD.

While all trials of SGLT2i have shown consistent benefits on cardiovascular and kidney outcomes, not all trials have demonstrated statistically significant benefits for all outcomes. A random effect meta-analysis that modeled heterogeneity in these trials [124], suggested that the cardiovascular and the kidney benefits are most likely a class, rather than an agent specific effect. Hence, the failure to meet statistical significance in some of the trials is most likely due to different baseline risks, short duration of treatment in the trials that enrolled lower risk patients and outcome definitions [124]. Nevertheless, the current indications on the label of the commercially available SGLT2i differ according to the prespecified outcomes of their registrational trials: while all four SGLT2i are indicated to improve glycemic control along with diet and exercise, ertugliflozin does not have a renoprotective or a cardioprotective indication, while canagliflozin, dapagliflozin and empagliflozin do. Canagliflozin's renoprotective indication is limited to patients with DKD, while dapagliflozin and empagliflozin are indicated for diabetic and non-diabetic forms of kidney disease. Dapagliflozin and empagliflozin are also indicated to reduce the risk for cardiovascular death and hospitalization in patients with reduced ejection fraction. At the time of this writing empagliflozin is the only SGLT2i approved by the FDA to reduce the risk of cardiovascular disease and hospitalization in patients with heart failure irrespective of their left ventricular systolic function (though it is likely that dapagliflozin will also receive this indication based on the results of the DELIVER trial). Importantly the cardiovascular and kidney benefit of these drugs do not vary by participant age, as has been shown in multiple meta-analyses to date [125, 126]. Table 8.5 summarizes the overall, and age subgroup results for the primary outcome in the cardiovascular, heart failure and kidney outcomes in the SGLT2i trials to date. Except for the EMPA-REG OUTCOME trial, in which the benefits of the drug appeared to be higher in the older subgroup of participants, the p-values for the interaction were not statistically significant, indicating that the benefit of the SGLT2i do not differ between younger and older individuals.

When prescribing SGLT2i it is important to keep in mind the biphasic effects on the eGFR, with an acute dip of between 2–5 mL/min/1.73 m^2 in the first 3–4 weeks after initiation [127–129] followed by stabilization thereafter. SGLT2i inhibitors are in general safe drugs, yet certain side effects such as diabetic ketoacidosis, and lower limb amputations have made practitioners somewhat cautious to prescribe over the years. A recent meta-analysis [130] that considered all major SGLT2i trials has quantified these risks in patients with and without diabetes. SGLT2i increase the risk of diabetic ketoacidosis in patients approximately two-fold (RR: 2.12, 95%CI 1.49–3.04) from a very low baseline (47 cases among 34,085 participants) and the risk of lower limb amputation by 15% (RR 1.15, 95%CI: 1.02–1.30) from a baseline of 460 events/34,082 participants among patients with diabetes. To put these numbers into perspective, in the same trials the SGLT2i reduced the death rate by 12% (RR: 0.88, 95% CI 0.84–0.93) from a very high baseline of 2901 events/34,113 participants and the risk for kidney disease progression by 40% (RR: 0.60, 95% CI: 0.53–0.69) from a baseline of 572 events/9755 participants. For patients with mortality and kidney disease risk profile similar to the participants in these trials, the Number Needed to Treat (NNT) to prevent one death [120] and one kidney disease progression event [48] were much smaller than the Number Needed to Harm (NNH) for the development of one lower limb amputation (309) or diabetic ketoacidosis event (636). For most patients, SGLT2i would present an acceptable tradeoff between benefits and risks, with the former being 3–10 times larger than the later

Table 8.5 SGLT2i and clinical outcomes in older vs. younger individuals (Hazard ratio and 95% confidence intervals)

Clinical trial	SGLT2 inhibitor	Outcome	Overall study effect	Definition of older subgroup	Effect on younger patients	Effect in older patients
CANVAS Program	Canagliflozin	MACE	0.86 0.75–0.97	≥ 65 vs < 65	0.91 0.76–1.10	0.80 0.67–0.95
CREDENCE	Canagliflozin	CRC	0.70 0.59–0.82	≥ 65 vs < 65	0.64 0.51–0.79	0.77 0.60–1.00
DECLARE-TIMI-58	Dapagliflozin	MACE	0.93 0.84–1.03	≥ 65 vs < 65‡	0.95 0.83–1.09	0.93 0.82–1.06
DAPA-HF	Dapagliflozin	HHF	0.74 0.65–0.85	≥ 65 vs < 65	0.78 0.63–0.96	0.72 0.60–0.85
DELIVER	Dapagliflozin	HHF	0.82 0.73–0.92	> 72 vs ≤ 72	0.82 0.69–0.97	0.81 0.69–0.96
DAPA-CKD	Dapagliflozin	CRC	0.61 0.51–0.72	≥ 65 vs < 65	0.64 0.51–0.80	0.58 0.43–0.77
EMPA-REG OUTCOME	Empagliflozin	MACE	0.86 0.74–0.99	≥ 65 vs < 65	1.04 0.84–1.29	0.71* 0.59–0.87
EMPEROR REDUCED	Empagliflozin	HHF	0.75 0.65–0.86	≥ 65 vs < 65	0.71 0.57–10.89	0.78 0.66–0.93
EMPEROR PRESERVED	Empagliflozin	HHF	0.79 0.69–0.90	≥ 70 vs <70	0.88 0.70–1.11	0.75 0.64–0.87
EMPA-KIDNEY	Empagliflozin	CRC	0.72 0.64–0.72	≥ 70 vs < 60†	0.72 0.59–0.88	0.65 0.52–0.81
VERTIS-CV	Ertugliflozin	MACE	0.97 0.85–1.11	≥ 65 vs < 65	0.90 0.73–1.10	1.03 0.86–1.22

CRC: Cardiorenal Composite (CREDENCE: death from kidney or cardiovascular causes, doubling of serum creatinine, or kidney failure defined as eGFR<15 mL/min/1.73 m², need for dialysis or transplant, DAPA-CKD: death from kidney or cardiovascular causes, decline of >50% of the eGFR from baseline and kidney failure, defined as need for dialysis, transplant, or sustained eGFR to less than 15 mL/min/1.73 m², EMPA-KIDNEY: death from cardiovascular cases or progression of kidney disease defined as ESKD, sustained decrease in eGFR <10 mL/min/1.73 m², decrease of eGFR >40% from baseline, death from kidney causes), HHF: Hospitalization for heart failure, MACE: Major Adverse Cardiovascular Events (composite of cardiovascular death, nonfatal myocardial infarction, or stroke)
*$p = 0.01$, p-values for all other subgroup analyses >0.05
†Three subgroups <60, 60–69 and > 70 were reported in the supplement of the study
‡Relative risk computed from the number of patients/events reported in the supplement of the primary publication of the study

depending on the specific pair of outcomes considered [130]. Other side effects include yeast and urinary tract infections, and volume depletion. However, acute kidney Injury risk was reduced by 23% (RR 0.77, 95% CI 0.70–0.84) by SGLT2i. A framework for managing these risks was recently put forward in a roundtable discussion involving physicians from three specialties (cardiology, endocrinology, and nephrology) and is summarized in Fig. 8.2.

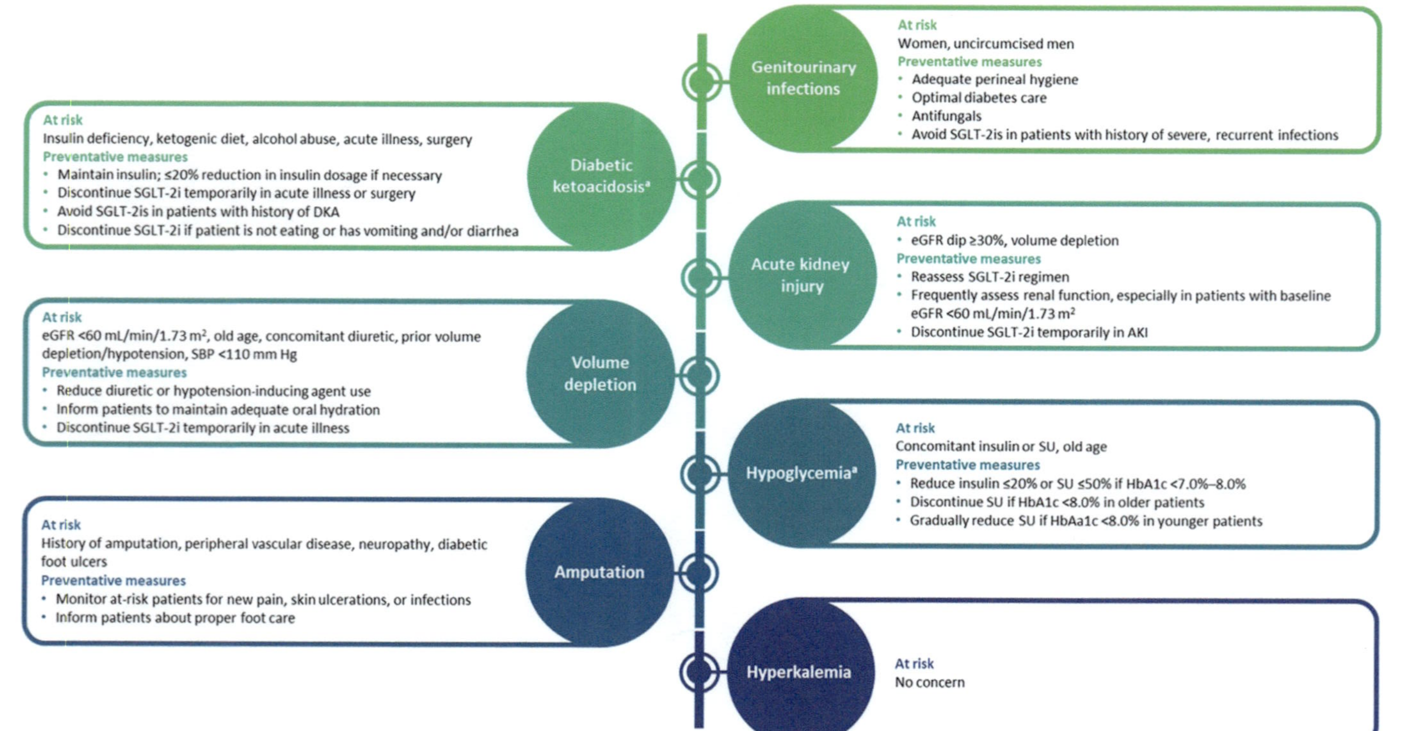

Fig. 8.2 Adverse events associated with SGLT-2i and proposed preventive measures. (The figure is available from [131] under the Creative Commons Attribution (CC BY) license)

Non-steroidal Mineralocorticoid Antagonists

Mineralocorticoid receptor antagonism (MRAs) using steroidal (e.g., spironolactone but also eplerenone) as an add-on therapy to ACEi or ARBs in diabetic and non-diabetic forms of CKD has been studied in multiple, small clinical trials. The use of MRAs in this condition is justified based on their effects on inflammation and fibrosis which may lead to improvement in tissue (kidney, blood vessel and heart damage). The effects of steroidal MRAs were recently summarized by the Cochrane group and include improvements in blood pressure by ~5 mmHg (95% CI 1.22 to 1.75 mmHg), reduction in protein excretion by 500 mg per day (95% CI 0.2 to 0.82 gm/day) and uncertain effects on kidney failure, cardiovascular and total mortality. In this meta-analysis of mostly spironolactone studies, there was a heightened risk for gynecomastia (NNH to ~14) and hyperkalemia (NNH to 41).

Newer, non-steroidal MRAs such as finerenone, esaxerenone and apararenone may offer distinct advantages over steroidal MRAs by achieving a balanced antagonism in the kidney and the heart, thus reducing the risk of hyperkalemia [31, 132]. Phase 2 clinical trials with esaxerenone [133] and apararenone [134] in DKD show that these agents may reduce proteinuria by 40–60% when added to maximum tolerated doses of inhibitors of the renin angiotensin system. Like the spironolactone studies, the improvement upon the proteinuria was accompanied by modest increases in the serum potassium level. At the time of this writing the only commercially available non-steroidal MRA in Northern America and Europe is finerenone, whose effects on cardiovascular and kidney-specific outcomes have been proven in two large randomized controlled trials: FIDELIO-DKD [135] and FIGARO-DKD [136] and a pre-specified patient-level meta-analysis of these two trials (FIDELITY) [137]. Both these studies followed a similar design, i.e. they enrolled patients with Type II DM and CKD who despite being on a maximum tolerated dose of an ACEi or an ARB (similar to the SGLT2i clinical trials) had evidence of residual albuminuria: FIGARO-DKD recruited patients with better-preserved kidney function (UACR >300 mg/g with eGFR >60 mL/min/1.73m^2 or UACR in 30–300 mg/g & eGFR in 25–90 mL/min/1.73m^2), while FIDELIO-DKD patients with more advanced CKD (UACR >300 mg/g and eGFR 25–75 mL/min/1.73m^2 or UACR in 30–300 mg/g and eGFR 25–60 mL/min/1.73m^2). Both studies recruited a sizable number of patients with non-proteinuric CKD. Participants had to have a serum potassium level less than 4.8 mEq/L and were excluded if they were on non-steroidal MRAs, renin inhibitors, had poorly controlled hypertension, or a class I indication for an MRA. The primary outcome for FIGARO-DKD was a composite of cardiovascular death, non-fatal myocardial infarction and stroke and hospitalization for heart failure (MACE/HHF). The primary outcome of FIDELIO-DKD was a composite of kidney failure (need of dialysis and transplant), sustained decrease of the eGFR by 40% relative to baseline and death from renal causes). The primary outcome of FIGARO-DKD was a secondary outcome of FIDELIO-DKD and vice versa, enabling the joint examination of the effects of finerenone on the cardiorenal risk in patients with DKD. While the primary outcome in FIDELITY was the same as the contributing trials, the composite renal outcome was defined based on a sustained drop in the eGFR by 57% (rather than 40%). The primary outcomes of the studies and the effects in subgroups of advanced age and younger individuals are shown in Table 8.6. Similar to the SGLT2i trials, finerenone was equally effective in younger and older patients.

These results led the FDA to grant one of the broadest indications to date for a drug in the cardiometabolic and kidney disease field. Finerenone is currently indicated to reduce the risk of sustained eGFR decline, ESKD, cardiovascular death, non-fatal myocardial infarction and hospitalization for heart failure in adult patients with CKD associated with type II DM.

In the pooled meta-analysis of the two trials, finerenone was associated with a substantial change of UACR from baseline to 4 months (ratio of least-squares mean change from baseline, 0.68; 95% CI, 0.66–0.70), an effect maintained throughout the trial. The effect of finerenone on eGFR is rather similar to those of the SGLT2i or inhibitors of the renin angiotensin system for that matter: an acute drop in the first 3–4 weeks of ~2 mL/min/1.73m^2 followed by a slower loss of kidney function between 0.7 (FIGARO-DKD, patients with UACR between 30–300 mg/g) to 1.3–1.5 mL/min (FIDELIO-DKD and participants in FIGARO-DKD with UACR >300 mg/g) [135, 138]. Patients receiving finerenone had a modest effect on blood pressure compared with patients receiving placebo [change in mean systolic blood pressure at 4 months was −3.2 ± 15.0 mmHg with finerenone and + 0.5 ± 14.6 mmHg) with placebo. Treatment emergent side effects were similar among the two study arms; while the incidence of AKI was the same between finerenone and placebo (3.5%), hyperkalemia was more frequent with finerenone, with an incidence

Table 8.6 Finerenone and clinical outcomes in older vs. younger individuals (Hazard Ratio and 95% Confidence Intervals)

Clinical trial	SGLT2 inhibitor	Outcome	Overall study effect	Definition of older subgroup	Effect in younger patients	Effect in older patients
FIGARO-DKD	Finerenone	MACE/HHF	0.87 0.76–0.98	≥65 vs < 65	0.90 0.74–1.10	0.85 0.72–1.00
FIGARO-DKD[a]	Finerenone	CR	0.77 0.60–0.99	≥65 vs < 65	0.72 0.52–0.99	0.92 0.61–1.38
FIDELIO-DKD	Finerenone	CR	0.82 0.73–0.93	≥65 vs < 65	0.85 0.72–1.01	0.79 0.67–0.94
FIDELITY	Finerenone	MACE/HHF	0.86 0.78–0.95	≥65 vs < 65	0.94 0.81–1.10	0.82 0.73–0.93
FIDELITY[b]	Finerenone	CR	0.77 0.67–0.88	–	–	–

CR: Composite Renal (variably defined for the three trials, see text for details), HHF: Hospitalization for heart failure, MACE: Major Adverse Cardiovascular Events (composite of cardiovascular death, non-fatal myocardial infarction, or stroke)

[a]The subgroup analysis was presented in a follow-up publication [138] and used a sustained reduction of eGFR>57%, rather than the 40% used in the primary analysis of the FIGARO-DKD study

[b]No subgroup analysis was reported for the CRC outcome in FIDELITY

rate of 0.66 events per 100 patient years vs. 0.22 events per 100 patient years on placebo. Stated otherwise, one would have to treat 150 patients for 1 year to see one episode of hyperkalemia. Across the entire study population, the mean change in potassium was modest +0.21 ± 0.47 mEq/L (finerenone) vs. 0.02 ± 0.43 mEq/L (placebo). Gynecomastia occurred with similar frequency in the finerenone and placebo arms (0.1–0.2%). Risk factors associated with hyperkalemia in FIDELIO-DKD were examined in a subsequent publication [139]. Independent risk factors for ≥mild hyperkalemia included serum potassium, lower eGFR, increased urine albumin-creatinine ratio, younger age, female sex, and β-blocker use. Individuals *older* than 75 years old had a 19% decreased risk for hyperkalemia (HR: 0.81, 95%CI: 0.65–0.99) relative to individuals between 65 and 74 years old. Diuretic or sodium-glucose co-transporter-2 inhibitor use reduced risk. In both groups, short-term increases in serum potassium and decreases in eGFR were associated with subsequent hyperkalemia. Other electrolyte abnormalities observed in the trials were hypotension (4.6% vs 3.9% in the placebo arm) and hyponatremia (1.3% vs. 0.7% in the placebo arm).

Considering the broad cardiorenal benefits of both finerenone and SGLT2s, one may wonder whether the drugs can be combined. A clinical trial (CONFIDENCE, NCT50254002) about this specific question is currently ongoing and will likely shed some light whether the combination of empagliflozin with finerenone works better than either finerenone or empagliflozin in reducing the surrogate marker of proteinuria, which is the primary outcome of the study. In the meantime, data from the existing studies provide reassurance that the combination of finerenone and SGLT2i does not reduce the therapeutic benefit of finerenone [137] and that the combination of dapagliflozin with steroidal MRA (mostly spironolactone) does not reduce the benefit of the dapagliflozin (DAPA-CKD trial) [140].

GLP1 and Dual GLP1/GIP1 Receptor Agonists

GLP1 and the emerging class of dual receptor agonists of the GLP1/GIP receptors are a class of antiglycemic agents that confer clinical benefits beyond the reduction of blood sugar levels. Several drugs belonging to the first class have been available for more than a decade, while the dual agonist tirzepatide was recently introduced for clinical use. These drugs work by activating the receptors of the endogenous incretins, glucagon-like peptide 1 and glucose-dependent insulinotropic polypeptide (GIP). GLP1RAs were initially introduced to manage diabetes and were found to be effective in lowering the HbA1c with a minimal risk for hypoglycemia, while also reducing weight. GLP1 RAs increase glucose-dependent insulin secretion, delay gastric emptying and increase satiety by activating the GLP1 receptor. Specific GLP1 RAs (liraglutide and semaglutide) have also been approved as anti-obesity medications even in patients with diabetes. Dual agonists also activate the GIP receptor, and lead to more pronounced weight loss and an enhanced antiglycemic effect relative to insulin or pure GLP1RAs in the SURPASS clinical trial [141–144].

Specific members of the GLP1 class (dulaglutide, liraglutide, semaglutide) have been shown to have cardiovascular benefits, and thus are indicated in the ADA standards of care for diabetes [145] for the management of patients with atherosclerotic cardiovascular disease (ASCVD), or with high-risk indicators of ASCVD. In a recent meta-analysis [146], GLP-1 receptor agonists in adults older than 65 years old, were associated with a 15.3% (OR 0.85, 95% CI 0.79 to 0.91) reduction in MACE events, similar to the 16% (OR 0.84, 95% CI 0.70 to 1.01) benefit seen in younger adults. Hence, GLP1RAs are equally beneficial in older and younger adults with type II DM for the management of their cardiovascular disease. To date, the clinical benefits of GLP1 and GLP1/GIP RA on kidney outcomes have been limited to examinations of surrogate markers of kidney function loss (eGFR loss) and markers of kidney damage (UACR) and explorations of kidney-specific outcomes [147–150] in their cardiovascular safety and primary efficacy trials. The definition of the kidney-specific outcomes adopted in the GLP1, GLP1/GIP RA trials were not uniform and the clinical benefit was largely driven by improvement in albuminuria in almost all studies.

GLP1(/GIP) drug	Trial	Composite kidney-specific outcome	Treatment effect
Semaglutide	SUSTAIN-6	New or worsening nephropathy defined as a new onset of persistent macroalbuminuria, or persistent doubling of serum creatinine level and eGFR <45 mL/min/1.73 m^2, need for dialysis or death from renal causes	0.64 0.46–0.88
Dulaglutide	REWIND	New macroalbuminuria, a sustained 30% or greater decline in eGFR or new chronic renal replacement therapy comprising dialysis or renal transplantation	0.85 0.77–0.93
Liraglutide	LEADER	New-onset persistent macroalbuminuria, persistent doubling of the serum creatinine level and an estimated GFR of ≤45 mL/min/ 1.73 m^2 of body-surface area, need for dialysis or death from renal disease	0.78 0.60–0.91
Tirzepatide	SURPASS-4	eGFR decline of at least 40% from baseline, Death due to kidney failure, progression to end-stage Kidney disease, or new-onset macroalbuminuria	0.58 0.43–0.80

Pooled analyses of the GLP1RA trials as well as the secondary analyses of SURPASS-4 show that this class of drugs may decrease the rate of loss of kidney function (eGFR slope) and albuminuria. REWIND was the only study to report a subgroup analysis of the kidney-specific outcome according to participant age. Older individuals (age ≥ 66 years) had a HR of 0.79 (95%CI 0.69–0.90) that was statistically not-different (p-value for the interaction 0.17) to individuals younger than 66 years (HR: 0.90, 95% CI: 0.79–1.02) [148]. In SURPASS-4, neither the rate of loss of eGFR, nor the percentage reduction of albuminuria differ in older (≥65 years old) and younger individuals and tirzepatide favorably impacted either.

References

1. Wild S, Roglic G, Green A, Sicree R, King H. Global prevalence of diabetes: estimates for the year 2000 and projections for 2030. Diabetes Care. 2004;27(5):1047–53.
2. Williams ME. Diabetic kidney disease in elderly individuals. Med Clin North Am. 2013;97(1):75–89.
3. McClure M, Jorna T, Wilkinson L, Taylor J. Elderly patients with chronic kidney disease: do they really need referral to the nephrology clinic? Clin Kidney J. 2017;10(5):698–702.
4. Liu P, Quinn RR, Lam NN, Al-Wahsh H, Sood MM, Tangri N, et al. Progression and regression of chronic kidney disease by age among adults in a population-based cohort in Alberta, Canada. JAMA Netw Open. 2021;4(6):e2112828.
5. Afkarian M, Zelnick LR, Hall YN, Heagerty PJ, Tuttle K, Weiss NS, et al. Clinical manifestations of kidney Disease among US adults with diabetes, 1988-2014. JAMA. 2016;316(6):602–10.
6. Halimi JM. The emerging concept of chronic kidney disease without clinical proteinuria in diabetic patients. Diabetes Metab. 2012;38(4):291–7.
7. Ho K, McKnight AJ. The changing landscape of diabetic kidney disease: new reflections on phenotype, classification, and disease progression to influence future investigative studies and therapeutic trials. Adv Chronic Kidney Dis. 2014;21(3):256–9.
8. Robles NR, Villa J, Gallego RH. Non-proteinuric diabetic nephropathy. J Clin Med. 2015;4(9):1761–73.
9. Lim AK. Diabetic nephropathy—complications and treatment. Int J Nephrol Renovasc Dis. 2014;7:361–81.
10. National Diabetes Statistics Report. Estimates of diabetes and its burden in the United States. CDC; 2020. p. 32.
11. Home, resources, diabetes L with, acknowledgement, FAQs, Contact, et al. IDF Diabetes Atlas|Tenth Edition [Internet]. [cited 2022 Dec 1]. https://diabetesatlas.org/.
12. Johansen KL, Chertow GM, Gilbertson DT, Herzog CA, Ishani A, Israni AK, et al. US renal data system 2021 annual data report: epidemiology of kidney disease in the United States. Am J Kidney Dis. 2022;79(4 Suppl 1):A8–12.
13. Russo GT, De Cosmo S, Viazzi F, Mirijello A, Ceriello A, Guida P, et al. Diabetic kidney disease in the elderly: prevalence and clinical correlates. BMC Geriatr. 2018;18(1):38.
14. McCullough KP, Morgenstern H, Saran R, Herman WH, Robinson BM. Projecting ESRD incidence and prevalence in the United States through 2030. J Am Soc Nephrol. 2019;30(1):127–35.
15. Rule AD, Amer H, Cornell LD, Taler SJ, Cosio FG, Kremers WK, et al. The association between age and nephrosclerosis on renal biopsy among healthy adults. Ann Intern Med. 2010;152(9):561–7.
16. Denic A, Lieske JC, Chakkera HA, Poggio ED, Alexander MP, Singh P, et al. The substantial loss of nephrons in healthy human kidneys with aging. J Am Soc Nephrol. 2017;28(1):313–20.
17. Denic A, Mathew J, Lerman LO, Lieske JC, Larson JJ, Alexander MP, et al. Single-nephron glomerular filtration rate in healthy adults. N Engl J Med. 2017;376(24):2349–57.
18. Tan JC, Busque S, Workeneh B, Ho B, Derby G, Blouch KL, et al. Effects of aging on glomerular function and number in living kidney donors. Kidney Int. 2010;78(7):686–92.
19. Brenner BM, Cooper ME, de Zeeuw D, Keane WF, Mitch WE, Parving HH, et al. Effects of losartan on renal and cardiovascular outcomes in patients with type 2 diabetes and nephropathy. N Engl J Med. 2001;345(12):861–9.
20. Brenner BM, Lawler EV, Mackenzie HS. The hyperfiltration theory: a paradigm shift in nephrology. Kidney Int. 1996;49(6):1774–7.
21. Tsaih SW, Pezzolesi MG, Yuan R, Warram JH, Krolewski AS, Korstanje R. Genetic analysis of albuminuria in aging mice and concordance with loci for human diabetic nephropathy found in a genome-wide association scan. Kidney Int. 2010;77(3):201–10.

22. Kasper M, Funk RH. Age-related changes in cells and tissues due to advanced glycation end products (AGEs). Arch Gerontol Geriatr. 2001 Jun;32(3):233–43.
23. Mei C, Zheng F. Chronic inflammation potentiates kidney aging. Semin Nephrol. 2009;29(6):555–68.
24. Vlassara H, Torreggiani M, Post JB, Zheng F, Uribarri J, Striker GE. Role of oxidants/inflammation in declining renal function in chronic kidney disease and normal aging. Kidney Int Suppl. 2009;114:S3–11.
25. Vlassara H, Uribarri J, Ferrucci L, Cai W, Torreggiani M, Post JB, et al. Identifying advanced glycation end products as a major source of oxidants in aging: implications for the management and/or prevention of reduced renal function in elderly persons. Semin Nephrol. 2009;29(6):594–603.
26. Guo J, Zheng HJ, Zhang W, Lou W, Xia C, Han XT, et al. Accelerated kidney aging in diabetes mellitus. Oxidative Med Cell Longev. 2020;2020:1234059.
27. Wang G, Ouyang J, Li S, Wang H, Lian B, Liu Z, et al. The analysis of risk factors for diabetic nephropathy progression and the construction of a prognostic database for chronic kidney diseases. J Transl Med. 2019;17(1):264.
28. Selye H, Hall CE, Rowley EM. Malignant hypertension produced by treatment with desoxycorticosterone acetate and sodium chloride. Can Med Assoc J. 1943;49(2):88–92.
29. Ferreira NS, Tostes RC, Paradis P, Schiffrin EL. Aldosterone, inflammation, immune system, and hypertension. Am J Hypertens. 2021;34(1):15–27.
30. Fuller PJ, Yang J, Young MJ. 30 years of the mineralocorticoid receptor: coregulators as mediators of mineralocorticoid receptor signalling diversity. J Endocrinol. 2017;234(1):T23–34.
31. Kawanami D, Takashi Y, Muta Y, Oda N, Nagata D, Takahashi H, et al. Mineralocorticoid receptor antagonists in diabetic kidney Disease. Front Pharmacol. 2021;12:754239. https://doi.org/10.3389/fphar.2021.754239.
32. Tuttle KR, Agarwal R, Alpers CE, Bakris GL, Brosius FC, Kolkhof P, et al. Molecular mechanisms and therapeutic targets for diabetic kidney disease. Kidney Int. 2022;102(2):248–60.
33. Tervaert TWC, Mooyaart AL, Amann K, Cohen AH, Cook HT, Drachenberg CB, et al. Pathologic classification of diabetic nephropathy. J Am Soc Nephrol. 2010;21(4):556–63.
34. Stout LC, Kumar S, Whorton EB. Insudative lesions—their pathogenesis and association with glomerular obsolescence in diabetes: a dynamic hypothesis based on single views of advancing human diabetic nephropathy. Hum Pathol. 1994;25(11):1213–27.
35. Mauer SM, Steffes MW, Ellis EN, Sutherland DE, Brown DM, Goetz FC. Structural-functional relationships in diabetic nephropathy. J Clin Invest. 1984;74(4):1143–55.
36. Alsaad KO, Herzenberg AM. Distinguishing diabetic nephropathy from other causes of glomerulosclerosis: an update. J Clin Pathol. 2007;60(1):18–26.
37. Brito PL, Fioretto P, Drummond K, Kim Y, Steffes MW, Basgen JM, et al. Proximal tubular basement membrane width in insulin-dependent diabetes mellitus. Kidney Int. 1998;53(3):754–61.
38. Nadasdy T, Laszik Z, Blick KE, Johnson DL, Silva FG. Tubular atrophy in the end-stage kidney: a lectin and immunohistochemical study. Hum Pathol. 1994;25(1):22–8.
39. Sawicki PT, Kaiser S, Heinemann L, Frenzel H, Berger M. Prevalence of renal artery stenosis in diabetes mellitus—an autopsy study. J Intern Med. 1991 Jun;229(6):489–92.
40. Moriya T, Omura K, Matsubara M, Yoshida Y, Hayama K, Ouchi M. Arteriolar Hyalinosis predicts increase in albuminuria and GFR decline in Normo-and Microalbuminuric Japanese patients with type 2 diabetes. Diabetes Care. 2017;40(10):1373–8.
41. Ekinci EI, Jerums G, Skene A, Crammer P, Power D, Cheong KY, et al. Renal structure in normoalbuminuric and albuminuric patients with type 2 diabetes and impaired renal function. Diabetes Care. 2013;36(11):3620–6.
42. Shimizu M, Furuichi K, Yokoyama H, Toyama T, Iwata Y, Sakai N, et al. Kidney lesions in diabetic patients with normoalbuminuric renal insufficiency. Clin Exp Nephrol. 2014;18(2):305–12.

43. Moriya T, Yamagishi T, Matsubara M, Ouchi M. Serial renal biopsies in normo-and micro-albuminuric patients with type 2 diabetes demonstrate that loss of renal function is associated with a reduction in glomerular filtration surface secondary to mesangial expansion. J Diabetes Complicat. 2019;33(5):368–73.

44. Palmer MB, Abedini A, Jackson C, Blady S, Chatterjee S, Sullivan KM, et al. The role of glomerular epithelial injury in kidney function decline in patients with diabetic kidney disease in the TRIDENT cohort. Kidney Int Rep. 2021;6(4):1066–80.

45. Klessens CQF, Woutman TD, Veraar KAM, Zandbergen M, Valk EJJ, Rotmans JI, et al. An autopsy study suggests that diabetic nephropathy is underdiagnosed. Kidney Int. 2016;90(1):149–56.

46. Delanaye P, Jager KJ, Bökenkamp A, Christensson A, Dubourg L, Eriksen BO, et al. CKD: a call for an age-adapted definition. J Am Soc Nephrol. 2019;30(10):1785–805.

47. Rudberg S, Persson B, Dahlquist G. Increased glomerular filtration rate as a predictor of diabetic nephropathy—an 8-year prospective study. Kidney Int. 1992;41(4):822–8.

48. Fioretto P, Steffes MW, Sutherland DE, Mauer M. Sequential renal biopsies in insulin-dependent diabetic patients: structural factors associated with clinical progression. Kidney Int. 1995;48(6):1929–35.

49. Mogensen CE, Vestbo E, Poulsen PL, Christiansen C, Damsgaard EM, Eiskjaer H, et al. Microalbuminuria and potential confounders. A review and some observations on variability of urinary albumin excretion. Diabetes Care. 1995;18(4):572–81.

50. Mogensen CE. Microalbuminuria as a predictor of clinical diabetic nephropathy. Kidney Int. 1987 Feb;31(2):673–89.

51. Messent JW, Elliott TG, Hill RD, Jarrett RJ, Keen H, Viberti GC. Prognostic significance of microalbuminuria in insulin-dependent diabetes mellitus: a twenty-three year follow-up study. Kidney Int. 1992;41(4):836–9.

52. Mogensen CE. Progression of nephropathy in long-term diabetics with proteinuria and effect of initial anti-hypertensive treatment. Scand J Clin Lab Invest. 1976;36(4):383–8.

53. Parving HH, Smidt UM, Friisberg B, Bonnevie-Nielsen V, Andersen AR. A prospective study of glomerular filtration rate and arterial blood pressure in insulin-dependent diabetics with diabetic nephropathy. Diabetologia. 1981;20(4):457–61.

54. Wasén E, Isoaho R, Mattila K, Vahlberg T, Kivelä SL, Irjala K. Renal impairment associated with diabetes in the elderly. Diabetes Care. 2004;27(11):2648–53.

55. Dai Q, Chen N, Zeng L, Lin XJ, Jiang FX, Zhuang XJ, et al. Clinical features of and risk factors for normoalbuminuric diabetic kidney disease in hospitalized patients with type 2 diabetes mellitus: a retrospective cross-sectional study. BMC Endocr Disord. 2021;21(1):104.

56. Retnakaran R, Cull CA, Thorne KI, Adler AI, Holman RR, UKPDS Study Group. Risk factors for renal dysfunction in type 2 diabetes: U.K. prospective diabetes study 74. Diabetes. 2006;55(6):1832–9.

57. Shi S, Ni L, Gao L, Wu X. Comparison of Nonalbuminuric and Albuminuric diabetic kidney Disease among patients with type 2 diabetes: a systematic review and meta-analysis. Front Endocrinol (Lausanne). 2022;13:871272.

58. Alicic RZ, Rooney MT, Tuttle KR. Diabetic kidney disease: challenges, Progress, and possibilities. Clin J Am Soc Nephrol. 2017;12(12):2032–45.

59. Umanath K, Lewis JB. Update on diabetic nephropathy: Core curriculum 2018. Am J Kidney Dis. 2018;71(6):884–95.

60. Brock M. Kidney health: a new HEDIS measure [internet]. NCQA 2020 [cited 2023 Apr 5]. https://www.ncqa.org/blog/kidneyhealth/.

61. Anders HJ, Huber TB, Isermann B, Schiffer M. CKD in diabetes: diabetic kidney disease versus nondiabetic kidney disease. Nat Rev Nephrol. 2018;14(6):361–77.

62. Iqbal Z, Meguira S, Friedman EA. Geriatric diabetic nephropathy: an analysis of renal referral in patients age 60 or older. Am J Kidney Dis. 1990;16(4):312–6.

63. Marshall SM, Alberti KG. Comparison of the prevalence and associated features of abnormal albumin excretion in insulin-dependent and non-insulin-dependent diabetes. Q J Med. 1989;70(261):61–71.
64. Parving HH, Gall MA, Skøtt P, Jørgensen HE, Løkkegaard H, Jørgensen F, et al. Prevalence and causes of albuminuria in non-insulin-dependent diabetic patients. Kidney Int. 1992;41(4):758–62.
65. Torffvit O, Agardh E, Agardh CD. Albuminuria and associated medical risk factors: a cross-sectional study in 476 type I (insulin-dependent) diabetic patients. Part 1. J Diabet Complications. 1991;5(1):23–8.
66. Joseph AJ, Friedman EA. Diabetic nephropathy in the elderly. Clin Geriatr Med. 2009;25(3):373–89.
67. Blicklé JF, Doucet J, Krummel T, Hannedouche T. Diabetic nephropathy in the elderly. Diabetes Metab. 2007;33(Suppl 1):S40–55.
68. Espinel E, Agraz I, Ibernon M, Ramos N, Fort J, Serón D. Renal biopsy in type 2 diabetic patients. J Clin Med. 2015;4(5):998–1009.
69. Fiorentino M, Bolignano D, Tesar V, Pisano A, Biesen WV, Tripepi G, et al. Renal biopsy in patients with diabetes: a pooled meta-analysis of 48 studies. Nephrol Dial Transplant. 2017;32(1):97–110.
70. Glassock RJ, Hirschman GH, Striker GE. Workshop on the use of renal biopsy in research on diabetic nephropathy: a summary report. Am J Kidney Dis. 1991;18(5):589–92.
71. Caramori ML. Should all patients with diabetes have a kidney biopsy? Nephrol Dial Transplant. 2017;32(1):3–5.
72. Oh SW, Kim S, Na KY, Chae DW, Kim S, Jin DC, et al. Clinical implications of pathologic diagnosis and classification for diabetic nephropathy. Diabetes Res Clin Pract. 2012;97(3):418–24.
73. Soni SS, Gowrishankar S, Kishan AG, Raman A. Non diabetic renal disease in type 2 diabetes mellitus. Nephrology (Carlton). 2006;11(6):533–7.
74. Beniwal P, Singh SK, Malhotra V, Agarwal D, Sharma M, Joshi P, et al. Gerontolizing nephrology: Spectrum of histopathological findings of kidney biopsy in the elderly. Indian J Nephrol. 2020;30(4):264–9.
75. Gupta P, Rana DS. Importance of renal biopsy in patients aged 60 years and older: experience from a tertiary care hospital. Saudi J Kidney Dis Transpl. 2018;29(1):140–4.
76. Perkowska-Ptasinska A, Deborska-Materkowska D, Bartczak A, Stompor T, Liberek T, Bullo-Piontecka B, et al. Kidney disease in the elderly: biopsy based data from 14 renal centers in Poland. BMC Nephrol. 2016;17(1):194.
77. Nair R, Bell JM, Walker PD. Renal biopsy in patients aged 80 years and older. Am J Kidney Dis. 2004;44(4):618–26.
78. Fedi M, Bobot M, Torrents J, Gobert P, Magnant É, Knefati Y, et al. Kidney biopsy in very elderly patients: indications, therapeutic impact and complications. BMC Nephrol. 2021;22(1):362.
79. Kohli HS, Jairam A, Bhat A, Sud K, Jha V, Gupta KL, et al. Safety of kidney biopsy in elderly: a prospective study. Int Urol Nephrol. 2006;38(3–4):815–20.
80. Uezono S, Hara S, Sato Y, Komatsu H, Ikeda N, Shimao Y, et al. Renal biopsy in elderly patients: a clinicopathological analysis. Ren Fail. 2006;28(7):549–55.
81. Ferriolli E, Pessanha FPAS, Marchesi JCLS. Diabetes and exercise in the elderly. Med Sport Sci. 2014;60:122–9.
82. Hoffmann TC, Maher CG, Briffa T, Sherrington C, Bennell K, Alison J, et al. Prescribing exercise interventions for patients with chronic conditions. CMAJ. 2016;188(7):510–8.
83. Izquierdo M, Rodriguez-Mañas L, Sinclair AJ. Editorial: what is new in exercise regimes for frail older people—how does the Erasmus Vivifrail project take us forward? J Nutr Health Aging. 2016;20(7):736–7.

84. Horikawa C, Aida R, Tanaka S, Kamada C, Tanaka S, Yoshimura Y, et al. Sodium intake and incidence of diabetes complications in elderly patients with type 2 diabetes-analysis of data from the Japanese elderly diabetes intervention study (J-EDIT). Nutrients. 2021;13(2):689.

85. Klahr S, Levey AS, Beck GJ, Caggiula AW, Hunsicker L, Kusek JW, et al. The effects of dietary protein restriction and blood-pressure control on the progression of chronic renal disease. Modification of diet in renal Disease study group. N Engl J Med. 1994;330(13):877–84.

86. Pijls LTJ, de Vries H, van Eijk JTM, Donker AJM. Protein restriction, glomerular filtration rate and albuminuria in patients with type 2 diabetes mellitus: a randomized trial. Eur J Clin Nutr. 2002;56(12):1200–7.

87. Kahn SE. Glucose control in type 2 diabetes: still worthwhile and worth pursuing. JAMA. 2009;301(15):1590–2.

88. Shorr RI, Franse LV, Resnick HE, Di Bari M, Johnson KC, Pahor M. Glycemic control of older adults with type 2 diabetes: findings from the third National Health and nutrition examination survey, 1988-1994. J Am Geriatr Soc. 2000;48(3):264–7.

89. Whitmer RA, Karter AJ, Yaffe K, Quesenberry CP, Selby JV. Hypoglycemic episodes and risk of dementia in older patients with type 2 diabetes mellitus. JAMA. 2009;301(15):1565–72.

90. Anon. Effect of intensive blood-glucose control with metformin on complications in overweight patients with type 2 diabetes (UKPDS 34). UK prospective diabetes study (UKPDS) group. Lancet. 1998;352(9131):854–65.

91. Anon. Intensive blood-glucose control with sulphonylureas or insulin compared with conventional treatment and risk of complications in patients with type 2 diabetes (UKPDS 33). UK prospective diabetes study (UKPDS) group. Lancet. 1998;352(9131):837–53.

92. Kidney Disease: Improving Global Outcomes (KDIGO) Blood Pressure Work Group. KDIGO. Clinical practice guideline for the management of blood pressure in chronic kidney disease. Kidney Int. 2021;99(3S):S1–87.

93. Sinclair AJ, Paolisso G, Castro M, Bourdel-Marchasson I, Gadsby R, Rodriguez Mañas L, et al. European diabetes working Party for Older People 2011 clinical guidelines for type 2 diabetes mellitus. Executive Summary Diabetes Metab. 2011;37(Suppl 3):S27–38.

94. American Diabetes Association Professional Practice Committee, Draznin B, Aroda VR, Bakris G, Benson G, Brown FM, et al. 13. Older adults: standards of medical Care in Diabetes-2022. Diabetes Care. 2022;45(Suppl 1):S195–207.

95. Gencer B, Marston NA, Im K, Cannon CP, Sever P, Keech A, et al. Efficacy and safety of lowering LDL cholesterol in older patients: a systematic review and meta-analysis of randomised controlled trials. Lancet. 2020;396(10263):1637–43.

96. Yourman LC, Cenzer IS, Boscardin WJ, Nguyen BT, Smith AK, Schonberg MA, et al. Evaluation of time to benefit of statins for the primary prevention of cardiovascular events in adults aged 50 to 75 years: a meta-analysis. JAMA Intern Med. 2021;181(2):179–85.

97. Baigent C, Landray MJ, Reith C, Emberson J, Wheeler DC, Tomson C, et al. The effects of lowering LDL cholesterol with simvastatin plus ezetimibe in patients with chronic kidney disease (study of heart and renal protection): a randomised placebo-controlled trial. Lancet. 2011;377(9784):2181–92.

98. Lewis EJ, Hunsicker LG, Clarke WR, Berl T, Pohl MA, Lewis JB, et al. Renoprotective effect of the angiotensin-receptor antagonist irbesartan in patients with nephropathy due to type 2 diabetes. N Engl J Med. 2001;345(12):851–60.

99. Lambers Heerspink HJ, Gansevoort RT, Brenner BM, Cooper ME, Parving HH, Shahinfar S, et al. Comparison of different measures of urinary protein excretion for prediction of renal events. J Am Soc Nephrol. 2010;21(8):1355–60.

100. de Zeeuw D, Remuzzi G, Parving HH, Keane WF, Zhang Z, Shahinfar S, et al. Proteinuria, a target for renoprotection in patients with type 2 diabetic nephropathy: lessons from RENAAL. Kidney Int. 2004;65(6):2309–20.

101. Fried LF, Petruski-Ivleva N, Folkerts K, Schmedt N, Velentgas P, Kovesdy CP. ACE inhibitor or ARB treatment among patients with diabetes and chronic kidney disease. Am J Manag Care. 2021;27(20 Suppl):S360–8.

102. Yang Y, Thumula V, Pace PF, Banahan BF, Wilkin NE, Lobb WB. High-risk diabetic patients in Medicare part D programs: are they getting the recommended ACEI/ARB therapy? J Gen Intern Med. 2010;25(4):298–304.

103. Rosen AB, Karter AJ, Liu JY, Selby JV, Schneider EC. Use of angiotensin-converting enzyme inhibitors and angiotensin receptor blockers in high-risk clinical and ethnic groups with diabetes. J Gen Intern Med. 2004;19(6):669–75.

104. Banerjee D, Winocour P, Chowdhury TA, De P, Wahba M, Montero R, et al. Management of hypertension and renin-angiotensin-aldosterone system blockade in adults with diabetic kidney disease: Association of British Clinical Diabetologists and the renal association UK guideline update 2021. BMC Nephrol. 2022;23(1):9.

105. Fried LF, Emanuele N, Zhang JH, Brophy M, Conner TA, Duckworth W, et al. Combined angiotensin inhibition for the treatment of diabetic nephropathy. N Engl J Med. 2013;369(20):1892–903.

106. Qiao Y, Shin JI, Chen TK, Inker LA, Coresh J, Alexander GC, et al. Association between renin-angiotensin system blockade discontinuation and all-cause mortality among persons with low estimated glomerular filtration rate. JAMA Intern Med. 2020;180(5):718–26.

107. Bhandari S, Ives N, Brettell EA, Valente M, Cockwell P, Topham PS, et al. Multicentre randomized controlled trial of angiotensin-converting enzyme inhibitor/angiotensin receptor blocker withdrawal in advanced renal disease: the STOP-ACEi trial. Nephrol Dial Transplant. 2016;31(2):255–61.

108. Bhandari S, Mehta S, Khwaja A, Cleland JGF, Ives N, Brettell E, et al. Renin-angiotensin system inhibition in advanced chronic kidney Disease. N Engl J Med. 2022;387(22):2021–32.

109. Tsapas A, Karagiannis T, Avgerinos I, Matthews DR, Bekiari E. Comparative effectiveness of glucose-lowering drugs for type 2 diabetes. Ann Intern Med. 2021;174(1):141.

110. Cherney DZI, Charbonnel B, Cosentino F, Dagogo-Jack S, McGuire DK, Pratley R, et al. Effects of ertugliflozin on kidney composite outcomes, renal function and albuminuria in patients with type 2 diabetes mellitus: an analysis from the randomised VERTIS CV trial. Diabetologia. 2021;64(6):1256–67.

111. Dekkers CCJ, Wheeler DC, Sjöström CD, Stefansson BV, Cain V, Heerspink HJL. Effects of the sodium-glucose co-transporter 2 inhibitor dapagliflozin in patients with type 2 diabetes and stages 3b-4 chronic kidney disease. Nephrol Dial Transplant. 2018;33(11):2005–11.

112. Wanner C, Inzucchi SE, Lachin JM, Fitchett D, von Eynatten M, Mattheus M, et al. Empagliflozin and progression of kidney disease in type 2 diabetes. N Engl J Med. 2016;375(4):323–34.

113. Zinman B, Wanner C, Lachin JM, Fitchett D, Bluhmki E, Hantel S, et al. Empagliflozin, cardiovascular outcomes, and mortality in type 2 diabetes. N Engl J Med. 2015;373(22):2117–28.

114. Cannon CP, Pratley R, Dagogo-Jack S, Mancuso J, Huyck S, Masiukiewicz U, et al. Cardiovascular outcomes with Ertugliflozin in type 2 diabetes. N Engl J Med. 2020;383(15):1425–35.

115. Neal B, Perkovic V, Matthews DR. Canagliflozin and cardiovascular and renal events in type 2 diabetes. N Engl J Med. 2017;377(21):2099.

116. Wiviott SD, Raz I, Bonaca MP, Mosenzon O, Kato ET, Cahn A, et al. Dapagliflozin and cardiovascular outcomes in type 2 diabetes. N Engl J Med. 2019;380(4):347–57.

117. McMurray JJV, Solomon SD, Inzucchi SE, Køber L, Kosiborod MN, Martinez FA, et al. Dapagliflozin in patients with heart failure and reduced ejection fraction. N Engl J Med. 2019;381(21):1995–2008.

118. Packer M, Anker SD, Butler J, Filippatos G, Pocock SJ, Carson P, et al. Cardiovascular and renal outcomes with Empagliflozin in heart failure. N Engl J Med. 2020;383(15):1413–24.

119. Solomon SD, McMurray JJV, Claggett B, de Boer RA, DeMets D, Hernandez AF, et al. Dapagliflozin in heart failure with mildly reduced or preserved ejection fraction. N Engl J Med. 2022;387(12):1089–98.

120. Anker SD, Butler J, Filippatos G, Ferreira JP, Bocchi E, Böhm M, et al. Empagliflozin in heart failure with a preserved ejection fraction. N Engl J Med. 2021;385(16):1451–61.

121. Perkovic V, Jardine MJ, Neal B, Bompoint S, Heerspink HJL, Charytan DM, et al. Canagliflozin and renal outcomes in type 2 diabetes and nephropathy. N Engl J Med. 2019;380(24):2295–306.

122. Heerspink HJL, Stefánsson BV, Correa-Rotter R, Chertow GM, Greene T, Hou FF, et al. Dapagliflozin in patients with chronic kidney Disease. N Engl J Med. 2020;383(15):1436–46.

123. EMPA-KIDNEY Collaborative Group, Herrington WG, Staplin N, Wanner C, Green JB, Hauske SJ, et al. Empagliflozin in patients with chronic kidney disease. N Engl J Med. 2022;388:117.

124. Johansen ME, Argyropoulos C. The cardiovascular outcomes, heart failure and kidney disease trials tell that the time to use sodium glucose cotransporter 2 inhibitors is now. Clin Cardiol. 2020;43(12):1376–87.

125. Bhattarai M, Salih M, Regmi M, Al-Akchar M, Deshpande R, Niaz Z, et al. Association of Sodium-Glucose Cotransporter 2 inhibitors with cardiovascular outcomes in patients with type 2 diabetes and other risk factors for cardiovascular disease: a meta-analysis. JAMA Netw Open. 2022;5(1):e2142078.

126. Strain WD, Griffiths J. A systematic review and meta-analysis of the impact of GLP-1 receptor agonists and SGLT-2 inhibitors on cardiovascular outcomes in biologically healthy older adults. Br J Diabet. 2021;21(1):30–5.

127. van Bommel EJM, Muskiet MHA, van Baar MJB, Tonneijck L, Smits MM, Emanuel AL, et al. The renal hemodynamic effects of the SGLT2 inhibitor dapagliflozin are caused by post-glomerular vasodilatation rather than pre-glomerular vasoconstriction in metformin-treated patients with type 2 diabetes in the randomized, double-blind RED trial. Kidney Int. 2020;97(1):202–12.

128. Heerspink HJL, Cherney DZI. Clinical implications of an acute dip in eGFR after SGLT2 inhibitor initiation. Clin J Am Soc Nephrol. 2021;16(8):1278–80.

129. Kraus BJ, Weir MR, Bakris GL, Mattheus M, Cherney DZI, Sattar N, et al. Characterization and implications of the initial estimated glomerular filtration rate "dip" upon sodium-glucose cotransporter-2 inhibition with empagliflozin in the EMPA-REG OUTCOME trial. Kidney Int. 2021;99(3):750–62.

130. Nuffield Department of Population Health Renal Studies Group. SGLT2 inhibitor meta-analysis cardio-renal Trialists' consortium. Impact of diabetes on the effects of sodium glucose co-transporter-2 inhibitors on kidney outcomes: collaborative meta-analysis of large placebo-controlled trials. Lancet. 2022;400(10365):1788–801.

131. Jabbour SA, Ibrahim NE, Argyropoulos CP. Physicians' considerations and practice recommendations regarding the use of sodium-glucose Cotransporter-2 inhibitors. J Clin Med. 2022;11(20):6051.

132. Barrera-Chimal J, Kolkhof P, Lima-Posada I, Joachim A, Rossignol P, Jaisser F. Differentiation between emerging non-steroidal and established steroidal mineralocorticoid receptor antagonists: head-to-head comparisons of pharmacological and clinical characteristics. Expert Opin Investig Drugs. 2021;30(11):1141–57.

133. Ito S, Kashihara N, Shikata K, Nangaku M, Wada T, Okuda Y, et al. Esaxerenone (CS-3150) in patients with type 2 diabetes and microalbuminuria (ESAX-DN): phase 3 randomized controlled clinical trial. CJASN. 2020;15(12):1715–27.

134. Wada T, Inagaki M, Yoshinari T, Terata R, Totsuka N, Gotou M, et al. Apararenone in patients with diabetic nephropathy: results of a randomized, double-blind, placebo-controlled phase 2 dose-response study and open-label extension study. Clin Exp Nephrol. 2021 Feb;25(2):120–30.

135. Bakris GL, Agarwal R, Anker SD, Pitt B, Ruilope LM, Rossing P, et al. Effect of Finerenone on chronic kidney disease outcomes in type 2 diabetes. N Engl J Med. 2020;383(23):2219–29.

136. Pitt B, Filippatos G, Agarwal R, Anker SD, Bakris GL, Rossing P, et al. Cardiovascular events with Finerenone in kidney disease and type 2 diabetes. N Engl J Med. 2021;385(24):2252–63.

137. Agarwal R, Filippatos G, Pitt B, Anker SD, Rossing P, Joseph A, et al. Cardiovascular and kidney outcomes with finerenone in patients with type 2 diabetes and chronic kidney disease: the FIDELITY pooled analysis. Eur Heart J. 2022;43(6):474–84.
138. Ruilope LM, Pitt B, Anker SD, Rossing P, Kovesdy CP, Pecoits-Filho R, et al. Kidney outcomes with finerenone: an analysis from the FIGARO-DKD study. Nephrol Dial Transplant. 2022;38:372.
139. Agarwal R, Joseph A, Anker SD, Filippatos G, Rossing P, Ruilope LM, et al. Hyperkalemia risk with Finerenone: results from the FIDELIO-DKD trial. J Am Soc Nephrol. 2022;33(1):225–37.
140. Provenzano M, Jongs N, Vart P, Stefánsson BV, Chertow GM, Langkilde AM, et al. The kidney protective effects of the sodium–glucose cotransporter-2 inhibitor, dapagliflozin, are present in patients with CKD treated with mineralocorticoid receptor antagonists. Kidney Int Rep. 2022;7(3):436–43.
141. Del Prato S, Kahn SE, Pavo I, Weerakkody GJ, Yang Z, Doupis J, et al. Tirzepatide versus insulin glargine in type 2 diabetes and increased cardiovascular risk (SURPASS-4): a randomised, open-label, parallel-group, multicentre, phase 3 trial. Lancet. 2021;398(10313):1811–24.
142. Frías JP, Davies MJ, Rosenstock J, Pérez Manghi FC, Fernández Landó L, Bergman BK, et al. Tirzepatide versus semaglutide once weekly in patients with type 2 diabetes. N Engl J Med. 2021;385(6):503–15.
143. Min T, Bain SC. The role of Tirzepatide, dual GIP and GLP-1 receptor agonist, in the Management of Type 2 diabetes: the SURPASS clinical trials. Diabetes Ther. 2021;12(1):143–57.
144. Rosenstock J, Wysham C, Frías JP, Kaneko S, Lee CJ, Fernández Landó L, et al. Efficacy and safety of a novel dual GIP and GLP-1 receptor agonist tirzepatide in patients with type 2 diabetes (SURPASS-1): a double-blind, randomised, phase 3 trial. Lancet. 2021;398(10295):143–55.
145. American Diabetes Association. Standards of medical Care in Diabetes-2022 abridged for primary care providers. Clin Diabetes. 2022;40(1):10–38.
146. Strain WD, Griffiths J. A systematic review and meta-analysis of the impact of GLP-1 receptor agonists and SGLT-2 inhibitors on cardiovascular outcomes in biologically healthy older adults. British J Diabet. 2021;21(1):30–5.
147. Gerstein HC, Colhoun HM, Dagenais GR, Diaz R, Lakshmanan M, Pais P, et al. Dulaglutide and renal outcomes in type 2 diabetes: an exploratory analysis of the REWIND randomised, placebo-controlled trial. Lancet. 2019;394(10193):131–8.
148. Heerspink HJL, Sattar N, Pavo I, Haupt A, Duffin KL, Yang Z, et al. Effects of tirzepatide versus insulin glargine on kidney outcomes in type 2 diabetes in the SURPASS-4 trial: post-hoc analysis of an open-label, randomised, phase 3 trial. Lancet Diabetes Endocrinol. 2022;10(11):774–85.
149. Mann JFE, Ørsted DD, Brown-Frandsen K, Marso SP, Poulter NR, Rasmussen S, et al. Liraglutide and renal outcomes in type 2 diabetes. N Engl J Med. 2017;377(9):839–48.
150. Marso SP, Bain SC, Consoli A, Eliaschewitz FG, Jódar E, Leiter LA, et al. Semaglutide and cardiovascular outcomes in patients with type 2 diabetes. N Engl J Med. 2016;375(19):1834–44.

Chapter 9
Cystic Kidney Diseases in the Elderly

Yeshwanter Radhakrishnan, Ioan-Andrei Iliuta, and Fouad T. Chebib

Introduction

There is no consensus on the classification of cystic kidney diseases in elderly patients. Cysts can be histologically classified based on their tubular or non-tubular origin. However, we propose a more clinically applicable algorithm that stratifies disorders based on family history and kidney function (Fig. 9.1). As this chapter is focused on patients aged ≥60 years, some of the inherited cystic diseases that typically present in childhood will not be discussed in detail.

Cases

1. A 64-year-old male patient presented to the clinic for evaluation of bilateral kidney cysts (Fig. 9.2a). He was asymptomatic. He had a past medical history of hypertension, which was well-controlled on hydrochlorothiazide. He had a family history significant for possible cystic kidney disease on his maternal side. His serum creatinine was elevated at 1.4 mg/dL with an estimated glomerular filtration rate (eGFR) of 56 mL/min/1.73m². An MRI revealed enlarged kidneys with numerous kidney cysts bilaterally (>10 on each side). Genetic testing was positive for a *PKD1* missense mutation. Imaging and genetics confirmed the

Y. Radhakrishnan
Division of Nephrology and Hypertension, Department of Medicine, Mayo Clinic, Rochester, MN, USA

I.-A. Iliuta · F. T. Chebib (⊠)
Division of Nephrology and Hypertension, Department of Medicine, Mayo Clinic, Jacksonville, FL, USA
e-mail: chebib.fouad@mayo.edu

H. Kramer et al. (eds.), *Kidney Disease in the Elderly*,
https://doi.org/10.1007/978-3-031-68460-9_9

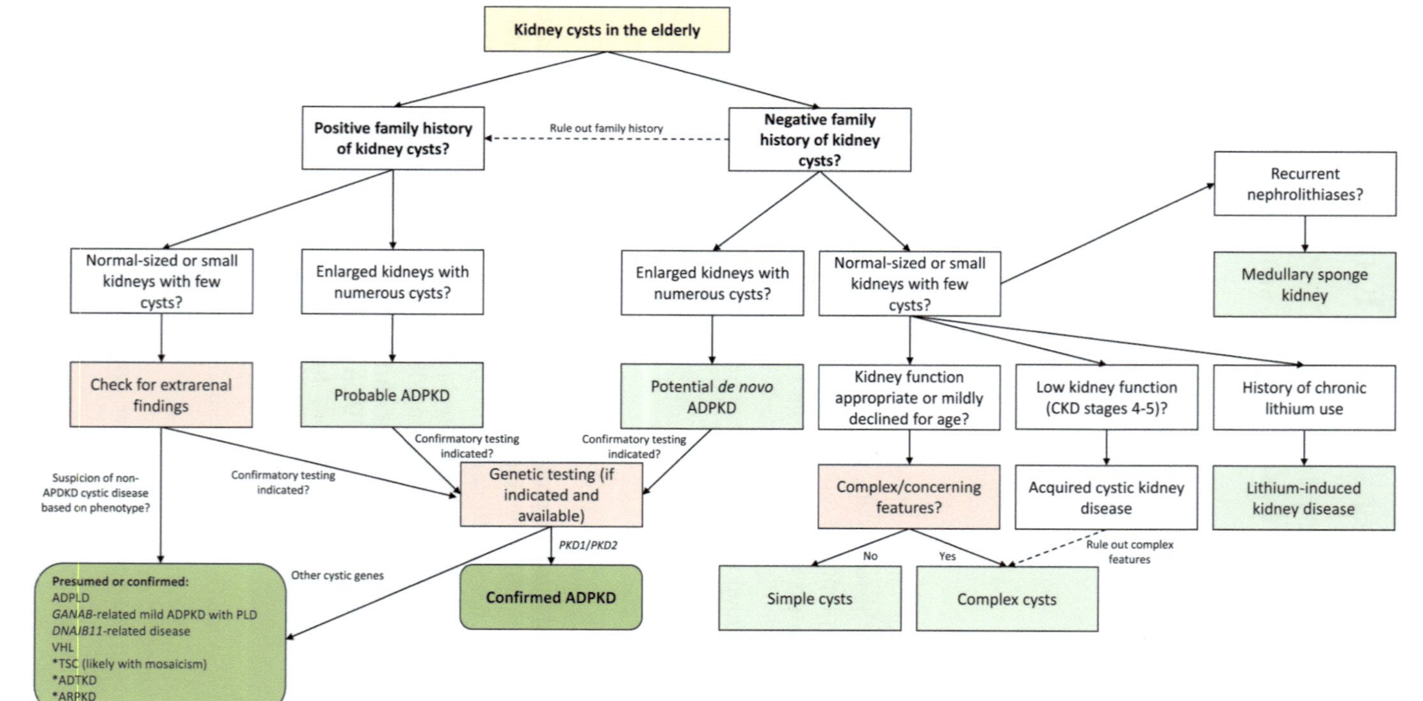

Fig. 9.1 Diagnostic approach to kidney diseases in the elderly. *ADPKD* autosomal dominant polycystic kidney disease, *ADPLD* autosomal dominant polycystic liver disease, *ADTKD* autosomal dominant tubulointerstitial kidney disease, *ARPKD* autosomal recessive polycystic kidney disease, *PLD* polycystic liver disease, *TSC* tuberous sclerosis complex, *VHL* von Hippel-Lindau. *Denotes cystic kidney diseases that usually present at an earlier age

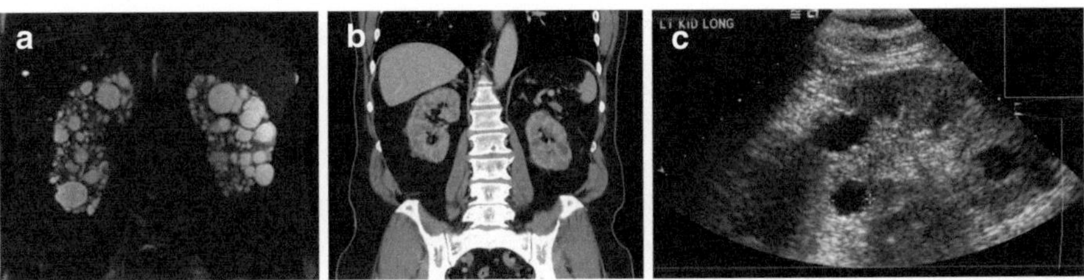

Fig. 9.2 Representative images for the clinical cases. (**a**) A 64-year old male with bilateral renal cysts, CKD stage 3a, family history of kidney cystic disease, and *PKD1* missense mutation. His TKV is 702 mL/m. (**b**) A 68-year old male with CKD stage 4, gout, bilateral renal cysts without renal enlargement and *DNAJB11* pathogenic mutation. (**c**) 69-year old female with 3 cysts in the right kidney and 4 cysts in the left kidney with normal kidney size and negative genetic testing.

diagnosis of ADPKD. His height-adjusted total kidney volume (ht-TKV) was 702 mL/m, which indicated a lower risk of progression to end-stage kidney disease (ESKD). Given his age and prognosis, he was initiated on conservative management with stricter blood pressure control (<120/80 mmHg), reduced sodium intake, and a higher water intake to target a urinary osmolality <280 mOsm/kg.

2. A 68-year-old male patient with a history of chronic kidney disease (CKD) stage 4 and gout presented to the clinic to discuss results of recent genetic testing. On his CT of the abdomen, he had numerous cysts with small kidneys (Fig. 9.2b). Genetic testing was positive for a pathogenic mutation in the *DNAJB11* gene. The patient was informed that monoallelic pathogenic variants in *DNAJB11* are highly penetrant, with more than 40% of affected patients reaching ESKD, with a median age of onset of 75 years. He was also advised to undergo screening for vascular complications (including intracranial aneurysms and dilatation of the thoracic aorta) and malignancy.

3. A 69-year-old female patient was referred to the clinic for evaluation of kidney cysts. She had no significant past medical history and had a negative family history of cystic kidney disease. Her serum creatinine was 1.1 mg/dL (eGFR of 51 mL/min/1.73 m^2). Kidney ultrasound imaging was significant for 3 cysts in the right kidney and 4 cysts in the left kidney with normal kidney size and no liver cysts (Fig. 9.2c). Genetic testing for renal cystic genes was unremarkable. Her lower GFR relative to her age would require investigating her for age-appropriate causes of CKD. In the event of extrarenal manifestations such as polycystic liver disease, whole exome sequencing may help rule out an inherited condition affecting both kidneys and liver.

Autosomal Dominant Polycystic Kidney Disease

Epidemiology

Autosomal dominant polycystic kidney disease (ADPKD) is a multi-system disorder that predominantly affects the kidneys with progressive cyst growth distorting the renal parenchyma and causing progressive loss of kidney function generally by the sixth decade of life [1, 2]. ADPKD has an estimated prevalence of 12.5 million cases worldwide [2]. It is the most common inherited kidney disease and the fourth most common cause of ESKD in the United States [3]. In a cohort with ADPKD from a large tertiary care center, 50% of patients progressed to kidney failure by 54 years of age and 75% by 62 years of age [4].

Pathogenesis

The molecular pathogenesis of ADPKD has not been completely elucidated, but involves the proteins polycystin-1 (PC1), encoded by *PKD1*, and polycystin-2 (PC2), encoded by *PKD2*. The polycystins modulate multiple signaling pathways, including calcium release from the endoplasmic reticulum, cyclic adenosine monophosphate (cAMP), mammalian target of rapamycin (mTOR), and vascular endothelial growth factor (VEGF), which together play an essential role in multiple processes, including extracellular matrix deposition and cell adhesion, cellular proliferation, metabolism, and fluid transport [5].

Genetic Mutations Associated with ADPKD

Patients with ADPKD have germline mutations in *PKD1* and *PKD2* that are inherited in an autosomal dominant manner [5]. The *PKD1* gene located on chromosome 16 encodes PC1, and mutations in *PKD1* can explain up to 78% of pedigrees of ADPKD. Another 15% of ADPKD pedigrees are due to mutations in the *PKD2* gene, located on chromosome 4, which encodes PC2. [5]. A small percentage (< 0.5%) of cases of ADPKD can be attributed to mutations in *GANAB*, which encodes the glucosidase II-α subunit responsible for the localization of polycystins [6]. Mutations in *GANAB* cause a milder phenotype of ADPKD in addition to polycystic liver disease ranging from mild to severe [6]. The remaining cases are genetically unresolved or associated with mutations in other cystic genes that produce an ADPKD-like phenotype (discussed below).

   ADPKD shows wide phenotypic variability ranging from indolent progression of CKD at an older age to rapid progression to kidney failure at a younger age [4]. In one study, patients with truncating *PKD1* mutations had an earlier onset of kidney failure with a median age of 55 years, followed by patients with non-truncating *PKD1* mutations (median age of 67 years), and patients with *PKD2* mutations (median age of 78 years) [7]. In addition to genetic heterogeneity (*PKD1* vs *PKD2* vs *GANAB*), other contributors to phenotypic variability include epigenetic, hormonal, and environmental factors such as decreased fluid intake, high dietary sodium intake, and high body mass index (BMI) [4].

Clinical Presentation

In a small study looking at clinical manifestations of ADPKD in patients aged 50 years and older, the most common presentation was hypertension (69%), followed by abdominal pain (47%) and urinary tract infection (41%) [8]. Other manifestations may include nephrolithiasis, defective urinary concentrating capacity, and progression of CKD. Hypertension, one of the earliest complications of ADPKD, develops in almost all affected patients. Uncontrolled blood pressure is associated with proteinuria and progression of CKD, left ventricular hypertrophy, and valvular diseases. Abdominal pain in patients with ADPKD can be caused by cystic complications such as cyst hemorrhage, cyst rupture, or cyst infection. In some patients with a higher cystic burden, abdominal discomfort or pain can become chronic. The differential diagnosis for patients presenting with fever, abdominal pain, and urinary tract symptoms should include both cyst infection and urinary tract infection [9]. In addition, the passage of kidney stones can present with colicky abdominal or flank pain. Risk factors for nephrolithiasis in patients with ADPKD include low urinary pH, low urinary citrate excretion, and urinary stasis from tubular obstruction by larger cysts, leading to the formation of calcium oxalate and uric acid stones. Although non-contrast CT imaging may demonstrate larger stones, contrast imaging is needed to differentiate parenchymal calcifications from smaller stones. Core measures to prevent nephrolithiasis comprise dietary sodium and animal protein restriction, and increased fluid intake. In the presence of hypocitraturia and low urinary pH, potassium citrate in a divided dose can be considered for urinary alkalinization [10]. Urologic interventions such as shock wave lithotripsy and percutaneous nephrolithotomy are appropriate in the setting of obstructive stones [10].

Extrarenal Manifestations

Extrarenal manifestations of ADPKD are shown in Table 9.1. Polycystic liver disease (PLD) is the most common extrarenal manifestation of ADPKD with a high prevalence of 80% [11]. The prevalence of PLD increases with age, with a stronger predisposition in females due to hormonal factors. Patients are usually asymptomatic and present with mild elevations in aminotransferases and alkaline phosphatase without overt loss of liver function [12]. Worsening PLD may manifest as

Table 9.1 Extrarenal manifestations of ADPKD

Complication	Prevalence	Manifestations	Screening
Polycystic liver disease	80%	Usually asymptomatic; mild elevations in AST/ALT/ALP, with no loss of liver function; **in severe cases**: Pain, nausea, vomiting, early satiety, jaundice, portal hypertension	At the time of the diagnosis of ADPKD, then every 1–2 years as indicated
Pancreatic cysts	10%	No loss of pancreatic function, reports of pancreatitis due to common bile duct obstruction from larger cysts	Routine screening not indicated
Intracranial aneurysms	8% (20% if family history of intracranial aneurysms)	Usually asymptomatic; headaches, subarachnoid hemorrhage	Indications: (a) Suggestive symptoms (b) Family history of intracranial aneurysm or aneurysm rupture (c) High-risk occupation (d) Planned major elective surgery (e) Personal history of intracerebral hemorrhage
Cardiac abnormalities	25%	Left ventricular hypertrophy, mitral valve prolapse, mitral regurgitation, aortic regurgitation, tricuspid valve prolapse	Screening only if symptoms or abnormal physical exam
Diverticular disease	Higher prevalence in patients with ADPKD and ESKD	Hematochezia, diverticulitis	Routine screening not indicated
Abdominal hernias	Increased prevalence compared to unaffected population	Usually asymptomatic; pain and discomfort; in severe cases: Incarceration of intestinal contents	Routine screening not indicated
Bronchiectasis	Threefold increased prevalence, compared with control patients with CKD	Cough, sputum production, dyspnea, rhinosinusitis, hemoptysis, bronchitis	Routine screening not indicated
Arachnoid cysts	8%	Generally asymptomatic; may increase the risk of developing subdural hematoma	Routine screening not indicated

ADPKD autosomal dominant polycystic kidney disease, *ALP* alkaline phosphatase, *ALT* alanine aminotransferase, *AST* aspartate aminotransferase, *CKD* chronic kidney disease, *ESKD* end-stage kidney disease abdominal distension, abdominal pain, early satiety, nausea, and vomiting. Compression of the portal vein and bile ducts may also result in jaundice and portal hypertension. Cystic complications such as cyst infection, cyst rupture, and hemorrhage are rare [13]. There are no established screening guidelines for PLD, but experts have recommended screening at the time of diagnosis of ADPKD, with periodic follow-up every 1–2 years if clinically indicated (e.g., in patients with severe PLD and large symptomatic cysts).

Less frequent cystic complications include pancreatic cysts, with an overall prevalence of 10%; they are associated with female sex and *PKD1* mutations [11]. Patients are diagnosed incidentally with abdominal imaging and do not lose pancreatic function. There have been reports of pancreatitis due to common bile duct obstruction from an enlarged cyst [13]. Routine screening is not indicated. Intracranial aneurysms (ICAs) are a significant complication of ADPKD that may result in high morbidity. The prevalence of ICAs is approximately 8% in all patients with ADPKD, but it increases to 20% in those with a family history of ICA [5]. Patients are usually asymptomatic and are diagnosed on screening with imaging modalities such as brain magnetic resonance angiography. Patients may present with thunderclap severe headache. ICA rupture can lead to subarachnoid hemorrhage, which is associated with elevated morbidity and mortality. ICA rupture in patients with ADPKD has been associated with a family history of rupture. As described in Table 9.1, screening for ICA should be performed in patients with a) concerning symptoms (e.g., sentinel headache); b) a family history of ICA or ICA rupture; c) high-risk occupation (e.g., airline pilot); d) planned major elective surgery such as kidney transplantation; or e) a personal history of intracerebral hemorrhage [11]. Other non-renal complications of ADPKD include cardiac abnormalities, diverticulosis, abdominal hernias, bronchiectasis, and arachnoid cysts; routine screening is generally not recommended (Table 9.1) [11, 14].

Diagnosis

Due to widespread availability and low cost, ultrasonography is the preferred initial imaging method with well-established diagnostic criteria in the setting of a family history of ADPKD [15]. In patients who are 60 years or older with a family history of ADPKD, the presence of 4 or more cysts in each kidney is diagnostic of ADPKD, with a sensitivity and positive predictive value of 100% [16, 17] . There are no established computed tomography (CT) or magnetic resonance imaging (MRI) criteria to diagnose ADPKD based on the number of cysts in the elderly. In patients younger than 40 years of age, a total of >10 renal cysts on CT or MRI are diagnostic for APDKD in the setting of positive family history [18]. However, the exact threshold in terms of cyst number has not been determined yet for older patients. In patients without a family history of ADPKD, enlarged kidneys with 10 or more cysts per kidney, along with extrarenal manifestations such as hepatic cysts, strongly suggest a diagnosis of ADPKD [1]. Confirmatory genetic testing can be considered in elderly patients for the following indications: (1) patients with no apparent family history or marked intrafamilial disease variability, (2) discordance between the cystic burden on imaging and renal function, (3) atypical patterns of cyst distribution (e.g., unilateral or asymmetric polycystic kidneys), (4) suspected somatic mosaicism, or (5) risk stratification to determine candidacy for disease-modifying therapy and enrollment into clinical trials [19].

ADPKD-Like Phenotypes that Can Mimic ADPKD

Autosomal Dominant Polycystic Liver Disease (ADPLD)

Patients with ADPLD have mutations in genes that encode proteins involved in endoplasmic reticulum function, protein folding, and protein translocation [12]. Causative mutations have been identified in *PRKCSH, SEC63, ALG8, SEC61B, GANAB*, and *LPR5,* resulting in dysfunctional protein folding and translocation, which lead to decreased expression and maturation of PC1[5, 12]. In a retrospective study, the point prevalence of definitive or likely ADPLD was 9.5 in 100,000 individuals [20]. ADPLD is characterized by the presence of numerous hepatic cysts with very few renal cysts and no progression to ESKD [21].

Autosomal Dominant Tubulointerstitial Kidney Disease (ADTKD)

Patients with ADTKD have mutations in genes that encode uromodulin (*UMOD*), renin (*REN*), and mucin (*MUC1*) [5], resulting in chronic tubulointerstitial disease with few cysts and non-enlarged kidneys, and frequent hyperuricemia and gout (especially with *UMOD*), [22]. ADTKD is discussed in detail later in this chapter.

Autosomal Recessive Polycystic Kidney Disease (ARPKD)

Patients with ARPKD have mutations in the *PKHD1* gene encoding fibrocystin, which is required for the normal functioning of renal cilia. Patients typically present at a very young age with marked cystic kidney disease and congenital hepatic fibrosis. ARPKD is very unlikely to be newly diagnosed in elderly patients due to typically severe and childhood-onset kidney and liver involvement. Hence, further discussion of ARPKD is beyond the scope of this chapter. However, individuals who are heterozygous for *PKHD1* mutations are predisposed for liver disease and renal involvement associated with increased medullary echogenicity on ultrasound [23].

DNAJB11-Associated Disease

Mutations in *DNAJB11*, a gene essential for the normal function of the endoplasmic reticulum, as well as protein folding, assembly, and maturation, lead to defects in PC1 and uromodulin, with subsequent cystogenesis in both kidneys and liver [24]. In addition, patients develop progressive CKD leading to ESKD after the sixth decade [25]. Extrarenal complications comprise vascular disease (including intracranial aneurysms, dilatation of the thoracic aorta, and carotid artery dissection) [25, 26] and a higher risk of malignancy (e.g., in the pancreas and thyroid); routine age-appropriate screening is advised [26–28].

Systemic Syndromes

Tuberous sclerosis and von Hippel-Lindau disease develop due to mutations in *TSC* and *VHL*, respectively. They are discussed in detail in the final section of this chapter.

Management of ADPKD

Conservative Nephroprotection in ADPKD

Targeting adequate blood pressure (BP) control, encouraging generous hydration, and restricting dietary sodium are cornerstones in the management of elderly patients with ADPKD to delay disease progression (Table 9.1) [2, 29].

Although intensive BP control ($\leq$110/75 mmHg) is associated with slower increase in TKV in individuals aged 18–50 years, in patients aged 50 years or older, BP targets should be individualized and a target of <120 mmHg may be more appropriate [29]. First-line therapy for hypertension in patients with ADPKD consists of renin-angiotensin-aldosterone blockade with angiotensin-converting enzyme inhibitors (ACEi) and angiotensin receptor blockers (ARB). Cardio-selective beta-blockers and combined alpha/beta-blockers may be used as second-line therapy in patients with comorbidities such as coronary artery disease and benign prostatic hyperplasia, respectively [29].

Since vasopressin is a mediator of cyst growth and CKD progression in patients with ADPKD, increased water intake to suppress vasopressin release and lower urine osmolality has been shown to slow TKV growth and GFR decline in some but not all rodent models [30]. However, a recent randomized controlled trial demonstrated that prescribed compared to *ad libitum* water intake did not affect TKV expansion over 3 years, possibly because of poor adherence to the 24-h urine osmolality target [31].

With respect to dietary and metabolic considerations, patients should consult with a dietitian and incorporate the Dietary Approaches to Stop Hypertension

(DASH) recommendations, which include restricting dietary sodium intake to 2.3–3 g per day [32]. In addition, targeting a normal BMI and treating dyslipidemia could also be important, as obesity and hyperlipidemia may be associated with faster cyst growth and GFR decline [29, 33].

Additional Considerations for the Management of CKD Specifically in the Elderly

In elderly patients, in conjunction with ADPKD, GFR decline can be accelerated by multiple comorbidities such as diabetes mellitus, suboptimally treated hypertension, vascular disease, and polypharmacy. General measures (e.g., dietary protein and phosphorus restriction, treatment of metabolic acidosis) can slow progression to ESKD (Table 9.2). Mild to moderate protein restriction can be nephroprotective in patients with advanced (stage 4–5) CKD [34]. Specifically in the ADPKD population, sub-analyses from the Consortium for Radiologic Imaging Studies of Polycystic Kidney Disease (CRISP) and Modification of Diet in Renal Disease (MDRD) cohort studies have highlighted an association between increased protein intake, and TKV growth and GFR decline [35, 36]. As protein restriction can be associated with bone mass loss and muscle wasting in the elderly, risks and benefits of modifying the dietary intake should be carefully discussed with the patient; moreover, multidisciplinary management of CKD should include assessment by a specialized renal dietitian. Other measures in advanced CKD include moderate restriction of dietary phosphorus to 800 mg daily to reduce progression of CKD mediated by fibroblast growth factor 23 (FGF-23). Treating metabolic acidosis with sodium bicarbonate supplements may also exert a nephroprotective effect (KDIGO guidelines recommend targeting a serum bicarbonate $\geq$22 mmol/L) [29].

Prognostic Markers to Assess the Progression of ADPKD

Patients with ADPKD who are at risk of rapid progression to kidney failure need to be initiated on disease-modifying therapy early to slow GFR decline. Various prognostic markers have been described to identify patients at risk of rapid progression [4].

In an ongoing, multicenter, prospective study assessing TKV with MRI, increasing TKV was reliably associated with a decline in GFR. Height-adjusted TKV (htTKV) is a validated prognostic marker to predict rapid disease progression [37–39]. HtTKV adjusted for age is used in the Mayo Imaging Classification (MIC), which divides ADPKD into typical (MIC1 or class 1) and atypical (MIC2 or class 2) cyst patterns based on kidney cyst distribution on imaging [40]. Typical refers to the homogenous distribution of cysts throughout the kidneys, with most cysts contributing evenly to TKV. By contrast, atypical patterns of cyst involvement include unilateral and asymmetric cystic disease, or ADPKD associated with kidney atrophy. Patients with typical imaging are further subdivided into classes 1A through 1E based on increasing estimated TKV growth rates. The higher-risk MIC classes (1C,

Table 9.2 Basic management of elderly patients with ADPKD

Intervention	Goal	Methods to achieve goal	Evidence
BP control	In patients >50 years, a target ≤120 mmHg is appropriate	By order of preference[a]: 1. ACEi/ARB 2. α/β or cardioselective β-blocker 3. Dihydropyridine CCB 4. Diuretic Dietary approaches to stop hypertension (DASH)-like diet at early stages	Grade 1B
Sodium	Moderate restriction (2.3–3 g/d) Adjust for extrarenal losses (e.g., hot climate, vomiting/diarrhea) if appropriate	Counseling Renal dietitian	Grade 1C
Hydration	Moderately enhanced hydration (mostly during the day, as risk of BPH and urinary incontinence higher with age) Maintain urine osmolality ≤280 mOsm/kg	Counseling Monitor first morning urine osmolality (and plasma copeptin if available)	Grade 1C
Protein	Consider 0.8–1.0 g/kg of ideal body weight (caution in the frail elderly)[b]	Renal dietitian	Grade 1C
Phosphorus	Moderate dietary phosphate restriction (800 mg/d)	Renal dietitian Read food labels and avoid food additives containing phosphates Phosphate binders in advanced CKD (calcium carbonate, non-calcium binders)	Grade 2C
Acid/base balance	Maintain plasma bicarbonate ≥22 mEq/L	Renal dietician Increase fruits/vegetables (2–4 cups/d) Oral sodium bicarbonate if needed	Grade 2B
Caloric intake	Maintain normal BMI Consider moderation in caloric intake	Renal dietician Regular exercise per tolerance	Grade 1C
Lipid control	Target serum LDL ≤100 mg/dL	Renal dietician Regular exercise per tolerance Statin if needed (ezetimibe if intolerant to statins)	Grade 2B

Table adapted from [29] Clin J Am Soc Neph
[a]Caution should be exercised with respect to higher doses of ACEi, ARBs, and diuretics (risk of acute kidney injury), α-blockers (increased risk of hypotension), and β-blockers (risk of arrythmia in patients with sick sinus syndrome)
[b]Protein intake can be monitored based on urine urea nitrogen: 6.25 x (urine urea nitrogen in g/d + [0.03 × weight in kg])

1D, and 1E) can help predict the decline in eGFR (2.63, 3.48, and 4.78 mL/min/1.73m^2 per year, respectively)[40]. The predictive accuracy of this classification was subsequently validated in prospective studies [41].

An alternative to the MIC, the Predicting Renal Outcome in ADPKD (PROPKD) scoring system uses a score > 6 to predict rapid progression to kidney failure before the age of 60 years, with a positive predictive value of 91%. This scoring system incorporates sex (males are assigned 1 point), hypertension before age of 35 years (assigned 2 points), urologic events before 35 years (assigned 2 points), and PKD mutation type (non-truncating *PKD1* mutations and truncating *PKD1* mutations are assigned 2 and 4 points, respectively; *PKD2* mutations are not assigned any points) [42].

A decline in eGFR $\geq$3 mL/min/1.73m^2 per year over 4 years or $\geq$ 5 mL/min/1.73m^2 in 1 year can also be used as evidence of rapid progression. When using the GFR slope as a stratification strategy, it is important to review other potential factors that could affect GFR (e.g., concomitant systemic diseases such as diabetes mellitus, hyperoxaluria, analgesic use, aging or vascular disease) [4]. Similarly, an annual TKV growth >5% is also considered a prognostic factor for rapidly progressive disease. Pitfalls of using TKV include the need for frequent measurements and the need for specialized training and equipment to measure TKV by planimetry or stereology, [4].

Disease-Modifying Treatment Options (V2 Receptor Antagonism)

In 2018, the Food and Drug Administration (FDA) approved the use of tolvaptan, an antagonist of vasopressin V2 receptors in the kidney tubule, as a disease-modifying treatment option in patients with ADPKD (18 to 55 years old) at risk of rapid progression [43]. This was based on two randomized controlled double-blind trials (TEMPO 3:4 and REPRISE) that demonstrated tolvaptan was effective in slowing the rate of decline in eGFR compared to placebo. TEMPO3:4 included patients aged from 18 to 50 years old with an eGFR >60 mL/min, while REPRISE included patients aged from 18 to 65 years old with an eGFR of 25 to 65 mL/min [44, 45]. In the REPRISE trial, patients aged >55 years did not benefit from tolvaptan, possibly because of slow disease progression, as suggested by their lower rate of eGFR decline on placebo (-2.34 mL/min per 1.73 m^2) compared with those aged $\leq$55 years (-4.60 mL/min per 1.73 m^2) [46]. At the time of writing this book chapter, current evidence suggests involving the patient with ADPKD aged 55–65 years in the decision-making process. This discussion should focus on assessing carefully for evidence of rapid progression (i.e., MIC 1C-E and/or an annual GFR rate of decline $\geq$3 mL/min/1.73 m^2). Tolvaptan is not indicated in patients above age 65, as patients above that age with GFR >25 mL/min/1.73 m^2 are likely to have slower disease.

Before initiating tolvaptan, clinicians should inform patients of potential risks and benefits, and consider patient lifestyle and preferences. Common adverse effects of tolvaptan therapy include increased thirst, polyuria, polydipsia, and nocturia [2, 44]. In the TEMPO3:4 and REPRISE trials, tolvaptan was associated with hepatocellular injury in 4.4% and 5.6% of participants, respectively. Hence, patients should be monitored for idiosyncratic hepatocellular injury with periodic liver function testing after initiation of tolvaptan (at a monthly interval for the first 18 months and then every 3 months thereafter) [44, 45].

Other Disease-Modifying Treatments Being Studied under Clinical Trials

As of 2022 at the time of writing this book chapter, several drugs have been in different phases of clinical trials. Bardoxolone methyl is a nuclear erythroid 2-related factor (NRF-2) activator that is currently being evaluated in a phase 3 trial (clinicaltrials.gov identifier: NCT03918447). Tesevatinib is a tyrosine kinase receptor inhibitor being evaluated in a phase 2 trial (NCT03203642). GLPG2737 is a cystic fibrosis transmembrane conductance regulator (CFTR) inhibitor being evaluated in a phase 2 trial (NCT04578548). Anti-micro RNAs (anti-MiRs) are a new class of drugs, currently investigated in ADPKD, which are being studied in Phase 1b (RGLS8429, NCT05521191). The landscape of current and upcoming clinical trials is evolving rapidly in ADPKD and likely to be different at the time of publishing this book chapter.

Management of Complications of ADPKD

Renal Cyst Hemorrhage

This common complication presents with an acute onset of flank pain with or without gross hematuria. Ruptured cysts, when connected to the urinary collecting system, may cause hematuria. Symptoms usually resolve within 7 days with conservative management including bed rest, analgesics, and adequate hydration [47]. Depending upon the severity of bleeding, patients may develop acute kidney injury. There have been reports of life-threatening hemorrhage leading to hemodynamic instability and hospitalization. In the setting of refractory bleeding and shock, interventional radiology-guided arterial embolization and surgery should be considered. In rare cases, if the bleeding remains refractory, nephrectomy may be required [47]. There are no randomized controlled trials investigating the efficacy of antifibrinolytic agents such as tranexamic acid, although case reports have shown some success in controlling refractory bleeding [48].

Chronic Flank Pain

Non-medical interventions such as physical therapy and the use of heating pads are typically considered as first-line therapy. Analgesics such as acetaminophen are preferred over non-steroidal anti-inflammatory drugs due to the latter's increased propensity to cause acute kidney injury and CKD with long-term use [49]. Opiates should generally be avoided for chronic pain due to the risk of abuse and dependence. Invasive approaches such as cyst aspiration with sclerotherapy or cyst fenestration can be considered in patients who do not respond to medical therapy or develop cystic complications [49]. In cases that are refractory to analgesics and cyst removal, renal denervation is also an option. In severe cases with advanced CKD, laparoscopic nephrectomy may be considered [49].

Cyst Infection

Cyst infection should be considered in patients presenting with recurrent fever and abdominal pain despite appropriate antibiotic therapy [9]. Ultrasonography, contrast-enhanced CT, and MRI are poorly sensitive in diagnosing cyst infection [50]. Positron emission tomography (PET) has been demonstrated to have better sensitivity, albeit with unclear specificity. Gram-negative bacteria are the most common pathogenic agents. A prolonged treatment course should be considered with antibiotics that penetrate the cyst such as fluoroquinolones or trimethoprim-sulfamethoxazole for 4–6 weeks. In cases of fluoroquinolone resistance, cephalosporins may be considered [50].

Simple Kidney Cysts

Epidemiology

Simple kidney cysts are the most common acquired cystic abnormalities, characterized by the presence of solitary or multiple cysts filled with clear or straw-colored fluid [51, 52]. Simple cysts are more common in males and increase in prevalence with age [53]. In a retrospective study of a healthy East Asian population using ultrasonography, simple cysts had a prevalence of 20% and 35% in the sixth and seventh decade of life, respectively [51]. In a review of abdominal CT imaging in 603 potential kidney donors between 50 to 75 years of age, at least one kidney cyst ≥ 2 mm and ≥ 5 mm in diameter was found in 63% and 43% of the patients, respectively [54]. In addition, a cortical, medullary, or parapelvic cyst ≥ 5 mm was present in 12%, 14%, or 2.8% of the patients, respectively. To distinguish between simple kidney cysts and other etiologies, the age-specific 97.5th percentile for the total number of both cortical and medullary cysts ≥ 5 mm can be used as the threshold (in the 60–69-year-old age group, 10 cysts for men and 4 for women) [54].

Pathogenesis

Simple cysts are thought to originate from renal ischemia leading to compensatory tubular hypertrophy and cyst formation [55]. Another hypothesis attributes the formation of these cysts to diverticula in the distal convoluted or collecting tubule due to weakening of the tubular basement membrane [51]. Histologically, these cysts are lined by a single layer of flattened or cuboidal epithelial cells that secrete a clear or straw-colored fluid.

Clinical Presentation

Simple cysts are usually asymptomatic and are therefore discovered incidentally with imaging. In rare cases, patients present with symptoms due to cyst enlargement leading to abdominal discomfort and flank pain. Complications such as cyst infection, rupture, hemorrhage, and renal pelvic obstruction are rare. Once clinical symptoms develop with simple cysts, patients should be evaluated further to rule out malignancy [56].

Diagnosis

Simple cysts are typically diagnosed incidentally during routine abdominal imaging with ultrasonography, contrast-enhanced CT, or MRI. On ultrasonography, they are anechoic, round, or oval-shaped with smooth margins and posterior enhancement without any septation or internal debris. Contrast-enhanced CT demonstrates non-enhancing and homogenous cysts [57]. According to the Bosniak classification of cystic masses >1 cm based on CT imaging, simple cysts are categorized as Bosniak I [58].

Treatment

Surveillance or treatment are not indicated in asymptomatic simple cysts [52]. Radiological interventions for symptomatic cysts include imaging-guided aspiration with or without sclerotherapy (using ethanol or newer sclerosing agents). Surgical interventions include excision via open, laparoscopic, or robotic surgery [59].

Complex Kidney Cyst

Complex kidney cysts refer to cystic abnormalities that do not show the imaging characteristics of simple cysts [56]. These cystic lesions need routine surveillance, as they may undergo malignant transformation. They can be further categorized on contrast-enhanced CT imaging using the Bosniak classification [56, 58].

Bosniak Classification

Based on the thickness and irregularity of the cyst wall, presence of septae, calcifications, and enhancement with contrast dye on CT imaging, kidney cysts can be classified into 5 categories, as summarized in Table 9.3 [60]. Due to atypical findings, some cystic lesions may need to be characterized further using additional imaging such as gadolinium-enhanced MRI or contrast-enhanced ultrasound. Discussing the MRI findings of unclassifiable cysts is beyond the scope of this chapter.

Bosniak I: Cysts with a thin wall and well-defined margins without any septations, calcifications, and enhancement with contrast administration. Simple kidney cysts are classified as Bosniak I [56]. The management of these cysts is described above. These cysts do not require periodic follow-up [52].

Bosniak II: Cysts with a few hairline septations, and fine punctate or linear calcifications in the wall or the septa. However, some cysts may appear homogenous with thin walls and well-defined margins, but with abnormally high imaging density [60]. Specifically, hyperdense cysts are characterized by higher Hounsfield density ($\geq$50 Hounsfield units or HU) compared to the adjacent renal parenchyma (30–40 HU) [57]. Hyperdense cysts that are subcapsular, <3 cm in size, and non-enhancing are also categorized as Bosniak II [57]. These cysts are considered benign and do not require further follow-up [61]. However, follow-up with ultrasound can be considered in younger patients if the size of the cyst is >3 cm [56].

Bosniak IIF: Cysts with 2–3 septations, thick calcifications in the septa or wall, without enhancement or with minimal enhancement are categorized as Bosniak IIF. The size of the wall or septa is <1 mm. In addition, hyperdense cysts that are intraparenchymal, > 3 cm in size, and non-enhancing also fall under this category [57]. Although these lesions are potentially benign, a malignancy risk of 5–15% has been reported [57]. Since Bosniak III cysts are at risk of malignant transformation and can be misclassified as IIF due to inter-operator variability, reviewing serial contrast-enhanced CT or MRI is recommended to ensure correct classification [62, 63]. Follow-up of IIF cysts with annual CT imaging is recommended to ensure they are stable or reclassify them to a higher-risk category [56, 57].

Table 9.3 Bosniak classification of cysts, management, and surveillance

Bosniak classification	Cyst wall	Septations	Calcifications	Enhancement	Management	Surveillance
Bosniak I	Thin, smooth, well-defined margins	None	None	No	Benign, asymptomatic	None
Bosniak II	Thin, smooth	Few, hairline thin septa	Few punctate/ linear	No	Benign, asymptomatic	None unless size >3 cm in young patients
Bosniak IIF	Minimal thickening	2–3 septa, minimal thickening <1 mm	Thick	Minimal enhancement	5–15% malignancy rate. Compare with previous images or obtain MRI	Annual CT imaging
Bosniak III	Thick wall, irregular margins	Thick, irregular septa >1 mm	Nodular, irregular	Yes, cyst wall	50% malignancy rate. Surgical intervention. Percutaneous biopsy and surveillance in high-risk patients.	Serial imaging with CT/ MRI every 3–6 months
Bosniak IV	Thick wall, irregular margins, nodular	Thick, irregular, septa	Nodular, irregular	Yes, soft tissue components	Surgical intervention	None recommended

Bosniak III: Cysts that have a thick wall and septations >1 mm, irregular calcifications, and enhancement of the cyst wall, without the presence of any soft tissue components in the cyst [57, 60]. This category includes both malignant neoplasms such as multilocular cystic renal cell carcinoma and tubulocystic carcinoma, and benign neoplasms such as cystic nephroma, or mixed epithelial and stromal tumors [64]. Surgical intervention/exploration is recommended for these cystic lesions due to the risk of malignancy of at least 50% [57, 61]. In patients with prohibitive surgical risk, clinicians may consider the use of percutaneous biopsy or active surveillance with frequent contrast-enhanced imaging to stratify risk and determine the need for further surgical intervention [57, 63]. However, percutaneous biopsy is considered controversial due to its inherent risk of hemorrhage and infection, sampling error, distortion of the lesion complicating imaging follow-up, and risk of tumor seeding [60].

Bosniak IV: Multilocular cysts, with thick irregular walls and nodularities, calcifications, and solid tissue components that enhance post-contrast. Around 90% of these lesions are malignant cystic neoplasms [64]. Surgical intervention is recommended for these cystic lesions due to the very high risk of malignancy [57, 61].

Acquired Cystic Kidney Disease

Epidemiology

Acquired cystic kidney disease (ACKD) is characterized by the development of bilateral kidney cysts ranging between 0.5 and 3 cm in size in patients with advanced CKD or ESKD on renal replacement therapy [65]. The prevalence of ACKD ranges between 7 and 80% depending on CKD stage and duration of dialysis, with a higher prevalence noted with longer exposure to dialysis [65, 66]. ACKD affects both sexes equally but has been noted to affect African-American individuals disproportionately [66].

Pathogenesis

The cysts in ACKD develop from the kidney tubule, mainly the proximal tubule. *In vivo* studies suggest that chemical injury to the renal epithelium, combined with loss of renal mass sufficient to produce azotemia, results in focal tubular dilation and expansion. In genetically susceptible individuals, tubular hypertrophy and hyperplasia, in addition to hormonal and environmental factors, may be sufficient to trigger latent oncogenes [55].

Clinical Presentation

The majority of patients with ACKD are asymptomatic [66]. However, a small proportion of patients with very large cysts can present with flank pain and hematuria due to cyst rupture, hemorrhage, or infection [67]. The most dreaded complication of ACKD is the development of renal cell carcinoma (RCC). Compared to the general population, patients with ACKD have an increased risk of RCC [66]. In prospective studies of ACKD, the incidence of RCC has been reported to vary between 4 and 7%, with a predisposition in males [68, 69]. In a prospective study of kidney transplant recipients, patients with ACKD had a higher prevalence of RCC compared to those without ACKD[70]. A review of RCC in elderly patients is discussed in a different chapter.

Diagnosis and Management

Since patients with ACKD are usually asymptomatic, cysts are diagnosed incidentally with abdominal imaging performed for a different indication. Small-sized kidneys with 3 or more cysts in each kidney in patients with advanced CKD or ESKD are diagnostic of ACKD [66]. Compared to ultrasonography, contrast-enhanced CT is more sensitive to detect ACKD and differentiate solid from cystic lesions. Based on the thickness and irregularity of the cyst wall, septations, calcifications, and contrast enhancement, cysts can be further categorized using the Bosniak classification [58]. Management of RCC is discussed in a different chapter.

Surveillance of ACKD

There are no established guidelines for the screening of ACKD in patients with CKD. As general guidance, screening for ACKD is not pursued in patients on dialysis with short life expectancy or with prohibitive surgical risk for future interventions [66]. Screening for ACKD is recommended for elderly patients on dialysis or with advanced CKD who are being evaluated for a kidney transplant. Potential kidney transplant recipients without ACKD can be screened every 3–5 years after the initial screening, while those with ACKD will need more frequent surveillance and their management will differ depending on the Bosniak class of the complex kidney cysts [66]. There is no established evidence behind choosing a particular imaging modality for screening. Ultrasonography can be considered as an initial modality due to its widespread availability, while contrast-based imaging modalities may be considered subsequently depending on the size and complexity of the cysts [66].

Medullary Sponge Kidney

Medullary sponge kidney (MSK) is a congenital malformation of the terminal collecting ducts leading to the development of diffuse cysts restricted to the medullary pyramids and a sponge-like appearance of the kidney on radiographic imaging [71]. MSK has a low prevalence of about 1% of the general population [72], and is usually diagnosed in the third decade of life, although the age at diagnosis can range from 12 to 69 years[72, 73].

Clinical Presentation

Patients with MSK present with recurrent symptomatic nephrolithiases composed of calcium phosphate and calcium oxalate [74]. Stone formation may also lead to urinary tract infections; in the presence of urease-splitting organisms, the stone composition may include struvite. Patients develop nephrocalcinosis over time, which is associated with chronic loin pain [73]. Other manifestations include painless hematuria that can be gross or microscopic, medullary concentration defects leading to nocturia, and urinary acidification defects leading to distal renal tubular acidosis [72]. Hypercalciuria and hypocitraturia associated with incomplete distal renal tubular acidosis underlie the recurrent formation of nephrolithiases [74]. Some patients remain asymptomatic during adulthood, and MSK is incidentally diagnosed during routine abdominal imaging for another indication.

Diagnosis

Plain radiographs will demonstrate calcium-containing stones and nephrocalcinosis. MSK has been previously diagnosed with intravenous pyelogram (IVP), which demonstrates nephrolithiasis, nephrocalcinosis, and pooling of contrast in dilated distal collecting ducts leading to the characteristic "paintbrush" or "bouquet of flowers" appearance [72]. However, the use of IVP has fallen out of favor due to the widespread availability of non-contrast CT ordered when patients present with renal colic. Non-contrast CT has a lower sensitivity in detecting MSK compared to IVP. However, CT urography with multidetector CT has been shown to have a sensitivity comparable to IVP and better sensitivity compared to non-contrast CT, but with the drawback of increased radiation [71, 75].

Treatment

There is no specific treatment option for MSK [71]. Management involves correcting the underlying metabolic abnormalities that increase stone formation. Treatment options include using potassium citrate 10–20 mmol in divided doses for patients with hypercalciuria and hypocitraturia, targeting a 24-h urinary citrate of 450 mg while keeping the urinary pH <7.5 [72]. Standard measures to prevent nephrolithiasis should also be implemented, such as increasing fluid intake and restricting dietary sodium and protein intake. The addition of thiazides can be considered in patients with hypercalciuria and recurrent stone disease despite the above approach [72].

Autosomal Dominant Tubulointerstitial Kidney Disease

Epidemiology

Autosomal dominant tubulointerstitial kidney disease (ADTKD) is a group of inherited kidney diseases characterized by autosomal dominant inheritance with tubulointerstitial fibrosis and CKD [22, 76, 77]. ADTKD remains underdiagnosed due to its nonspecific clinical presentation and the need for confirmatory genetic testing. The prevalence of ADTKD cannot be accurately determined. However, it is estimated to underlie CKD in 0.3–1% of individuals worldwide [78]. ADTKD is characterized by mutations in the genes *UMOD*, *REN*, *MUC1*, or *HNF1B*. Patients with mutations in *UMOD* and *MUC1* tend to present with progressive CKD during their teenage years or early adulthood, while mutations in *REN* and *HNF1B* tend to present in infancy and childhood [22]. Despite the early age of presentation, ADTKD should be part of the differential diagnosis in an elderly patient presenting with progressive CKD of unclear etiology.

Pathogenesis

ADTKD is characterized by mutations in the genes *UMOD*, *REN*, *MUC1*, and *HNF1B* in 50–60% of the cases. The remaining cases are genetically unresolved [77].

In ADTKD-UMOD, *UMOD* encodes uromodulin, which is secreted by the tubular epithelial cells of the thick ascending limb of the loop of Henle. Mutations in uromodulin lead to protein misfolding and accumulation in the endoplasmic reticulum. Downstream effects include apoptosis of tubular epithelial cells, defects in the trafficking of cellular transporters such as Na-K-2Cl (NKCC2), and mitochondrial dysfunction. This leads to defects in the function of the loop of Henle that manifest as urinary concentration defects, interstitial fibrosis, and tubular atrophy [22].

In ADTKD-MUC1, the *MUC1* gene encodes mucin 1, which is expressed by the tubular epithelial cells (specifically, the loop of Henle, distal tubule, and collecting duct). Frameshift mutations in *MUC1* affect cellular signaling and lubrication of the tubular epithelia [22]. In ADTKD-REN, the *REN* gene encodes preprorenin, mutations in which lead to defective renin production, hyporeninemic hypoaldosteronism, and apoptosis [22, 76].

In ADTKD-HNF1B, the *HNF1B* gene encodes the transcription factor hepatocyte nuclear factor 1β. Mutations in *HNF1B* lead to defective regulation and increased production of transforming growth factor-β. This subsequently activates genes involved in extracellular matrix deposition, which leads to interstitial fibrosis [22].

Clinical Presentation

Patients with ADTKD present with progressive CKD that may lead to kidney failure, with a family history of CKD and gout. Patients with mutations in *UMOD* and less frequently *MUC1*, *REN*, and *HNF1B* develop hyperuricemia and gout at an earlier age [22, 77]. The progression of CKD and age at the onset of kidney failure show considerable genotypic and phenotypic variability. The age at the onset of kidney failure in ADTKD-UMOD ranges between 25 and 80 years, with a mean of 50 years in men and 60 years in women [22]. ADTKD-associated with mutations in *REN* and *HNF1B* is frequently diagnosed in childhood and early adulthood, and hence may not be relevant to the geriatric population. ADTKD-REN presents with childhood-onset anemia, hyperkalemia, and hypotension due to hyporeninemic hypoaldosteronism. Conversely, ADTKD-HNF1B presents with congenital anomalies of the urinary tract (CAKUT), maturity-onset diabetes of the young (MODY), and hypomagnesemia. [22]

Diagnosis

Urinalysis demonstrates a bland urinary sediment with or without mild proteinuria, and low urinary osmolality reflecting a urinary concentrating defect [22]. The fractional excretion of urea is also reduced [77]. On imaging, patients with ADTKD may present with normal-sized or small kidneys, in addition to kidney cysts [22, 77]. The presence of many cysts with enlarged kidneys should raise the possibility of alternative diagnoses such as ADPKD[2]. Genetic testing in suspected individuals is confirmatory; however, it might be limited by availability and cost. Histopathology demonstrates non-specific diffuse tubulointerstitial fibrosis with secondary glomerular changes such as focal and segmental glomerulosclerosis [22].

Treatment

There is no specific therapy for the management of ADTKD. The mainstay of treatment focuses on reducing the progression of CKD, managing gout and diabetes mellitus as needed, and referring for kidney transplant evaluation. ADTKD does not recur in kidney allografts. Genetic testing of family members being considered for donation is important [71]. General measures to reduce CKD progression include BP control, dietary restriction of protein intake depending on the CKD stage, and treatment of complications such as metabolic acidosis, anemia, hyperkalemia, and bone mineral disorders [22]. Patients with ADTKD and hypertension should be treated with blockade of the renin-angiotensin-aldosterone system (i.e., ACEi and ARBs). Diuretics should be avoided as they can worsen hyperuricemia and natriuresis, leading to volume depletion [77]. It is unclear whether xanthine oxidase inhibitors such as allopurinol reduce CKD progression. However, allopurinol is recommended as the first choice for the prevention of gout in patients with ADTKD [77].

Tuberous Sclerosis

Epidemiology

Tuberous sclerosis (TSC) is a multisystem disorder characterized by mutations in tumor suppressor genes *TSC1* and *TSC2* with an incidence of 1 in 10,000 live births [64]. It has an autosomal dominant inheritance pattern in one-third of the cases, while in the remainder *de novo* mutations are responsible for the clinical features [79]. In the kidneys, TSC is associated with the development of angiomyolipoma, clear cell RCC, and multiple cysts [64]. Due to somatic mosaicism (i.e., the co-existence of mixed cell populations consisting of a wild-type and mutant genotype, occurring with de novo mutations at early stages of embryogenesis), TSC may present with very mild findings and remain undiagnosed until later in life [80].

Pathogenesis

TSC1, located on chromosome 9, and *TSC2,* located on chromosome 16, encode hamartin and tuberin, respectively[79]. Hamartin and tuberin form the TSC protein complex that inhibits the mTOR pathway, which is essential for cellular growth and proliferation. Mutations in these tumor suppressor genes lead to continuous activation of mTOR, enhancing cellular proliferation and protein synthesis [81].

Clinical Features

Cystic kidney disease is the most common renal manifestation after angiomyolipoma and has a prevalence ranging from 14 to 45% [64, 82]. Cysts are more common in patients with mutations in *TSC2* [82]. Cysts associated with TSC are generally described as simple cysts and tend to be asymptomatic. Cystic complications including hemorrhage and rupture are rare [82]. Extrarenal features comprise retinal hamartomas, benign cerebral lesions (e.g., tubers and subependymal giant cell astrocytoma), pulmonary lymphangioleiomyomatosis, cardiac rhabdomyomas, and various skin lesions such as facial angiofibromas and hypopigmented macules [83]. In about 5% of the patients, mutations in *TSC2* can be associated with mutations in the adjacent *PKD1* gene (known as the *TSC2/PKD1* contiguous gene syndrome), resulting in diffuse cystic kidney disease. However, this syndrome typically presents with early-onset kidney failure and kidney malignancy [64].

Diagnosis

The presence of bilateral cysts along with angiomyolipoma lesions should increase suspicion of TSC. Contrast- or non-contrast-based imaging usually demonstrates simple cysts. Multisystem diagnostic criteria were devised by the International TSC Consensus Group [84]. Genetic testing identifying mutations in *TSC1* and *TSC2* is confirmatory [79].

Management

Treatment or surveillance is not indicated for uncomplicated cysts in TSC. Cystic complications can be managed as described above (cf. Simple Kidney Cysts). Yearly MRI surveillance of the angiomyolipomas is recommended. Some patients might require nephron-sparing interventions (e.g., selective arterial embolization or partial nephrectomy) and administration of mTOR inhibitors [85]. Patients with TSC should also be referred to the appropriate specialists for the management of extrarenal features.

Von Hippel-Lindau Syndrome

Epidemiology

Von Hippel-Lindau (VHL) syndrome is a multisystem disorder characterized by mutations in the tumor suppressor gene *VHL* with an incidence of 1 in 35,000 live births [64]. It has an autosomal dominant inheritance pattern in 80% of the cases, with sporadic de novo mutations accounting for the remaining 20% [86].

Pathogenesis

The *VHL* gene, located in chromosome 3, encodes the VHL protein, which plays a regulatory role in the breakdown of the transcription factor hypoxia-inducible factor-1 (HIF-1). Mutations in *VHL* stabilize HIF-1 and stimulate the expression of growth factors such as vascular endothelial growth factor, platelet-derived growth factor, and transforming growth factor-α. These growth factors cause cellular growth, proliferation, and tumorigenesis [86]. Histopathology can demonstrate simple cysts with one layer of cuboidal epithelium, hyperplastic cysts with multiple epithelial cell layers, and clear cell RCC [87].

Clinical Features, Diagnosis, and Treatment

In the kidneys, VHL syndrome is associated with the development of multiple cysts and RCC [64]. A range of 50–70% of patients with VHL syndrome develop numerous kidney cysts bilaterally [86]. These simple cysts are usually asymptomatic without loss of kidney function, and cystic complications are rare. Observational studies have demonstrated that 90% of patients with VHL syndrome over 60 years of age will present with kidney cysts and RCC, which contributes to increased mortality in this subgroup [88]. Imaging modalities with contrast are preferred for the surveillance of complex cysts and monitoring for RCC in patients diagnosed with VHL syndrome [89]. Cysts in VHL syndrome have an indolent clinical course with slow growth over the individual's lifetime. However, periodic surveillance with imaging is important due to the high incidence of RCC in the elderly [88].

Lithium-Induced Nephropathy

Lithium is one of the most common mood stabilizers prescribed for the management of bipolar disorder worldwide. However, long-term use of lithium has been associated with various kidney adverse effects in the ageing population, such as nephrogenic diabetic insipidus, chronic tubulointerstitial nephritis, and increased risk of ESKD [90]. In addition, on histopathology, small bilateral microcysts (1–2 mm) originating from the distal tubules and collecting ducts have been reported in about 60% of biopsies [91]. MRI with gadolinium contrast is very sensitive to identify microcysts [91, 92]. Lithium-induced microcysts remain asymptomatic and do not need further monitoring.

References

1. Chebib FT, Torres VE. Autosomal dominant polycystic kidney disease: core curriculum 2016. Am J Kidney Dis. 2016;67(5):792–810. https://doi.org/10.1053/j.ajkd.2015.07.037.
2. Radhakrishnan Y, Duriseti P, Chebib FT. Management of autosomal dominant polycystic kidney disease in the era of disease-modifying treatment options. Kr J Nephrol. 2022;0:422. https://doi.org/10.23876/j.krcp.21.309.
3. Aung TT, Bhandari SK, Chen Q, Malik FT, Willey CJ, Reynolds K, Jacobsen SJ, Sim JJ. Autosomal dominant polycystic kidney disease prevalence among a racially diverse United States population, 2002 through 2018. Kidney360. 2021;2(12):2010–5. https://doi.org/10.34067/kid.0004522021.
4. Chebib FT, Torres VE. Assessing risk of rapid progression in autosomal dominant polycystic kidney disease and special considerations for disease-modifying therapy. Am J Kidney Dis. 2021;78(2):282–92. https://doi.org/10.1053/j.ajkd.2020.12.020.
5. Bergmann C, Guay-Woodford LM, Harris PC, Horie S, Peters DJM, Torres VE. Polycystic kidney disease. Nat Rev Dis Prim. 2018;4(1):50. https://doi.org/10.1038/s41572-018-0047-y.
6. Porath B, Gainullin VG, Cornec-Le Gall E, Dillinger EK, Heyer CM, Hopp K, Edwards ME, Madsen CD, Mauritz SR, Banks CJ, Baheti S, Reddy B, Herrero JI, Bañales JM, Hogan MC, Tasic V, Watnick TJ, Chapman AB, Vigneau C, Harris PC. Mutations in GANAB, encoding the glucosidase IIα subunit, cause autosomal-dominant polycystic kidney and liver disease. Am J Hum Genet. 2016;98(6):1193–207. https://doi.org/10.1016/j.ajhg.2016.05.004.
7. Cornec-Le Gall E, Audrézet M-P, Chen J-M, Hourmant M, Morin M-P, Perrichot R, Charasse C, Whebe B, Renaudineau E, Jousset P, Guillodo M-P, Grall-Jezequel A, Saliou P, Férec C, Le Meur Y. Type of PKD1 mutation influences renal outcome in ADPKD. J Am Soc Nephrol. 2013;24(6):1006–13. https://doi.org/10.1681/ASN.2012070650.
8. Milutinovic J, Fialkow PJ, Agodoa LY, Phillips LA, Rudd TG, Sutherland S. Clinical manifestations of autosomal dominant polycystic kidney disease in patients older than 50 years. Am J Kidney Dis. 1990;15(3):237–43. https://doi.org/10.1016/s0272-6386(12)80768-2.
9. Jouret F, Hogan MC, Chebib FT. A practical guide for the management of acute abdominal pain with fever in patients with autosomal dominant polycystic kidney disease. Nephrol Dial Transplant. 2022;37(8):1426–8. https://doi.org/10.1093/ndt/gfab040.
10. Torres VE, Wilson DM, Hattery RR, Segura JW. Renal stone disease in autosomal dominant polycystic kidney disease. Am J Kidney Dis. 1993;22(4):513–9. https://doi.org/10.1016/S0272-6386(12)80922-X.

11. Luciano RL, Dahl NK. Extra-renal manifestations of autosomal dominant polycystic kidney disease (ADPKD): considerations for routine screening and management. Nephrol Dial Transplant. 2013;29(2):247–54. https://doi.org/10.1093/ndt/gft437.
12. Qian Q. Isolated polycystic liver disease. Adv Chronic Kidney Dis. 2010;17(2):181–9. https://doi.org/10.1053/j.ackd.2009.12.005.
13. Pirson Y. Extrarenal manifestations of autosomal dominant polycystic kidney disease. Adv Chronic Kidney Dis. 2010;17(2):173–80. https://doi.org/10.1053/j.ackd.2010.01.003.
14. Chedid M, Kaidbay HD, Wigerinck S, Mkhaimer Y, Smith B, Zubidat D, Sekhon I, Prajwal R, Duriseti P, Issa N, Zoghby ZM, Hanna C, Senum SR, Harris PC, Hickson LJ, Torres VE, Nkomo VT, Chebib FT. Cardiovascular outcomes in kidney transplant recipients with ADPKD. Kidney Int Rep. 2022;7(9):1991–2005. https://doi.org/10.1016/j.ekir.2022.06.006.
15. Pei Y, Watnick T. Diagnosis and screening of autosomal dominant polycystic kidney disease. Adv Chronic Kidney Dis. 2010;17(2):140–52. https://doi.org/10.1053/j.ackd.2009.12.001.
16. Gradzik M, Niemczyk M, Gołębiowski M, Pączek L. Diagnostic imaging of autosomal dominant polycystic kidney disease. Pol J Radiol. 2016;81:441–53. https://doi.org/10.12659/PJR.894482.
17. Pei Y, Obaji J, Dupuis A, Paterson AD, Magistroni R, Dicks E, Parfrey P, Cramer B, Coto E, Torra R, San Millan JL, Gibson R, Breuning M, Peters D, Ravine D. Unified criteria for Ultrasonographic diagnosis of ADPKD. J Am Soc Nephrol. 2009;20(1):205–12. https://doi.org/10.1681/asn.2008050507.
18. Pei Y, Hwang YH, Conklin J, Sundsbak JL, Heyer CM, Chan W, Wang K, He N, Rattansingh A, Atri M, Harris PC, Haider MA. Imaging-based diagnosis of autosomal dominant polycystic kidney disease. J Am Soc Nephrol. 2015;26(3):746–53. https://doi.org/10.1681/ASN.2014030297.
19. Lanktree MB, Iliuta IA, Haghighi A, Song X, Pei Y. Evolving role of genetic testing for the clinical management of autosomal dominant polycystic kidney disease. Nephrol Dial Transplant. 2019;34(9):1453–60. https://doi.org/10.1093/ndt/gfy261.
20. Suwabe T, Chamberlain AM, Killian JM, King BF, Gregory AV, Madsen CD, Wang X, Kline TL, Chebib FT, Hogan MC, Kamath PS, Harris PC, Torres VE. Epidemiology of autosomal-dominant polycystic liver disease in Olmsted county. JHEP Rep. 2020;2(6):100166. https://doi.org/10.1016/j.jhepr.2020.100166.
21. Gevers TJ, Drenth JP. Diagnosis and management of polycystic liver disease. Nat Rev Gastroenterol Hepatol. 2013;10(2):101–8. https://doi.org/10.1038/nrgastro.2012.254.
22. Devuyst O, Olinger E, Weber S, Eckardt K-U, Kmoch S, Rampoldi L, Bleyer AJ. Autosomal dominant tubulointerstitial kidney disease. Nat Rev Dis Prim. 2019;5(1):60. https://doi.org/10.1038/s41572-019-0109-9.
23. Gunay-Aygun M, Turkbey BI, Bryant J, Daryanani KT, Gerstein MT, Piwnica-Worms K, Choyke P, Heller T, Gahl WA. Hepatorenal findings in obligate heterozygotes for autosomal recessive polycystic kidney disease. Mol Genet Metab. 2011;104(4):677–81. https://doi.org/10.1016/j.ymgme.2011.09.001.
24. Cornec-Le Gall E, Olson RJ, Besse W, Heyer CM, Gainullin VG, Smith JM, Audrézet M-P, Hopp K, Porath B, Shi B, Baheti S, Senum SR, Arroyo J, Madsen CD, Férec C, Joly D, Jouret F, Fikri-Benbrahim O, Charasse C, Harris PC. Monoallelic mutations to DNAJB11 cause atypical autosomal-dominant polycystic kidney disease. Am J Hum Genet. 2018;102(5):832–44. https://doi.org/10.1016/j.ajhg.2018.03.013.
25. Huynh VT, Audrézet MP, Sayer JA, Ong AC, Lefevre S, Le Brun V, Després A, Senum SR, Chebib FT, Barroso-Gil M, Patel C, Mallett AJ, Goel H, Mallawaarachchi AC, Van Eerde AM, Ponlot E, Kribs M, Le Meur Y, Harris PC, Cornec-Le Gall E. Clinical spectrum, prognosis and estimated prevalence of DNAJB11-kidney disease. Kidney Int. 2020;98(2):476–87. https://doi.org/10.1016/j.kint.2020.02.022.
26. Pisani I, Allinovi M, Palazzo V, Zanelli P, Gentile M, Farina MT, Giuliotti S, Cravedi P, Delsante M, Maggiore U, Fiaccadori E, Manenti L. More dissimilarities than affinities between

DNAJB11-PKD and ADPKD. Clin Kidney J. 2022;15(6):1179–87. https://doi.org/10.1093/ckj/sfac032.

27. Liu P, Zu F, Chen H, Yin X, Tan X. Exosomal DNAJB11 promotes the development of pancreatic cancer by modulating the EGFR/MAPK pathway. Cell Mol Biol Lett. 2022;27(1):87. https://doi.org/10.1186/s11658-022-00390-0.

28. Sun R, Yang L, Wang Y, Zhang Y, Ke J, Zhao D. DNAJB11 predicts a poor prognosis and is associated with immune infiltration in thyroid carcinoma: a bioinformatics analysis. J Int Med Res. 2021;49(11):3000605211053722. https://doi.org/10.1177/03000605211053722.

29. Chebib FT, Torres VE. Recent advances in the Management of Autosomal Dominant Polycystic Kidney Disease. Clin J Am Soc Nephrol. 2018;13(11):1765–76. https://doi.org/10.2215/cjn.03960318.

30. Hopp K, Wang X, Ye H, Irazabal MV, Harris PC, Torres VE. Effects of hydration in rats and mice with polycystic kidney disease. Am J Physiol Renal Physiol. 2015;308(3):F261–6. https://doi.org/10.1152/ajprenal.00345.2014.

31. Rangan GK, Wong ATY, Munt A, Zhang JQJ, Saravanabavan S, Louw S, Allman-Farinelli M, Badve SV, Boudville N, Chan J, Coolican H, Coulshed S, Edwards ME, Erickson BJ, Fernando M, Foster S, Gregory AV, Haloob I, Hawley CM, Harris DCH. Prescribed water intake in autosomal dominant polycystic kidney disease. NEJM Evidence. 2022;1(1):EVIDoa2100021. https://doi.org/10.1056/EVIDoa2100021.

32. Kramers BJ, Koorevaar IW, Drenth JPH, de Fijter JW, Neto AG, Peters DJM, Vart P, Wetzels JF, Zietse R, Gansevoort RT, Meijer E. Salt, but not protein intake, is associated with accelerated disease progression in autosomal dominant polycystic kidney disease. Kidney Int. 2020;98(4):989–98. https://doi.org/10.1016/j.kint.2020.04.053.

33. Nowak KL, You Z, Gitomer B, Brosnahan G, Torres VE, Chapman AB, Perrone RD, Steinman TI, Abebe KZ, Rahbari-Oskoui FF, Yu ASL, Harris PC, Bae KT, Hogan M, Miskulin D, Chonchol M. Overweight and obesity are predictors of progression in early autosomal dominant polycystic kidney disease. J Am Soc Nephrol. 2018;29(2):571–8. https://doi.org/10.1681/ASN.2017070819.

34. Carriazo S, Perez-Gomez MV, Cordido A, García-González MA, Sanz AB, Ortiz A, Sanchez-Niño MD. Dietary care for ADPKD patients: current status and future directions. Nutrients. 2019;11(7):1576. https://doi.org/10.3390/nu11071576.

35. Klahr S, Breyer JA, Beck GJ, Dennis VW, Hartman JA, Roth D, Steinman TI, Wang SR, Yamamoto ME. Dietary protein restriction, blood pressure control, and the progression of polycystic kidney disease. Modification of diet in renal disease study group. J Am Soc Nephrol. 1995;5(12):2037–47. https://doi.org/10.1681/asn.V5122037.

36. Torres VE, Grantham JJ, Chapman AB, Mrug M, Bae KT, King BF, Wetzel LH, Martin D, Lockhart ME, Bennett WM, Moxey-Mims M, Abebe KZ, Lin Y, Bost JE, Consortium for Radiologic Imaging Studies of Polycystic Kidney, D. Potentially modifiable factors affecting the progression of autosomal dominant polycystic kidney disease. Clin J Am Soc Nephrol. 2011;6(3):640–7. https://doi.org/10.2215/cjn.03250410.

37. Chapman AB. Approaches to testing new treatments in autosomal dominant polycystic kidney disease: insights from the CRISP and HALT-PKD studies. Clin J Am Soc Nephrol. 2008;3(4):1197–204. https://doi.org/10.2215/cjn.00060108.

38. Chapman AB, Bost JE, Torres VE, Guay-Woodford L, Bae KT, Landsittel D, Li J, King BF, Martin D, Wetzel LH, Lockhart ME, Harris PC, Moxey-Mims M, Flessner M, Bennett WM, Grantham JJ. Kidney volume and functional outcomes in autosomal dominant polycystic kidney disease. Clin J Am Soc Nephrol. 2012;7(3):479–86. https://doi.org/10.2215/CJN.09500911.

39. Grantham JJ, Torres VE, Chapman AB, Guay-Woodford LM, Bae KT, King BF, Wetzel LH, Baumgarten DA, Kenney PJ, Harris PC, Klahr S, Bennett WM, Hirschman GN, Meyers CM, Zhang X, Zhu F, Miller JP. Volume progression in polycystic kidney disease. N Engl J Med. 2006;354(20):2122–30. https://doi.org/10.1056/NEJMoa054341.

40. Irazabal MV, Rangel LJ, Bergstralh EJ, Osborn SL, Harmon AJ, Sundsbak JL, Bae KT, Chapman AB, Grantham JJ, Mrug M, Hogan MC, El-Zoghby ZM, Harris PC, Erickson BJ, King BF, Torres VE, Investigators, t. C. Imaging classification of autosomal dominant polycystic kidney disease: a simple model for selecting patients for clinical trials. J Am Soc Nephrol. 2015;26(1):160–72. https://doi.org/10.1681/asn.2013101138.

41. Yu ASL, Shen C, Landsittel DP, Grantham JJ, Cook LT, Torres VE, Chapman AB, Bae KT, Mrug M, Harris PC, Rahbari-Oskoui FF, Shi T, Bennett WM, Consortium for Radiologic Imaging Studies of Polycystic Kidney, D. Long-term trajectory of kidney function in autosomal-dominant polycystic kidney disease. Kidney Int. 2019;95(5):1253–61. https://doi.org/10.1016/j.kint.2018.12.023.

42. Cornec-Le Gall, E., Audrézet, M.-P., Rousseau, A., Hourmant, M., Renaudineau, E., Charasse, C., Morin, M.-P., Moal, M.-C., Dantal, J., Wehbe, B., Perrichot, R., Frouget, T., Vigneau, C., Potier, J., Jousset, P., Guillodo, M.-P., Siohan, P., Terki, N., Sawadogo, T., . . . Le Meur, Y. (2016). The PROPKD score: a new algorithm to predict renal survival in autosomal dominant polycystic kidney disease. J Am Soc Nephrol, 27(3), 942–951. https://doi.org/10.1681/asn.2015010016.

43. Administration, U. F. a. D. 2018. https://www.accessdata.fda.gov/drugsatfda_docs/nda/2018/204441Orig1s000Approv.pdf. Accessed 24 Oct.

44. Torres VE, Chapman AB, Devuyst O, Gansevoort RT, Grantham JJ, Higashihara E, Perrone RD, Krasa HB, Ouyang J, Czerwiec FS. Tolvaptan in patients with autosomal dominant polycystic kidney disease. N Engl J Med. 2012;367(25):2407–18. https://doi.org/10.1056/NEJMoa1205511.

45. Torres VE, Chapman AB, Devuyst O, Gansevoort RT, Perrone RD, Koch G, Ouyang J, McQuade RD, Blais JD, Czerwiec FS, Sergeyeva O. Tolvaptan in later-stage autosomal dominant polycystic kidney disease. N Engl J Med. 2017;377(20):1930–42. https://doi.org/10.1056/NEJMoa1710030.

46. Chebib FT, Perrone RD, Chapman AB, Dahl NK, Harris PC, Mrug M, Mustafa RA, Rastogi A, Watnick T, Yu ASL, Torres VE. A practical guide for treatment of rapidly progressive ADPKD with Tolvaptan. J Am Soc Nephrol. 2018;29(10):2458–70. https://doi.org/10.1681/asn.2018060590.

47. Cheng CI, Karvelas NB, Aronowitz P. Retroperitoneal cyst hemorrhage in polycystic kidney disease. Cleve Clin J Med. 2015;82(1):20–1. https://doi.org/10.3949/ccjm.82a.14007.

48. Vujkovac B, Sabovic M. A successful treatment of life-threatening bleeding from polycystic kidneys with antifibrinolytic agent tranexamic acid. Blood Coagul Fibrinolysis. 2006;17(7):589–91. https://doi.org/10.1097/01.mbc.0000245293.41774.c8.

49. Hogan MC, Norby SM. Evaluation and management of pain in autosomal dominant polycystic kidney disease. Adv Chronic Kidney Dis. 2010;17(3):e1–e16. https://doi.org/10.1053/j.ackd.2010.01.005.

50. Sallée M, Rafat C, Zahar J-R, Paulmier B, Grünfeld J-P, Knebelmann B, Fakhouri F. Cyst infections in patients with autosomal dominant polycystic kidney disease. Clin J Am Soc Nephrol. 2009;4(7):1183–9. https://doi.org/10.2215/CJN.01870309.

51. Chang C-C, Kuo J-Y, Chan W-L, Chen K-K, Chang LS. Prevalence and clinical characteristics of simple renal cyst. J Chin Med Assoc. 2007;70(11):486–91. https://doi.org/10.1016/S1726-4901(08)70046-7.

52. Simms RJ, Ong ACM. How simple are 'simple renal cysts'? Nephrol Dialy Transplant. 2014;29(suppl_4):iv106-iv112. https://doi.org/10.1093/ndt/gfu106.

53. Terada N, Ichioka K, Matsuta Y, Okubo K, Yoshimura K, Arai Y. The natural history of simple renal cysts. J Urol. 2002;167(1):21–3.

54. Rule AD, Sasiwimonphan K, Lieske JC, Keddis MT, Torres VE, Vrtiska TJ. Characteristics of renal cystic and solid lesions based on contrast-enhanced computed tomography of potential kidney donors. Am J Kidney Dis. 2012;59(5):611–8. https://doi.org/10.1053/j.ajkd.2011.12.022.

55. Grantham JJ. Acquired cystic kidney disease. Kidney Int. 1991;40(1):143–52. https://doi.org/10.1038/ki.1991.192.
56. Eknoyan G. A clinical view of simple and complex renal cysts. J Am Soc Nephrol. 2009;20(9):1874–6. https://doi.org/10.1681/asn.2008040441.
57. Hélénon O, Crosnier A, Verkarre V, Merran S, Méjean A, Correas JM. Simple and complex renal cysts in adults: classification system for renal cystic masses. Diagn Interv Imaging. 2018;99(4):189–218. https://doi.org/10.1016/j.diii.2017.10.005.
58. Bosniak MA. The current radiological approach to renal cysts. Radiology. 1986;158(1):1–10. https://doi.org/10.1148/radiology.158.1.3510019.
59. Skolarikos A, Laguna MP, de la Rosette JJ. Conservative and radiological management of simple renal cysts: a comprehensive review. BJU Int. 2012;110(2):170–8. https://doi.org/10.1111/j.1464-410X.2011.10847.x.
60. Israel GM, Bosniak MA. An update of the Bosniak renal cyst classification system. Urology. 2005;66(3):484–8. https://doi.org/10.1016/j.urology.2005.04.003.
61. Whelan TF. Guidelines on the management of renal cyst disease. Canadian Urol Assoc J. 2010;4(2):98–9. https://doi.org/10.5489/cuaj.10023.
62. Israel GM, Hindman N, Bosniak MA. Evaluation of cystic renal masses: comparison of CT and MR imaging by using the Bosniak classification system. Radiology. 2004;231(2):365–71. https://doi.org/10.1148/radiol.2312031025.
63. McGuire BB, Fitzpatrick JM. The diagnosis and management of complex renal cysts. Curr Opin Urol. 2010;20(5):349–54. https://doi.org/10.1097/MOU.0b013e32833c7b04.
64. Bonsib SM. Renal cystic diseases and renal neoplasms: a mini-review. Clin J Am Soc Nephrol. 2009;4(12):1998–2007. https://doi.org/10.2215/cjn.02020309.
65. Narasimhan N, Golper TA, Wolfson M, Rahatzad M, Bennett WM. Clinical characteristics and diagnostic considerations in acquired renal cystic disease. Kidney Int. 1986;30(5):748–52. https://doi.org/10.1038/ki.1986.251.
66. Rahbari-Oskoui F, O'Neill WC. Diagnosis and management of acquired cystic kidney disease and renal tumors in ESRD patients. Semin Dial. 2017;30(4):373–9. https://doi.org/10.1111/sdi.12605.
67. Truong LD, Krishnan B, Cao JT, Barrios R, Suki WN. Renal neoplasm in acquired cystic kidney disease. Am J Kidney Dis. 1995;26(1):1–12. https://doi.org/10.1016/0272-6386(95)90146-9.
68. Ishikawa I, Saito Y, Shikura N, Kitada H, Shinoda A, Suzuki S. Ten-year prospective study on the development of renal cell carcinoma in dialysis patients. Am J Kidney Dis. 1990;16(5):452–8. https://doi.org/10.1016/s0272-6386(12)80058-8.
69. Levine E, Slusher SL, Grantham JJ, Wetzel LH. Natural history of acquired renal cystic disease in dialysis patients: a prospective longitudinal CT study. AJR Am J Roentgenol. 1991;156(3):501–6. https://doi.org/10.2214/ajr.156.3.1899744.
70. Schwarz A, Vatandaslar S, Merkel S, Haller H. Renal cell carcinoma in transplant recipients with acquired cystic kidney disease. Clin J Am Soc Nephrol. 2007;2(4):750–6. https://doi.org/10.2215/cjn.03661106.
71. Imam TH, Patail H, Patail H. Medullary sponge kidney: current perspectives. Int J Nephrol Renovasc Dis. 2019;12:213–8. https://doi.org/10.2147/ijnrd.S169336.
72. Fabris A, Anglani F, Lupo A, Gambaro G. Medullary sponge kidney: state of the art. Nephrol Dial Transplant. 2012;28(5):1111–9. https://doi.org/10.1093/ndt/gfs505.
73. Forster JA, Taylor J, Browning AJ, Biyani CS. A review of the natural progression of medullary sponge kidney and a novel grading system based on intravenous urography findings. Urol Int. 2007;78(3):264–9. https://doi.org/10.1159/000099350.
74. Gambaro G, Danza FM, Fabris A. Medullary sponge kidney. Curr Opin Nephrol Hypertens. 2013;22(4):421–6. https://doi.org/10.1097/MNH.0b013e3283622b86.
75. Koraishy FM, Ngo TT, Israel GM, Dahl NK. CT urography for the diagnosis of medullary sponge kidney. Am J Nephrol. 2014;39(2):165–70. https://doi.org/10.1159/000358496.
76. Ayasreh N, Miquel R, Matamala A, Ars E, Torra R. A review on autosomal dominant tubulointerstitial kidney disease. Nefrología (English Edition). 2017;37(3):235–43. https://doi.org/10.1016/j.nefroe.2017.05.012.

77. Eckardt KU, Alper SL, Antignac C, Bleyer AJ, Chauveau D, Dahan K, Deltas C, Hosking A, Kmoch S, Rampoldi L, Wiesener M, Wolf MT, Devuyst O. Autosomal dominant tubulointerstitial kidney disease: diagnosis, classification, and management—a KDIGO consensus report. Kidney Int. 2015;88(4):676–83. https://doi.org/10.1038/ki.2015.28.

78. Gast C, Marinaki A, Arenas-Hernandez M, Campbell S, Seaby EG, Pengelly RJ, Gale DP, Connor TM, Bunyan DJ, Hodaňová K, Živná M, Kmoch S, Ennis S, Venkat-Raman G. Autosomal dominant tubulointerstitial kidney disease-UMOD is the most frequent non polycystic genetic kidney disease. BMC Nephrol. 2018;19(1):301. https://doi.org/10.1186/s12882-018-1107-y.

79. Randle SC. Tuberous sclerosis complex: a review. Pediatr Ann. 2017;46(4):e166–71. https://doi.org/10.3928/19382359-20170320-01.

80. Tyburczy ME, Dies KA, Glass J, Camposano S, Chekaluk Y, Thorner AR, Lin L, Krueger D, Franz DN, Thiele EA, Sahin M, Kwiatkowski DJ. Mosaic and Intronic mutations in TSC1/TSC2 explain the majority of TSC patients with no mutation identified by conventional testing. PLoS Genet. 2015;11(11):e1005637. https://doi.org/10.1371/journal.pgen.1005637.

81. Uysal SP, Şahin M. Tuberous sclerosis: a review of the past, present, and future. Turk J Med Sci. 2020;50(Si-2):1665–76. https://doi.org/10.3906/sag-2002-133.

82. Rakowski SK, Winterkorn EB, Paul E, Steele DJ, Halpern EF, Thiele EA. Renal manifestations of tuberous sclerosis complex: incidence, prognosis, and predictive factors. Kidney Int. 2006;70(10):1777–82. https://doi.org/10.1038/sj.ki.5001853.

83. Nair N, Chakraborty R, Mahajan Z, Sharma A, Sethi SK, Raina R. Renal manifestations of tuberous sclerosis complex. J Kidney Cancer VHL. 2020;7(3):5–19. https://doi.org/10.15586/jkcvhl.2020.131.

84. Northrup H, Aronow ME, Bebin EM, Bissler J, Darling TN, de Vries PJ, Frost MD, Fuchs Z, Gosnell ES, Gupta N, Jansen AC, Jóźwiak S, Kingswood JC, Knilans TK, McCormack FX, Pounders A, Roberds SL, Rodriguez-Buritica DF, Roth J, Krueger DA. Updated international tuberous sclerosis complex diagnostic criteria and surveillance and management recommendations. Pediatr Neurol. 2021;123:50–66. https://doi.org/10.1016/j.pediatrneurol.2021.07.011.

85. Restrepo J, Millan DAC, Sabogal CAR, Bernal AFP, Donoso WD. New trends and evidence for the Management of Renal Angiomyolipoma: a comprehensive narrative review of the literature. J Kidney Cancer VHL. 2022;9(1):33–41. https://doi.org/10.15586/jkcvhl.v9i1.177.

86. Varshney N, Kebede AA, Owusu-Dapaah H, Lather J, Kaushik M, Bhullar JS. A review of Von Hippel-Lindau syndrome. J Kidney Cancer VHL. 2017;4(3):20–9. https://doi.org/10.15586/jkcvhl.2017.88.

87. Choyke PL, Glenn GM, Walther MM, Zbar B, Weiss GH, Alexander RB, Hayes WS, Long JP, Thakore KN, Linehan WM. The natural history of renal lesions in von Hippel-Lindau disease: a serial CT study in 28 patients. AJR Am J Roentgenol. 1992;159(6):1229–34. https://doi.org/10.2214/ajr.159.6.1442389.

88. Chauveau D, Duvic C, Chrétien Y, Paraf F, Droz D, Melki P, Hélénon O, Richard S, Grünfeld JP. Renal involvement in von Hippel-Lindau disease. Kidney Int. 1996;50(3):944–51. https://doi.org/10.1038/ki.1996.395.

89. Untanas A, Trakymas M, Lekienė I, Briedienė R. Von Hippel-Lindau syndrome and renal tumours: radiological diagnostic and treatment options. A case report and literature review. Acta Med Litu. 2020;27(1):25–32. https://doi.org/10.6001/actamedica.v27i1.4263.

90. Alsady M, Baumgarten R, Deen PMT, de Groot T. Lithium in the kidney: friend and foe? J Am Soc Nephrol. 2016;27(6):1587. https://doi.org/10.1681/ASN.2015080907.

91. McCartney Y, Browne C, Little DM, Gulmann C. Lithium-induced nephrotoxicity: a case report of renal cystic disease presenting as a mass lesion. Urol Case Rep. 2014;2(6):186–8. https://doi.org/10.1016/j.eucr.2014.08.002.

92. Anthonissen B, Danse E, Goffin E. An unexpected imaging finding in a CKD patient on lithium therapy. Kidney360. 2021;2(1):180–1. https://doi.org/10.34067/kid.0003642020.

Chapter 10
Glomerular Disease in the Elderly

Jeffrey Kott, Nitzy Muñoz Casablanca, and Samuel Mon-Wei Yu

Take Home Points
- Diagnosing acute kidney injury including glomerular diseases in the elderly require comprehensive history taking and careful laboratory data review. A native kidney biopsy can assist with accurate diagnosis and should not be delayed to initiate treatments.
- Renin-angiotensin-aldosterone system blockade remains the standard-of-care for proteinuria. The use of immunological agents should be individualized according to patients' underlying condition and comorbidities.
- Closer monitoring of side effects and infections from corticosteroid use or cytotoxic agents is important. Newer agents with less cytotoxic effects might be of particular interest for elderly patients with glomerular diseases.

Clinical Scenario

An 80-year-old woman was referred by her primary care physician (PCP) to the outpatient nephrology clinic for elevated serum creatinine (SCr). She had a past medical history of hypertension, and chronic kidney disease (CKD) stage 3 with subnephrotic proteinuria. Her baseline SCr was 1.29 mg/dL with an estimated glomerular filtrate rate (eGFR) of 40 mL/min/1.73 m^2. At the time of referral, her SCr was elevated to 1.91 mg/dL (eGFR: 24 mL/min/1.73 m^2). Urinalysis showed 3+

J. Kott · S. M.-W. Yu (✉)
Nephrology Division, Department of Medicine, Mount Sinai Hospital, New York, NY, USA
e-mail: mon-wei.yu@mountsinai.org

N. M. Casablanca
Nephrology Division, Department of Medicine, Elmhurst Hospital, Queens, New York, NY, USA

© The Author(s), under exclusive license to Springer Nature Switzerland AG 2024
H. Kramer et al. (eds.), *Kidney Disease in the Elderly*,
https://doi.org/10.1007/978-3-031-68460-9_10

protein, large blood, moderate leukocytes, and few epithelial cells. Serum albumin was 3.6 mg/dL. Her primary care physician suggested patient stop enalapril and furosemide, which were used for blood pressure control. Her repeated SCr improved slightly after stopping the medications. Despite the clinical improvement, the nephrologist sent out serological tests for glomerulonephritis (GN) workup and asked the patient to return the following week.

General Consideration of Glomerular Disease in the Elderly Patients

As life expectancy continues to increase worldwide, understanding kidney diseases in the elderly population to provide better clinical care has become an area of vigorous research. One of the challenges to prompt recognition of kidney diseases in elderly patients is the confounding effects of nephron loss and associated eGFR declines with aging. In one study performed on community-dwelling older adults, the rates of eGFR decline of men and women without diabetes were 0.8 and 1.4 mL/min/1.73 m^2 per year [1], respectively, and the eGFR decline was faster in the presence of chronic kidney disease (CKD). Podocyte loss has been implicated in kidney aging and is associated with increasing proteinuria in elderly patients [2]. Common comorbidities in the elderly, including diabetes mellitus (DM) and hypertension (HTN), also lead to proteinuria. Since clinical clues of active glomerular diseases (decline of eGFR and proteinuria) might be present at the time of diagnosis, nephrologists will need to obtain a comprehensive history and diligently compare previous laboratory data, if available, to correctly diagnose glomerular disease with acute pathology in the elderly patients.

Indication of Kidney Biopsy in the Elderly Patients

The misconception that advanced age is unfavorable for kidney biopsy has been disputed after a landmark study by Moutzouris et al. [3], in which the authors found that the results of a kidney biopsy potentially changed the clinical management for two-thirds of cohort patients. In addition, the risks of bleeding after kidney biopsy in the elderly did not differ from younger patients in a small prospective study [4]. Nevertheless, cessation of anti-platelet or anti-coagulation agents is needed perioperatively based on clinical history.

Table 10.1 summarizes the proposed general criteria for kidney biopsy and common indications for considering kidney biopsy in the geriatric population. Given the limited kidney biopsy data in elderly patients, the true prevalence of each diagnosis might vary depending on the indication of biopsy and inclusion criteria. For instance, pauci-immune glomerulonephritis (GN) was the most common diagnosis among

Table 10.1 General indications for kidney biopsy in geriatric population

Criteria for kidney biopsy	Common indication for kidney biopsy in the elderly
• A kidney biopsy is required to make a diagnosis or provide information that guides treatment	• Acute eGFR decline out of proportion to natural loss from aging
• The natural history of suspected diseases is associated with significant morbidity and/or mortality	• Proteinuria and/or hematuria
• The natural history of these diseases can be improved with therapy	• Active urinary sediment
• The treatments for these diseases differ between diagnosis that are made by kidney biopsy	
• The treatments' adverse event profiles are acceptable to your patients in his/her current state of health	
• The risk of the procedure is acceptable to your patient in his/her current state of health	

Adapted from Berns et al. [5] and Abrass [6]

Table 10.2 Indications for kidney biopsy and most common findings in the very elderly patients (more than 80 years of age)

Indications for kidney biopsy	Most common pathological diagnosis
Acute kidney injury (46.4%)	Pauci-immune GN
Chronic kidney injury (23.8%)	FSGS secondary to HTN/aging
Nephrotic syndrome (13.2%)	Membranous nephropathy
Acute kidney injury and nephrotic syndrome (9.4%)	Minimal change disease
Proteinuria (5.5%)	HTN nephrosclerosis
Proteinuria and hematuria (1.3%)	Membranous nephropathy

Data adapted from Moutzouris et al. [3]

patients with acute kidney injury (AKI). In contrast, focal segmental glomerulosclerosis (FSGS), likely caused by chronic HTN, was frequently seen in patients with CKD (Table 10.2) [3]. In this chapter, we will divide glomerular diseases in the elderly into nephrotic and nephritic syndromes, followed by a summary of the use of immunosuppression in elderly patients.

Glomerular Diseases with Nephrotic Syndrome

Diabetic Kidney Disease

The prevalence of diabetes mellitus (DM) with kidney complications, or diabetic kidney disease (DKD), are estimated to affect 41.3% of those aged >65 and more than 60% of those aged >75 [7]. Diagnosis of DKD is based on history and laboratory findings and usually does not require a kidney biopsy. However, a kidney biopsy might be necessary to rule out other glomerular diseases in patients with atypical features such as proteinuria without proliferative retinopathy, sudden onset proteinuria, or rapid progression of kidney impairment. Similar to younger adult patients, the treatment goal of DKD is to ameliorate disease progression to ESKD via appropriate glycemic and blood pressure control. However, it is important to consider other risk factors such as increased frailty, risks of hypoglycemia, and polypharmacy in this unique population. Some experts suggested that a higher glycemic target with hemoglobin A1c (HbA1c) <8.0% might be appropriate for elderly patients [8]. Therefore, clinicians should recognize underlying risk factors before treatment initiation and adjust the goals accordingly.

With regard to the treatment, the use of renin-angiotensin-aldosterone system (RAAS) blockade, including angiotensin-converting enzyme inhibitors (ACEi) and angiotensin receptor blockers (ARB), remains the standard of care for DKD. After a long pause of approved new treatment for kidney diseases, sodium-glucose cotransporter 2 inhibitors (SGLT2i) have demonstrated substantial renoprotective and cardiovascular benefits, in addition to improving glycemic control. In older patients, the use of SGLT2i achieved a 0.4% reduction in hemoglobin A1c [9]. In addition, subgroup analysis based on age in the EMPA-REG OUTCOME [10] and DECLARE-TIMI 58 [11] trials confirmed the preventive effects of SGLT2i on cardiovascular outcomes regardless of age, and there were no increased incidences of ketoacidosis among patients aged >65 years. However, data regarding the risks of genital and urinary tract infection (UTI) among elderly patients were conflicting [12], consistent with a later finding from a large cohort that no apparent increased risks of UTI among all adult patients [13]. Lastly, concurrent use of diuretics with SGLT2i should be carefully monitored for AKI mediated by overt volume depletion.

FSGS/HTN

Focal segmental glomerulosclerosis (FSGS) is a group of diseases histologically characterized by podocyte foot process effacement and one or more glomerulosclerosis seen in one kidney biopsy sample. FSGS is considered one of the leading causes of nephrotic syndromes in adults of all ages and a major cause of ESKD [14, 15]. To date, FSGS is classified by the etiologies (primary, secondary, genetic, and FSGS of unknown cause) [16] or by the histological findings according to the Columbia classification [17]. However, the true prevalence of each category remains unclear largely due to different nomenclature used in the literature.

Among the elderly, a series of kidney biopsies reported that primary FSGS is present in only 5.4% of patients over 60 years with nephrotic syndrome [18] and approximately 3.9% among patients aged 80 years or older [3]. The major form of FSGS in older adults is secondary, caused by chronic adaptive changes from hypertension, vascular disease, and obesity. In addition, prior exposure to interferons or intravenous bisphosphonates (especially pamidronate) can also lead to drug-induced

FSGS [19]. Histologically, tip lesions are more prevalent in older adults, particularly individuals with white race/ethnicity [17, 20]. Tip lesions tend to have diffuse foot process effacement but the least amount of tubular atrophy and interstitial fibrosis. Thus, patients with tip lesions usually respond to glucocorticoid therapy well and have the lowest risk for disease progression. On the contrary, collapsing FSGS tends to have a more aggressive course and more tubulointerstitial injury, leading to poor response and prognosis [21]. A retrospective study in patients aged 65 or older with biopsy-proven collapsing glomerulopathy showed a median of 40% globally and 16% segmentally sclerotic glomeruli, which was higher than the average of the younger counterpart [22]. It is important to note that the risk alleles of *APOL1* are associated with collapsing FSGS and might partly explain hypertensive glomerulosclerosis, especially in patients of African descent [23].

The general approach to patients with primary or secondary FSGS includes RAAS blockade, dietary sodium restriction, and blood pressure control. High-dose glucocorticoids could be considered for those with primary FSGS and nephrotic range proteinuria or nephrotic syndrome [16]. To minimize the potential toxicity of daily high-dose steroids, Nagai et al. [24] assessed high-dose alternate-day steroid therapy in a group of 61 to 78-year-old patients ($n = 17$) with "idiopathic FSGS" and found that 44% of participants attained a complete remission after 3–5 months of therapy. CNI could be used as the alternative if high-dose corticosteroid is contraindicated.

Membranous Nephropathy

Membranous nephropathy (MN) is the most common cause of nephrotic syndrome in adults of all ages, with a predominance in white and male patients. The prevalence peaks in adults between 50 and 60 years of age, and about 20–40% of kidney biopsies obtained from elderly patients with nephrotic syndrome showed MN [25–27]. Therefore, it is important to rule out MN secondary to malignancy, especially from solid tumors, due to high incidences of secondary MN in elderly patients [28]. Regardless of primary or secondary etiology, the pathological findings are characterized by the presence of diffuse granular electron-dense immune-complex deposits along the subepithelial surface of the glomerular capillary wall. In primary MN, several podocyte antigenic targets with circulating autoantibodies have been identified. Of these, M-type phospholipase A2 receptor (PLA2R) and thrombospondin type 1 domain–containing 7A (THSD7A) account for approximately 70% and 1–5% of MN cases, respectively [25]. For the remaining 15–20% of cases, efforts have been made to identify the causal antigens/antibodies. Of interest, some of the other putative antigens have been found to be mostly in older adults, namely protocadherin 7 (PCDH7) and serine protease high-temperature requirement A1 (HTRA1). A study by Sethi et al. estimated that the prevalence of PCDH7-associated MN is approximately 1.6–2% and that the mean age for this subtype was 61 (SD ± 11.7) years [29]. Similarly, HTRA1-associated MN may explain 1–2% of all suspected primary MN cases, and the mean age for this cohort was 67.3 years [30]. Thus, the recognition of novel antibody/antigenic targets has not only provided insight into the pathophysiology of this disease but also aided in the diagnosis of MN.

Clinically, elderly patients with primary MN have a similar presentation compared with younger adults, apart from decreased GFR and a higher prevalence of hypertension. It has been estimated that between 65% and 87% of elderly patients with membranous nephropathy present with nephrotic syndrome, and 25–50% have hypertension [31, 32]. Interestingly, while in the elderly there is a decreased kidney reserve at the onset of MN, which may impact their risk stratification for disease progression, the rate of decline in kidney function was similar to younger patients [33]. Therapeutic options and outcomes were also similar in older and younger individuals [34]. According to current KDIGO guidelines, all patients with MN and proteinuria should receive conservative therapy with dietary salt and protein restriction, maximally tolerated dose of ACEIs or ARBs, diuretics, and antihyperlipidemic agents [16]. These measures are especially pertinent for the elderly with multiple medical comorbidities, and risks of adverse effects from immunosuppression use are higher. For those at higher risks for disease progression, namely patients with eGFR <45 mL/min/1.73 m^2, increase in serum creatinine >25%, or persistent nephrotic syndrome (proteinuria >3.5 g/day and no decrease >50% after 6 months of conservative treatment), immunosuppressive treatment should be considered, especially if life expectancy is more than 5 years [19, 32]. The general practice for immunosuppression is to use rituximab or cyclophosphamide and alternate month glucocorticoids for 6 months, or calcineurin inhibitor (CNI)-based therapy for ≥6 months, with the choice of treatment depending on the risk estimate [16].

Minimal Change Disease

Minimal change disease (MCD) accounts for approximately 10–25% of adult-onset nephrotic syndrome [35]. A kidney biopsy is typically required to diagnose MCD in adult patients, given its lower prevalence compared to the pediatric population. The presence of diffuse effacement of podocyte foot processes on electron microscopy with negative immunofluorescence staining usually characterizes pathological findings. Yet, superimposed lesions such as arteriolonephrosclerosis or global glomerulosclerosis are commonly seen in adult and elderly patients due to concomitant diseases such as hypertension and diabetes [27]. Similar to MN, MCD is also associated with malignancy but more in hematological disorders such as lymphoma and leukemia [36]. The exact pathogenesis of primary MCD remains unclear but is possibly related to the dysregulated immune system [37]. Thus, in the adult MCD, clinicians should perform a careful history taking and review of medications to diagnose secondary MCD, which can be elicited by various causes including drugs (nonsteroidal anti-inflammatory drugs, antibiotics, lithium), infection, and hematologic malignancies.

Adult-onset MCD frequently presents with AKI, microscopic hematuria, and hypertension [38]. A retrospective review by Waldman et al. [39] on 95 patients with biopsy-proven primary adult-onset MCD (ages 19–78 years, mean age was 45.1 ± 1.6 years) at a single tertiary center showed that the subset of patients with "acute renal failure" (ARF; rise in serum creatinine to >50% baseline) were more likely to be male, older (mean age 54.5 ± 3.4 years), hypertensive with lower serum albumin, and greater protein excretion than those without ARF. Stefan et al. [40] demonstrated that in adults older than 50 with MCD, the presence of vascular lesions (i.e. renal artery atherosclerosis and/or small arterial and arteriolar lesions) and tubulointerstitial fibrosis further increased the susceptibility to AKI.

The treatment for elderly patients with MCD is similar to adult-onset MCD with high-dose oral glucocorticoids. If there are contraindications for glucocorticoid use as the first-line treatment, cyclophosphamide or CNI may be considered [16]. Growing evidence also supports rituximab used as first-line therapy, but data in adult patients are limited [41]. In general, the relapse rate in adult-onset MCD remains high. Approximately 50–75% of all adults who respond to glucocorticoids have a relapsing episode, 10–25% become frequent relapsers (defined as two or more relapses within 6 months or four or more times within 12 months), and 14–30% become steroid-dependent (relapsing within 2 weeks of glucocorticoid therapy). Interestingly, some reports have suggested that relapsing episodes were lower in the older (above 40- or 50-year-old) versus younger patients [42, 43]. Adults who do relapse are usually retreated with the initial regimen of glucocorticoids. For frequently relapsing or steroid-dependent MCD, the recommendation is to use either cyclophosphamide (preferred second-line agent based on extrapolation of studies in children; remission rate 50–80%), CNIs, mycophenolate, or rituximab. Finally, a repeat biopsy might be necessary to rule out other pathological processes such as FSGS, which confers a worse prognosis [38, 44].

Glomerular Diseases with Nephritic Syndrome

ANCA-Associated Vasculitis

ANCA-associated vasculitis (AAV) is a constellation of diseases that involve inflammation and damage to small or medium-sized vessels in the presence of circulating ANCA autoantibodies. Based on the involved vessels, autoantibodies, and clinical presentations, AAV is classified into three major diagnoses: granulomatosis with polyangiitis (GPA), microscopic polyangiitis (MPA), and eosinophilic GPA (EGPA, previously known as Churg-Strauss syndrome) (Table 10.3) [45]. The incidence of AAV is approximately 20/million and has a heavy regional distribution. MPA is more common in Southern Europe and Asia, while GPA bias toward Europe [47]. Of note, the prevalence of AAV substantially increases with age, likely due to certain environmental exposure triggering autoimmunity [48]. The highest risk age

Table 10.3 Common features of ANCA-associated casculitis disease [45, 46]

	Disease features
Microscopic polyangiitis (MPA)	– Necrotizing glomerulonephritis – Pulmonary capillaritis – Non-granulomatous inflammation – MPO+: 58%, PR3+ 26%
Granulomatosis with polyangiitis (GPA)	– Necrotizing glomerulonephritis – Pulmonary capillaritis – Ocular vasculitis – Upper respiratory tract involvement – Granulomatous and non-granulomatous inflammation – PR3+: 66%, MPO+: 24%
Eosinophilic granulomatosis with polyangiitis (EGPA)	– Eosinophilic rich and necrotizing granulomatous inflammation – Typically involves the upper respiratory tract – Asthma is common – Eosinophilia present – Glomerular disease associated with ANCA positivity

of developing AAV occurs in the population aged 65–74, with an incidence as high as 60.1/million [47]. Consistent with the epidemiological data, AAV (or pauci-immune vasculitis) is the most common finding of kidney biopsy among older patients, especially in those who presented with AKI and nephritis [3, 20, 49]. Clinical manifestations between elderly and young patients are largely similar, though elderly patients are more frequently diagnosed with MPA (with the positivity of MPO autoantibody) rather than GPA and more severe kidney involvement [50, 51]. As such, elderly patients have a higher risk of death after 6 months of diagnosis [52], and older age, higher creatinine, and lower Birmingham Vasculitis Activity Score were associated with poor outcomes [53].

Given the significant mortality and high likelihood of progression to ESKD [46], induction therapy that typically combines pulse glucocorticoids with cyclophospha-mide- or rituximab-based treatment should be immediately initiated if no contrain-dications. An important study by Weiner et al. reported that in patients aged 75 years or older with the diagnosis of GPA or MPA, receipt of standard immunosuppressive regimens (cyclophosphamide or rituximab-based induction therapy) was associated with significantly better outcomes compared to no immunosuppression treatment [53]. However, the mortality within the first 3 months remained high and was related to the complications of immunosuppression such as infections (Table 10.4). Thietart et al. recently evaluated the outcome of rituximab-based induction and maintenance therapy in patients older than 75 [57]. Despite the promising high remission and low relapse rate, the incidence of serious infections and death remained high in patients who received combined glucocorticoid and rituximab. Therefore, balancing suffi-cient immunosuppression and preventing treatment-related complications continues to be a clinical challenge in treating elderly patients with AAV. Newer agents, such as the C5a receptor antagonist, was non-inferior to standard corticosteroid tapering

Table 10.4 Clinical outcomes for treated elderly patients with ANCA-associated vasculitis

	Harper and Savage [51]	Pagnoux et al. [54]	Chen et al. [50]	Bomback et al. [55]	Harris et al. [56]	Weiner et al. [53]	Thietart et al. [57]
N	114	22	99	50	43	151	93
Age (mean, median)	70 (65–90)	79 ± 3	72 ± 5.6	83 ± 2.7	72 ± 6	79 (77–82)	79 (76.7–83.1)
Creatinine	7.5	2.5	4.5	4.5	6.7	3.2	2.0
Death (1 year)	29	32	–	47	39	29	–
Death (2 years)	–	36	48	56	–	35	9.5
ESRD (1 year)	30	–	31	36	32	25	–
Remission (%)	26	–	15	49	78	–	86.4
Relapse (%)	26	–	15	4.3	19		3
Infection (%)	40	–	–	38	39	–	19.7%

Adapted from "Treating Elderly Patients with ANCA-Associated Vasculitis" by Jefferson [58]

after initial cyclophosphamide or rituximab treatment [59]. Given their milder immunosuppressive effects and more specific targets, the C5a receptor antagonist might be of future interest, particularly in elderly patients, to avoid prolonged exposure to corticosteroids.

Systemic Lupus Erythematosus

Systemic lupus erythematosus (SLE) is an autoimmune disease that disproportionately presents in women of childbearing age, with a six-to-tenfold female predominance in the ages of 16–64. Still, 6–19% of SLE cases are diagnosed after 50, with a consistent female predominance (5:1) [60–63]. In the elderly, the presentation of SLE is more insidious. Most patients present with non-specific symptoms such as fever, lymphadenopathy, and weight loss, which could be misdiagnosed with other diseases such as malignancy [64–67]. Meanwhile, lupus nephritis, malar rash, and discoid lupus, considered characteristic in younger patients, are relatively rare in the elderly. Clinicians should also consider drug-induced SLE, particularly in older patients with polypharmacy [68]. Like SLE in the elderly, drug-induced SLE typically presents with arthritis or serositis and less commonly manifests as nephritis.

SLE in the elderly is diagnosed through similar serological features, including anti-nuclear antibody (ANA), anti-double stranded DNA (anti-dsDNA), and hypocomplementemia. ANA tends to be present in 67–100% of elderly onset SLE patients. However, ANA has poor sensitivity, as seen in the younger population and other rheumatological diseases such as rheumatoid arthritis (RA). Contrary to the younger population of individuals with SLE, anti-dsDNA and hypocomplementemia are less common. Overall, lupus nephritis remains a rare condition in the elderly. In the epidemiologic biopsy series performed on elderly patients, lupus nephritis was found as the pathologic lesion between 1.5% and 4% of biopsies in individuals with either nephrotic or nephritic syndrome [20, 49]. Given the paucity of data, treatment for lupus nephritis among the elderly remains the same as for younger individuals, with combined pulse glucocorticoids and cyclophosphamide or mycophenolate mofetil [69].

IgA Nephropathy

IgA nephropathy (IgAN) is the most common form of GN worldwide, with an estimated prevalence of 0.2–5 persons per 100,000 per year. The disease has a higher prevalence in East Asian countries, with large biopsy series demonstrating IgAN representing around 50% of newly diagnosed GN and a lower prevalence in North America [70, 71]. The incidence of IgAN in the elderly has increased over the past 25 years. However, this may be confounded by increasing lifespans and better tolerance for kidney biopsy [72]. The exact pathogenesis of IgAN remains elusive and more likely to be multifactorial. More data suggested that the aberrant glycosylation of IgA secreted by B cells located in the mucosal-associated lymphoid tissue (MALT) forms immune complexes with circulating IgA autoantibodies. These immune complexes subsequently deposit in the kidneys and ultimately activate complement pathways leading to glomerular injury [73]. IgAN can be primary or secondary due to diseases such as inflammatory bowel disease, malignancies (e.g., lymphoma, lung cancer, IgA multiple myeloma), autoimmune diseases (e.g., ankylosing spondylitis, rheumatoid arthritis), or pulmonary diseases (e.g., sarcoidosis, idiopathic pulmonary fibrosis). Patients typically present with microscopic hematuria and proteinuria. AKI is common, and rarely rapidly progressive GN (RPGN) can occur in patients with crescentic lesions on the kidney biopsy [74].

In the elderly, IgAN tends to be associated with more severe kidney disease than in the younger population. Several studies have compared the clinical findings of IgAN in the elderly versus the younger population [20, 75, 76]. Clinically, the elderly population presents with more hypertension, nephrotic range proteinuria, and AKI than younger populations. Although some biopsy series reported a higher degree of globally sclerotic glomeruli and tubular injury in the elderly without a significant increase in crescents [76], IgAN in the elderly can still be necrotizing and crescentic GN [77]. Ultimately, the risk factor for progression to ESKD was almost twice as likely for the elderly, with increased risks of infection and mortality [72]. The treatment of IgAN in the elderly is similar to that in younger patients. RAAS blockade should be initiated for blood pressure control and proteinuria, yet the benefit of RAAS blockade is unclear in patients with normotension or proteinuria <0.5 g/day [19, 78]. SGLT2 inhibitors can be considered based on a recent subgroup analysis evaluating kidney outcomes of those with IgAN. However, only 16% of this subgroup was older than 64; therefore, more studies are needed to verify the findings [79]. Targeted-released budesonide, a form of corticosteroid released in the distal ileum, was recently approved to treat patients with IgAN. However, the initial study population's average age was between 30 and 40 years old [80]. The most recent report included patients with a wider range of ages, although more than 50% of the study patients were younger than 45 [81]. Thus, whether budesonide could achieve similar responses in elderly patients needs further validation. Lastly, for patients presenting with RPGN, pulse glucocorticoids and additional immuno-suppression should be considered similar to other RPGNs such as AAV [19, 20].

Use of Immune Modulating Agents in Elderly Patients

Immunosuppressive medications are the mainstay of treatment for virtually all immune-mediated GN. In this section, we will outline the major immunosuppression medications, as well as several novel treatments currently undergoing clinical trials. In general, immunosuppressive agents increase the risks of infections, and antimicrobial prophylaxis is required to prevent opportunistic infections. Elderly patients are particularly susceptible to adverse effects from immunosuppression, careful evaluation is warranted prior to treatment initiation [58].

Glucocorticoid

High-dose glucocorticoids are used as the initial treatment for various GN. By inhibiting leukocyte trafficking and function, glucocorticoids can quickly suppress the overactive immune system to ameliorate acute damage [82]. However, major adverse effects from chronic glucocorticoid exposure substantially limit its prolonged use, and therefore rapid tapering followed by a glucocorticoid-sparing agent is usually necessary. For example, the TESTING trial revealed the potential kidney benefits of treating patients with IgAN (proteinuria of 1 g/day or greater) with glucocorticoids compared to supportive therapy. However, the excessively severe infections led to the early termination of the trial, albeit in a fairly young population [83]. Two clinical trials of AAV [rituximab in ANCA-associated vasculitis (RAVE) [84] and rituximab versus cyclophosphamide in ANCA-associated vasculitis (RITUXVAS) [85] used a standard glucocorticoid regimen (1–3 g of methylpred-nisolone followed by 1 mg/kg prednisone tapered to 5 mg over 6 months) combined with other immunosuppressants as the induction therapy. The patient population of the RITUXIVAS trial was older than the RAVE trial, with a median age of 67 and early 50s, respectively. Despite the relatively low rates of adverse events in both studies, high-dose glucocorticoids remained the major cause of adverse events. Most recently, the PEXIVAS trial (evaluating the use of plasmapheresis and reduced-dose glucocorticoids in AAV) adapted a more rapid tapering of glucocorticoids and demonstrated that the reduced-dose regimen was non-inferior to the standard-dose regimen in death and ESKD [86]. Meanwhile, the investigators of the initial TESTING trial redesigned the study with a reduced-dose glucocorticoid regiment (TESTING Low-Dose Study). Compared to the placebo, glucocorticoid treatment for patients with IgAN at high risk of progression resulted in a consistent and improved kidney outcome [87]. In addition, the side effects and major infection were less common in patients receiving reduced-dose glucocorticoids. Although the currently available data on elderly patients are scarce, promising results from the more rapid tapering protocols should be considered when treating elderly patients. Lastly, other prophylactic measures to prevent opportunistic infections, vitamin D supplements, and anti-acid therapy should be routinely given similarly to younger patients.

Cyclophosphamide

Cyclophosphamide, a cytotoxic alkylating agent, is historically the first-line treatment for severe rheumatologic diseases such as AAV and lupus nephritis. Given the rise of alternative, less toxic immunosuppressive medications, cyclophosphamide has gradually fallen out of favor as the first-line immunosuppressant. It is now occasionally reserved for severe disease refractory to other immunosuppressants. If needed, the total cumulative dose per patient should not exceed 10 g. A prior cohort study demonstrated that patients who received a total cumulative dose of >10 g had an increased risk of malignancy compared to the general population [88]. Prominent adverse reactions of cyclophosphamide use include cytopenia, infection, gonadal toxicity, teratogenicity, hemorrhagic cystitis, and hyponatremia. In addition, observational studies on a cohort of the elderly have shown an increased rate of malignancy compared to the general population, with significantly high risks of bladder cancer and pancreatic cancer [88]. Most importantly, the dose of cyclophosphamide needs to be adjusted according to GFR, which is typically lower in elderly patients.

Rituximab

Rituximab is a monoclonal antibody against CD20 (a transmembrane protein found on pre and mature B-lymphocytes), which leads to apoptosis of these cells and, ultimately, B cell depletion lasting around 24 weeks [89]. Given its mechanism of action, rituximab induces prolonged B cell depletion and pan-hypogammaglobulinemia, putting individuals at higher risks for opportunistic infections such as pneumocystis, as well as reactivation of tuberculosis (TB) and hepatitis B. Thus, prior to its use, individuals should be screened for TB and hepatitis B infection [90]. Given the severe side effects with cyclophosphamide and glucocorticoids, rituximab has been evaluated as primary treatment for glomerular diseases such as AAV, in which studies have shown non-inferiority as the induction therapy in both general and elderly populations [84, 85, 91–93]. However, it is important to point out that despite a lower incidence of leukopenia in patients receiving rituximab, the infection rate remained similar between cyclophosphamide and rituximab arms in both RAVE and RITUXVAS trials. In addition, rituximab has been used as the first-line treatment for membranous nephropathy [94, 95]. Some case reports demonstrated encouraging results using rituximab to treat glucocorticoid-resistant minimal change disease, focal segmental glomerulosclerosis, and lupus nephritis. Nevertheless, this data was reported in younger populations given the disease demographics, and more data is required to assess its efficacy in elderly patients [41, 96].

Calcineurin Inhibitors

Calcineurin Inhibitors (CNI) such as tacrolimus and cyclosporine are T-cell inhibitors that have longstanding use in the organ transplant population. CNIs are mostly used as a glucocorticoid-sparing agent in glucocorticoid-dependent or resistant patients or as a multitarget therapy in lupus nephritis [97]. Animal studies also demonstrated the non-immunological effects of CNIs that facilitate podocyte remodeling and proteinuria mitigation [98]. Typically, CNIs are dosed orally once to twice daily depending on formulation, and doses need to be adjusted according to the serum trough level. In a cohort of kidney transplant recipients, the CNI trough levels were higher in older patients than that of younger patients, likely due to reduced metabolism from CYP3A4 [99]. Therefore, more frequent monitoring and adjustment might be warranted in elderly patients receiving CNI for primary glomerular diseases.

Mycophenolate Mofetil

Mycophenolate Mofetil (MMF) targets inosine monophosphate dehydrogenase and inhibits guanosine nucleotide synthesis necessary for lymphocyte proliferation. MMF is effective as induction therapy in lupus nephritis [100, 101], and its use for maintenance therapy has better outcome compared to azathioprine [102]. Similar effects have been demonstrated in a recent meta-analysis for ANCA-associated vasculitis [103]. Given its use in lupus nephritis, typically found in younger patients, data for the use of MMF in the elderly with glomerulonephritis is limited. However, in transplant patients, 66% of the elderly transplant patients required a dose reduction of MMF at 1 year, with almost half developing either leukopenia or gastrointestinal side effects [104].

Clinical Scenario Follow-Up

The patient returned to the clinic the following week and denied any new symptoms. Repeated SCr was stable at 1.87 mg/dL (eGFR: 25 mL/min/1.73 m^2). The serological tests were positive for anti-myeloperoxidase (anti-MPO) >100.0 U/mL. She underwent an urgent kidney biopsy demonstrating crescentic GN, acute tubular injury, FSGS, and moderate parenchymal scarring. She was tested negative for QuantiFERON, hepatitis B core antibody, and surface antigen. Given no apparent contraindication and stable physical condition, the nephrologist discussed with the patient and her family and agreed on immunosuppression treatment. She received four doses of rituximab infusion, pulse glucocorticoids according to RAVE trial, and appropriate prophylactic medications without complications.

Conclusion

Despite the rapidly aging population worldwide, research and clinical trials focusing on the geriatric population remain scarce, and recommended treatments are largely extrapolated from the data analyzed in the younger population. DKD remains the most common cause of nephrotic range proteinuria in elderly patients. Yet, clinicians should look out for any atypical presentations such as hematuria and rapid decline of kidney function. Given the high likelihood of frailty, cognitive impairment, and other comorbidities, it is important to carefully evaluate patients' general conditions and individualize therapeutic plans. Close monitoring of adverse effects from glucocorticoids or other immunosuppressants is particularly necessary to prevent severe infections. More targeted therapy and generalized patient selection in clinical trials might shed light in treating elderly patients with glomerular diseases in the future.

References

1. Hemmelgarn BR, Zhang J, Manns BJ, Tonelli M, Larsen E, Ghali WA, et al. Progression of kidney dysfunction in the community-dwelling elderly. Kidney Int. 2006;69(12):2155–61.
2. Shankland SJ, Wang Y, Shaw AS, Vaughan JC, Pippin JW, Wessely O. Podocyte aging: why and how getting old matters. J Am Soc Nephrol. 2021;32(11):2697–713.
3. Moutzouris DA, Herlitz L, Appel GB, Markowitz GS, Freudenthal B, Radhakrishnan J, et al. Renal biopsy in the very elderly. Clin J Am Soc Nephrol. 2009;4(6):1073–82.
4. Kohli HS, Jairam A, Bhat A, Sud K, Jha V, Gupta KL, et al. Safety of kidney biopsy in elderly: a prospective study. Int Urol Nephrol. 2006;38(3–4):815–20.
5. Hogan JJ, Mocanu M, Berns JS. The native kidney biopsy: update and evidence for best practice. Clin J Am Soc Nephrol. 2016;11(2):354–62.
6. Abrass CK. Chapter 10: Glomerular disease in the elderly; 2009.

7. Russo GT, De Cosmo S, Viazzi F, Mirijello A, Ceriello A, Guida P, et al. Diabetic kidney disease in the elderly: prevalence and clinical correlates. BMC Geriatr. 2018;18(1):38.
8. Strain WD, Hope SV, Green A, Kar P, Valabhji J, Sinclair AJ. Type 2 diabetes mellitus in older people: a brief statement of key principles of modern day management including the assessment of frailty. A national collaborative stakeholder initiative. Diabet Med. 2018;35(7):838–45.
9. Cintra R, Moura FA, Carvalho LSF, Barreto J, Tambascia M, Pecoits-Filho R, et al. Inhibition of the sodium-glucose co-transporter 2 in the elderly: clinical and mechanistic insights into safety and efficacy. Rev Assoc Med Bras (1992). 2019;65(1):70–86.
10. Monteiro P, Bergenstal RM, Toural E, Inzucchi SE, Zinman B, Hantel S, et al. Efficacy and safety of empagliflozin in older patients in the EMPA-REG OUTCOME(R) trial. Age Ageing. 2019;48(6):859–66.
11. Cahn A, Mosenzon O, Wiviott SD, Rozenberg A, Yanuv I, Goodrich EL, et al. Efficacy and safety of dapagliflozin in the elderly: analysis from the DECLARE-TIMI 58 Study. Diabetes Care. 2020;43(2):468–75.
12. Varshney N, Billups SJ, Saseen JJ, Fixen CW. Sodium-glucose cotransporter-2 inhibitors and risk for genitourinary infections in older adults with type 2 diabetes. Ther Adv Drug Saf. 2021;12:2042098621997703.
13. Dave CV, Schneeweiss S, Kim D, Fralick M, Tong A, Patorno E. Sodium-glucose cotransporter-2 inhibitors and the risk for severe urinary tract infections: a population-based cohort study. Ann Intern Med. 2019;171(4):248–56.
14. Kitiyakara C, Eggers P, Kopp JB. Twenty-one-year trend in ESRD due to focal segmental glomerulosclerosis in the United States. Am J Kidney Dis. 2004;44(5):815–25.
15. Haas M, Meehan SM, Karrison TG, Spargo BH. Changing etiologies of unexplained adult nephrotic syndrome: a comparison of renal biopsy findings from 1976-1979 and 1995-1997. Am J Kidney Dis. 1997;30(5):621–31.
16. Kidney Disease: Improving Global Outcomes (KDIGO) Glomerular Diseases Work Group. KDIGO 2021 clinical practice guideline for the management of glomerular diseases. Kidney Int. 2021;100(4S):S1–S276.
17. D'Agati VD, Kaskel FJ, Falk RJ. Focal segmental glomerulosclerosis. N Engl J Med. 2011;365(25):2398–411.
18. Hogg R, Middleton J, Vehaskari VM. Focal segmental glomerulosclerosis—epidemiology aspects in children and adults. Pediatr Nephrol. 2007;22(2):183–6.
19. Qian Q, Nasr SH. Diagnosis and treatment of glomerular diseases in elderly patients. Adv Chronic Kidney Dis. 2014;21(2):228–46.
20. Sumnu A, Gursu M, Ozturk S. Primary glomerular diseases in the elderly. World J Nephrol. 2015;4(2):263–70.
21. Meliambro K, Schwartzman M, Cravedi P, Campbell KN. The impact of histologic variants on FSGS outcomes. Int Sch Res Notices. 2014;2014:913690.
22. Kukull B, Avasare RS, Smith KD, Houghton DC, Troxell ML, Andeen NK. Collapsing glomerulopathy in older adults. Mod Pathol. 2019;32(4):532–8.
23. Friedman DJ, Pollak MR. APOL1 nephropathy: from genetics to clinical applications. Clin J Am Soc Nephrol. 2021;16(2):294–303.
24. Nagai R, Cattran DC, Pei Y. Steroid therapy and prognosis of focal segmental glomerulosclerosis in the elderly. Clin Nephrol. 1994;42(1):18–21.
25. Couser WG. Primary membranous nephropathy. Clin J Am Soc Nephrol. 2017;12(6):983–97.
26. Yokoyama H, Sugiyama H, Sato H, Taguchi T, Nagata M, Matsuo S, et al. Renal disease in the elderly and the very elderly Japanese: analysis of the Japan Renal Biopsy Registry (J-RBR). Clin Exp Nephrol. 2012;16(6):903–20.
27. Glassock RJ. An update on glomerular disease in the elderly. Clin Geriatr Med. 2013;29(3):579–91.

28. Lefaucheur C, Stengel B, Nochy D, Martel P, Hill GS, Jacquot C, et al. Membranous nephropathy and cancer: epidemiologic evidence and determinants of high-risk cancer association. Kidney Int. 2006;70(8):1510–7.

29. Sethi S, Madden B, Debiec H, Morelle J, Charlesworth MC, Gross L, et al. Protocadherin 7-associated membranous nephropathy. J Am Soc Nephrol. 2021;32(5):1249–61.

30. Al-Rabadi LF, Caza T, Trivin-Avillach C, Rodan AR, Andeen N, Hayashi N, et al. Serine protease HTRA1 as a novel target antigen in primary membranous nephropathy. J Am Soc Nephrology. 2021;32:1666.

31. O'Callaghan CA, Hicks J, Doll H, Sacks SH, Cameron JS. Characteristics and outcome of membranous nephropathy in older patients. Int Urol Nephrol. 2002;33(1):157–65.

32. Deegens JK, Wetzels JF. Membranous nephropathy in the older adult: epidemiology, diagnosis and management. Drugs Aging. 2007;24(9):717–32.

33. Zent R, Nagai R, Cattran DC. Idiopathic membranous nephropathy in the elderly: a comparative study. Am J Kidney Dis. 1997;29(2):200–6.

34. Abrass CK. Treatment of membranous nephropathy in the elderly. Semin Nephrol. 2003;23(4):373–8.

35. Cameron JS. Nephrotic syndrome in the elderly. Semin Nephrol. 1996;16(4):319–29.

36. Audard V, Larousserie F, Grimbert P, Abtahi M, Sotto JJ, Delmer A, et al. Minimal change nephrotic syndrome and classical Hodgkin's lymphoma: report of 21 cases and review of the literature. Kidney Int. 2006;69(12):2251–60.

37. Kim SH, Park SJ, Han KH, Kronbichler A, Saleem MA, Oh J, et al. Pathogenesis of minimal change nephrotic syndrome: an immunological concept. Korean J Pediatr. 2016;59(5):205–11.

38. Hogan J, Radhakrishnan J. The treatment of minimal change disease in adults. J Am Soc Nephrol. 2013;24(5):702–11.

39. Waldman M, Crew RJ, Valeri A, Busch J, Stokes B, Markowitz G, et al. Adult minimal-change disease: clinical characteristics, treatment, and outcomes. Clin J Am Soc Nephrol. 2007;2(3):445–53.

40. Stefan G, Busuioc R, Stancu S, Hoinoiu M, Zugravu A, Petre N, et al. Adult-onset minimal change disease: the significance of histological chronic changes for clinical presentation and outcome. Clin Exp Nephrol. 2021;25(3):240–50.

41. Xue C, Yang B, Xu J, Zhou C, Zhang L, Gao X, et al. Efficacy and safety of rituximab in adult frequent-relapsing or steroid-dependent minimal change disease or focal segmental glomerulosclerosis: a systematic review and meta-analysis. Clin Kidney J. 2021;14(4):1042–54.

42. Nakayama M, Katafuchi R, Yanase T, Ikeda K, Tanaka H, Fujimi S. Steroid responsiveness and frequency of relapse in adult-onset minimal change nephrotic syndrome. Am J Kidney Dis. 2002;39(3):503–12.

43. Tse KC, Lam MF, Yip PS, Li FK, Choy BY, Lai KN, et al. Idiopathic minimal change nephrotic syndrome in older adults: steroid responsiveness and pattern of relapses. Nephrol Dial Transplant. 2003;18(7):1316–20.

44. Korbet SM, Whittier WL. Management of adult minimal change disease. Clin J Am Soc Nephrol. 2019;14(6):911–3.

45. Jennette JC, Falk RJ, Bacon PA, Basu N, Cid MC, Ferrario F, et al. 2012 revised international Chapel Hill consensus conference nomenclature of vasculitides. Arthritis Rheum. 2013;65(1):1–11.

46. Lyons PA, Rayner TF, Trivedi S, Holle JU, Watts RA, Jayne DR, et al. Genetically distinct subsets within ANCA-associated vasculitis. N Engl J Med. 2012;367(3):214–23.

47. Watts RA, Lane SE, Bentham G, Scott DG. Epidemiology of systemic vasculitis: a ten-year study in the United Kingdom. Arthritis Rheum. 2000;43(2):414–9.

48. Kitching AR, Anders HJ, Basu N, Brouwer E, Gordon J, Jayne DR, et al. ANCA-associated vasculitis. Nat Rev Dis Primers. 2020;6(1):71.

49. Perkowska-Ptasinska A, Deborska-Materkowska D, Bartczak A, Stompor T, Liberek T, Bullo-Piontecka B, et al. Kidney disease in the elderly: biopsy based data from 14 renal centers in Poland. BMC Nephrol. 2016;17(1):194.

50. Chen M, Yu F, Zhang Y, Zhao MH. Antineutrophil cytoplasmic autoantibody-associated vasculitis in older patients. Medicine (Baltimore). 2008;87(4):203–9.
51. Harper L, Savage CO. ANCA-associated renal vasculitis at the end of the twentieth century—a disease of older patients. Rheumatology (Oxford). 2005;44(4):495–501.
52. Hoganson DD, From AM, Michet CJ. ANCA vasculitis in the elderly. J Clin Rheumatol. 2008;14(2):78–81.
53. Weiner M, Goh SM, Mohammad AJ, Hruskova Z, Tanna A, Bruchfeld A, et al. Outcome and treatment of elderly patients with ANCA-associated vasculitis. Clin J Am Soc Nephrol. 2015;10(7):1128–35.
54. Pagnoux C, Hogan SL, Chin H, Jennette JC, Falk RJ, Guillevin L, et al. Predictors of treatment resistance and relapse in antineutrophil cytoplasmic antibody-associated small-vessel vasculitis: comparison of two independent cohorts. Arthritis Rheum. 2008;58(9):2908–18.
55. Bomback AS, Appel GB, Radhakrishnan J, Shirazian S, Herlitz LC, Stokes B, et al. ANCA-associated glomerulonephritis in the very elderly. Kidney Int. 2011;79(7):757–64.
56. Haris A, Polner K, Aranyi J, Braunitzer H, Kaszas I, Mucsi I. Clinical outcomes of ANCA-associated vasculitis in elderly patients. Int Urol Nephrol. 2014;46(8):1595–600.
57. Thietart S, Karras A, Augusto JF, Philipponnet C, Carron PL, Delbrel X, et al. Evaluation of rituximab for induction and maintenance therapy in patients 75 years and older with antineutrophil cytoplasmic antibody-associated vasculitis. JAMA Netw Open. 2022;5(7):e2220925.
58. Jefferson JA. Treating elderly patients with ANCA-associated vasculitis. Clin J Am Soc Nephrol. 2015;10(7):1110–3.
59. Jayne DRW, Merkel PA, Schall TJ, Bekker P, Group AS. Avacopan for the treatment of ANCA-associated vasculitis. N Engl J Med. 2021;384(7):599–609.
60. Voulgari PV, Katsimbri P, Alamanos Y, Drosos AA. Gender and age differences in systemic lupus erythematosus. A study of 489 Greek patients with a review of the literature. Lupus. 2002;11(11):722–9.
61. Formiga F, Moga I, Pac M, Mitjavila F, Rivera A, Pujol R. Mild presentation of systemic lupus erythematosus in elderly patients assessed by SLEDAI. SLE Disease Activity Index. Lupus. 1999;8(6):462–5.
62. Catoggio LJ, Skinner RP, Smith G, Maddison PJ. Systemic lupus erythematosus in the elderly: clinical and serological characteristics. J Rheumatol. 1984;11(2):175–81.
63. Domenech I, Aydintug O, Cervera R, Khamashta M, Jedryka-Goral A, Vianna JL, et al. Systemic lupus erythematosus in 50 year olds. Postgrad Med J. 1992;68(800):440–4.
64. Maddison PJ. Systemic lupus erythematosus in the elderly. J Rheumatol Suppl. 1987;14(Suppl 13):182–7.
65. Ho CT, Mok CC, Lau CS, Wong RW. Late onset systemic lupus erythematosus in southern Chinese. Ann Rheum Dis. 1998;57(7):437–40.
66. Pu SJ, Luo SF, Wu YJ, Cheng HS, Ho HH. The clinical features and prognosis of lupus with disease onset at age 65 and older. Lupus. 2000;9(2):96–100.
67. Gossat DM, Walls RS. Systemic lupus erythematosus in later life. Med J Aust. 1982;1(7):297–9.
68. Greitemann B, Mues B, Polster J, Pauly T, Sorg C. Inflammatory reactions in primary osteoarthritis of the hip and total hip prosthesis loosening. Arch Orthop Trauma Surg. 1992;111(3):138–41.
69. Lazaro D. Elderly-onset systemic lupus erythematosus: prevalence, clinical course and treatment. Drugs Aging. 2007;24(9):701–15.
70. McGrogan A, Franssen CF, de Vries CS. The incidence of primary glomerulonephritis worldwide: a systematic review of the literature. Nephrol Dial Transplant. 2011;26(2):414–30.
71. Zhou FD, Zhao MH, Zou WZ, Liu G, Wang H. The changing spectrum of primary glomerular diseases within 15 years: a survey of 3331 patients in a single Chinese centre. Nephrol Dial Transplant. 2009;24(3):870–6.
72. Sevillano AM, Diaz M, Caravaca-Fontan F, Barrios C, Bernis C, Cabrera J, et al. IgA nephropathy in elderly patients. Clin J Am Soc Nephrol. 2019;14(8):1183–92.
73. Lai KN. Pathogenesis of IgA nephropathy. Nat Rev Nephrol. 2012;8(5):275–83.

74. Pattrapornpisut P, Avila-Casado C, Reich HN. IgA nephropathy: core curriculum 2021. Am J Kidney Dis. 2021;78(3):429–41.

75. Oshima Y, Moriyama T, Itabashi M, Takei T, Nitta K. Characteristics of IgA nephropathy in advanced-age patients. Int Urol Nephrol. 2015;47(1):137–45.

76. Wen YK, Chen ML. Differences in new-onset IgA nephropathy between young adults and the elderly. Ren Fail. 2010;32(3):343–8.

77. Heras M, Saiz A, Pardo J, Fernandez-Reyes MJ, Sanchez R, Alvarez-Ude F. [Rapidly progressive renal failure as the onset of an IgA nephropathy in an elderly patient]. Nefrologia. 2011;31(2):234–6.

78. Li PK, Kwan BC, Chow KM, Leung CB, Szeto CC. Treatment of early immunoglobulin A nephropathy by angiotensin-converting enzyme inhibitor. Am J Med. 2013;126(2):162–8.

79. Wheeler DC, Toto RD, Stefansson BV, Jongs N, Chertow GM, Greene T, et al. A pre-specified analysis of the DAPA-CKD trial demonstrates the effects of dapagliflozin on major adverse kidney events in patients with IgA nephropathy. Kidney Int. 2021;100(1):215–24.

80. Fellstrom BC, Barratt J, Cook H, Coppo R, Feehally J, de Fijter JW, et al. Targeted-release budesonide versus placebo in patients with IgA nephropathy (NEFIGAN): a double-blind, randomised, placebo-controlled phase 2b trial. Lancet. 2017;389(10084):2117–27.

81. Barratt J, Lafayette R, Kristensen J, Stone A, Cattran D, Floege J, et al. Results from part A of the multi-center, double-blind, randomized, placebo-controlled NefIgArd trial, which evaluated targeted-release formulation of budesonide for the treatment of primary immunoglobulin A nephropathy. Kidney Int. 2023;103(2):391–402.

82. Strehl C, Ehlers L, Gaber T, Buttgereit F. Glucocorticoids-all-rounders tackling the versatile players of the immune system. Front Immunol. 2019;10:1744.

83. Lv J, Zhang H, Wong MG, Jardine MJ, Hladunewich M, Jha V, et al. Effect of oral methylprednisolone on clinical outcomes in patients with IgA nephropathy: the TESTING Randomized Clinical Trial. JAMA. 2017;318(5):432–42.

84. Stone JH, Merkel PA, Spiera R, Seo P, Langford CA, Hoffman GS, et al. Rituximab versus cyclophosphamide for ANCA-associated vasculitis. N Engl J Med. 2010;363(3):221–32.

85. Jones RB, Tervaert JW, Hauser T, Luqmani R, Morgan MD, Peh CA, et al. Rituximab versus cyclophosphamide in ANCA-associated renal vasculitis. N Engl J Med. 2010;363(3):211–20.

86. Walsh M, Merkel PA, Peh CA, Szpirt WM, Puechal X, Fujimoto S, et al. Plasma exchange and glucocorticoids in severe ANCA-associated vasculitis. N Engl J Med. 2020;382(7):622–31.

87. Lv J, Wong MG, Hladunewich MA, Jha V, Hooi LS, Monaghan H, et al. Effect of oral methylprednisolone on decline in kidney function or kidney failure in patients with IgA nephropathy: the TESTING Randomized Clinical Trial. JAMA. 2022;327(19):1888–98.

88. Heijl C, Westman K, Hoglund P, Mohammad AJ. Malignancies in patients with antineutrophil cytoplasmic antibody-associated vasculitis: a population-based cohort study. J Rheumatol. 2020;47(8):1229–37.

89. Onrust SV, Lamb HM, Balfour JA. Rituximab. Drugs. 1999;58(1):79–88; discussion 9–90.

90. Nixon A, Ogden L, Woywodt A, Dhaygude A. Infectious complications of rituximab therapy in renal disease. Clin Kidney J. 2017;10(4):455–60.

91. Keogh KA, Wylam ME, Stone JH, Specks U. Induction of remission by B lymphocyte depletion in eleven patients with refractory antineutrophil cytoplasmic antibody-associated vasculitis. Arthritis Rheum. 2005;52(1):262–8.

92. Specks U, Merkel PA, Seo P, Spiera R, Langford CA, Hoffman GS, et al. Efficacy of remission-induction regimens for ANCA-associated vasculitis. N Engl J Med. 2013;369(5):417–27.

93. Guillevin L, Pagnoux C, Karras A, Khouatra C, Aumaitre O, Cohen P, et al. Rituximab versus azathioprine for maintenance in ANCA-associated vasculitis. N Engl J Med. 2014;371(19):1771–80.

94. Fervenza FC, Appel GB, Barbour SJ, Rovin BH, Lafayette RA, Aslam N, et al. Rituximab or cyclosporine in the treatment of membranous nephropathy. N Engl J Med. 2019;381(1):36–46.

95. van den Brand J, Ruggenenti P, Chianca A, Hofstra JM, Perna A, Ruggiero B, et al. Safety of rituximab compared with steroids and cyclophosphamide for idiopathic membranous nephropathy. J Am Soc Nephrol. 2017;28(9):2729–37.

96. Diaz-Lagares C, Croca S, Sangle S, Vital EM, Catapano F, Martinez-Berriotxoa A, et al. Efficacy of rituximab in 164 patients with biopsy-proven lupus nephritis: pooled data from European cohorts. Autoimmun Rev. 2012;11(5):357–64.

97. Zhang H, Liu Z, Zhou M, Liu Z, Chen J, Xing C, et al. Multitarget therapy for maintenance treatment of lupus nephritis. J Am Soc Nephrol. 2017;28(12):3671–8.

98. Peleg Y, Bomback AS, Radhakrishnan J. The evolving role of calcineurin inhibitors in treating lupus nephritis. Clin J Am Soc Nephrol. 2020;15(7):1066–72.

99. Jacobson PA, Schladt D, Oetting WS, Leduc R, Guan W, Matas AJ, et al. Lower calcineurin inhibitor doses in older compared to younger kidney transplant recipients yield similar troughs. Am J Transplant. 2012;12(12):3326–36.

100. Ginzler EM, Dooley MA, Aranow C, Kim MY, Buyon J, Merrill JT, et al. Mycophenolate mofetil or intravenous cyclophosphamide for lupus nephritis. N Engl J Med. 2005;353(21):2219–28.

101. Appel GB, Contreras G, Dooley MA, Ginzler EM, Isenberg D, Jayne D, et al. Mycophenolate mofetil versus cyclophosphamide for induction treatment of lupus nephritis. J Am Soc Nephrol. 2009;20(5):1103–12.

102. Dooley MA, Jayne D, Ginzler EM, Isenberg D, Olsen NJ, Wofsy D, et al. Mycophenolate versus azathioprine as maintenance therapy for lupus nephritis. N Engl J Med. 2011;365(20):1886–95.

103. Kuzuya K, Morita T, Kumanogoh A. Efficacy of mycophenolate mofetil as a remission induction therapy in antineutrophil cytoplasmic antibody: associated vasculitis—a meta-analysis. RMD Open. 2020;6(1):e001195.

104. Witek S, Malat G, Sawinski D, Sammons C, LaFratte C, Forte A, et al. Tolerability of mycophenolate mofetil in elderly kidney transplant recipients: a retrospective cohort study. Clin Transpl. 2022;36(7):e14671.

Chapter 11
CKD in Elderly: Bone and Mineral Metabolism

Marriam Ali and Pauline Camacho

Case Presentation

A 73-year-old woman with a history of hypertension, osteoarthritis and chronic kidney disease stage 3 presents for evaluation and management of osteoporosis following a compression fracture. The patient noted a history of back pain following a fall from standing height. Subsequent radiographs revealed a subacute L2 vertebral compression fracture which was managed conservatively with pain control. She denies previous fractures but notes her mother suffered a hip fracture at a similar age. She describes a 1-in height loss in the past year. She avoids exercise due to joint pain. She is lactose intolerant and does not take any supplements. She denies a history of smoking or alcohol use. She does not have acid reflux. Her medications include amlodipine and lisinopril. On exam, she is a thin, frail female with a cautious gate. Oropharynx reveals no dental abnormalities. There is minimal scoliosis and absence of vertebral point tenderness.

A bone density obtained prior to her visit reveals a *T*-score of −2.8 at the lumbar spine and −2.5 at mean femoral necks.

Additional serum and urine workup is below:

Serum calcium 9.0
Serum phosphorus 3.6
Serum creatinine 1.9
GFR 44 mL/min/1.73 m^2 (>60)
Vitamin D 19 (30–80)
Intact parathyroid hormone 80 (11–65)

M. Ali · P. Camacho (✉)
Endocrinology and Metabolism, Loyola Medicine Center, Maywood, IL, USA
e-mail: marriam.ali@lumc.edu

© The Author(s), under exclusive license to Springer Nature Switzerland AG 2024

H. Kramer et al. (eds.), *Kidney Disease in the Elderly*,
https://doi.org/10.1007/978-3-031-68460-9_11

SPEP without monoclonal spike
Bone-specific alkaline phosphatase 25 (11.6–42.7 unit/L)
Urine calcium 80 mg/24 h (100–300 mg/day)

Calcium Regulation and Bone Mineral Metabolism in CKD

Both aging and chronic kidney disease (CKD) can impact calcium and phosphate homeostasis and bone mineral metabolism through dysregulation of pathways involving vitamin D, parathyroid hormone (PTH), and fibroblast growth factor-23 (FGF-23) and increase risk for fractures, morbidity and mortality [1]. Below, we review the physiologic roles and interplay of these elements and the pathologic impact of CKD and/or aging on their function, as summarized in Table 11.1. This dysregulation ultimately leads to disrupted bone turnover and the, development of bone disease including chronic kidney disease–mineral and bone disorder (CKD-MBD) and osteoporosis.

The physiologic interplay of bone-related factors and the net impact of CKD on this homeostasis. FGF-23, fibroblast growth factor-23; CKD, chronic kidney disease; PTH, parathyroid hormone.

Calcium

Calcium is largely obtained through the normal adult diet and exists in circulation as ionized (~51%), protein-bound (~40%) and complexed (~10%) [2]. Calcium is obtained via intestinal absorption from dietary sources, through kidney reabsorption and bone resorption or turnover. These pathways are influenced by parathyroid hormone, vitamin D status and glomerular filtration rate as well as medications, volume status and lifestyle effects. In the kidney, calcium is filtered through the glomeruli and is primarily reabsorbed in the proximal tubule with about 10% via the distal convoluted tubule [3]. Vitamin D, parathyroid hormone, volume contraction and thiazide diuretics increase while loop diuretics and FGF-23 decreases the reabsorption of calcium by the kidney.

Table 11.1 Factors affecting calcium and phosphate levels

	Calcium	Phosphate	Parathyroid hormone	Vitamin D 1,25	FGF-23	Effect of CKD
Vitamin D 1,25	↑	↑	↓	–	↑	↓
Parathyroid hormone	↑	↓	–	↑	↑	↑
FGF-23	↓	↓	↓	↓	–	↑
CKD net effect	↓	↑	↑	↓	↑	–

Kidney function decline leads to decrease in active vitamin D (1,25 vitamin D), and increases in FGF-23, parathyroid hormone and protein-bound calcium loss. The net effect of kidney function decline is reduced circulating calcium and pathologically increased or decreased bone turnover, i.e. osteoporosis or adynamic bone disease, respectively.

Phosphate

Phosphate is primarily obtained through dietary absorption which is promoted by active vitamin D. Phosphate is primarily distributed within the bone and cells and excreted by the kidneys. Reabsorption is regulated by vitamin D which increases phosphate reabsorption in the kidneys. Contrarily, parathyroid hormone and FGF-23 promote excretion [4].

Decline in glomerular filtration rate (age-related and pathologic) leads to phosphate retention and hyperphosphatemia. To maintain balance, in early CKD, FGF-23 levels increase to promote renal phosphate excretion. In late stages of CKD, however, this compensation of higher FGF-23 levels is insufficient to maintain phosphate levels within a normal range. Additionally, hyperphosphatemia itself raises PTH and FGF-23 and suppresses hydroxylation of 25-OH vitamin D as well as decreases circulatory calcium [2]. This cascade of effects contribute to parathyroid hyperplasia and bone mineral dysregulation.

Vitamin D

Unlike calcium, western diets are a poor source of vitamin D. Without supplementation, the major source of vitamin D is through conversion of 7-deoxycholesterol to cholecalciferol (vitamin D_3) by ultraviolet radiation in sunlight. Insufficient sun exposure and absence of supplementation can lead to vitamin D deficiency or insufficiency. Diets can be supplemented with either cholecalciferol or ergocalciferol (vitamin D_2) which are subsequently converted to 25-hydroxyvitamin D by the liver, and further hydroxylated to the highly active form, 1,25 dihydroxyvitamin D (calcitriol) by 1,25-alpha hydroxylase in the kidney. This process is enhanced by PTH and inhibited by FGF-23 and hyperphosphatemia. Vitamin D promotes intestinal calcium and phosphate absorption while mediating PTH-induced bone resorption [5].

CKD reduces vitamin D activation through inhibition of 1 alpha hydroxylase, increased FGF-23 which further inhibits 1,25 vitamin D, and increased protein-bound vitamin D losses through the urine. Additionally, aging reduces skin renewal and intestinal absorption of vitamin D. In this manner, elderly patients can reduce fracture risk by 14–30% with vitamin D [6]. Similarly, supplementation with 1,25 vitamin D (calcitriol) is often indicated in patients with CKD.

Parathyroid Hormone

Intact parathyroid hormone (PTH) is produced by the four parathyroid glands located in the neck. PTH is metabolized in the liver and the inactive portion is excreted by the kidneys. When released into circulation, PTH is responsible for increasing serum calcium through accelerated bone turnover, simulation of 1-alpha-hydoxylation of vitamin D and increased renal tubular calcium reabsorption. It also decreases renal tubular phosphate reabsorption and increases FGF-23 gene expression [7]. The net effect of elevated PTH is increased serum calcium and decreased serum phosphorus. PTH synthesis is activated by hypocalcemia which is sensed by a calcium-sensing receptor on the parathyroid cells. It can also be stimulated by low circulating vitamin D levels or hyperphosphatemic states.

Parathyroid hormone can pathologically rise due to a parathyroid adenoma, defined as primary hyperparathyroidism, which has a higher occurrence with age. Decline in kidney function is associated with impaired phosphate excretion, reduced calcium reabsorption, and decreased vitamin D activation, all of which stimulate parathyroid hormone release, known as secondary hyperparathyroidism. As CKD advances, there is increased bone resistance to parathyroid hormone and ongoing secondary hyperparathyroidism, by which PTH levels rise to 150–300 p/mL (normal <65) to maintain healthy bone turnover [2]. In CKD, a level >300 pg/mL is an indication for treatment to suppress PTH synthesis. PTH suppression can be undertaken by supplementation of vitamin D 25-OH and 1,25 vitamin D as well as drugs that activate calcium-sensing receptors on the parathyroid gland, thereby reducing PTH synthesis or drugs that bind excess phosphate. This must be balanced in such a way to prevent oversuppression of PTH (PTH <150 pg/mL) resulting in adynamic bone disease or suppressed bone turnover.

Fibroblast Growth Factor-23 (FGF-23)

FGF-23 is a protein produced by osteoclasts and osteoblasts in bone and primarily influences phosphate homeostasis with an indirect role in calcium regulation. FGF-23 when bound to its receptor, stimulates renal tubular phosphate excretion, reduces 1a-hydroxylation of vitamin D, and suppresses PTH release [8]. The net effect of circulating FGF-23 is reduced phosphate and calcium levels in the blood. FGF-23 production is stimulated by active vitamin D, hyperphosphatemia, and parathyroid hormone. FGF-23 levels also rise in CKD.

In the elderly, abnormal levels of FGF-23 and resultant phosphate wasting can rarely be seen in mesenchymal tumors and lead to a form of bone disease known as tumor-induced osteomalacia. More commonly, elevated FGF-23 is seen in early and late stages of CKD and is associated with refractory secondary hyperparathyroidism. As noted earlier, secondary hyperparathyroidism is associated with dysregulated bone turnover (Fig. 11.1).

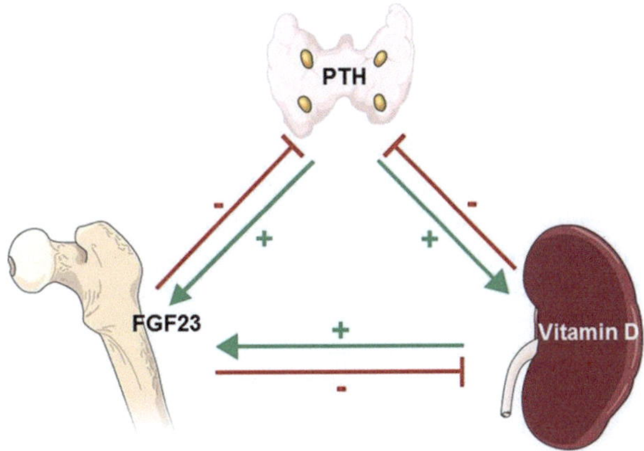

Fig. 11.1 Interplay of PTH, FGF-23 and active Vitamin D. (Adapted from Nutrients. 2013 May 29)

CKD-MBD

Bone disease in elderly patients with CKD occurs due to dysregulated calcium and phosphate balance through interplay between calcium, phosphate, parathyroid hormone, FGF-23 and calcitriol. Chronic kidney disease-mineral and bone disease is a systemic disorder that encompasses these bone metabolic abnormalities and is characterized by at least one of the following [9]:

- Abnormalities in serum calcium, phosphate, PTH, FGF-23 or vitamin D
- Abnormal bone turnover, mineralization, volume, and strength
- Vascular or soft tissue (extra skeletal) calcification

CKD-MBD then contributes to increased fracture risk, vascular calcifications, and ultimately all-cause mortality. The elderly CKD population is particularly vulnerable as CKD impacts premature aging and causes resultant age-associated cardiovascular and metabolic disease [10].

KDIGO recommends that CKD-MBD be categorized based on bone turnover, mineralization, and volume known as the TMV system.

Bone turnover describes the balance between bone formation and resorption and is dictated by PTH. The gold standard to assess bone turnover and the specific bone disorder involved in patients with CKD is via a bone biopsy. However, as bone biopsies are not readily available or cost effective, bone biomarkers are used as a surrogate for diagnosing and monitoring bone turnover. PTH in conjunction with bone-specific alkaline phosphatase can indicate underlying bone turnover and predict the underlying bone disease.

Bone turnover is defined the rate of bone resorption. Abnormalities in CKD-MBD range from high turnover states such as osteitis fibrosa cystica to low-turnover states such as adynamic bone disease. Mixed bone disease is characterized by features of high and low bone turnover. In the high turnover bone disease, known as osteitis fibrosa cystica, high levels of PTH increase bone turnover by activating

RANK on osteoclasts which, in turn, promotes bone resorption and inhibits osteoprotegerin which suppresses osteoclast activity [3]. In contrast, adynamic bone disease, characterized by low bone formation rates, is a state with reduced PTH levels, typically <150 pg/mL, decreased bone cellular activity and decreased turnover [11]. Adynamic bone disease is more often seen in those individuals with underlying diabetes and/or who are on peritoneal dialysis [3].

Both high and low turnover disorders of CKD-MBD are associated with increased fracture risk, calcium-phosphate product elevation, extraskeletal calcification as well as overall mortality [12, 13]. Another bone disorder known as osteomalacia is characterized by large amounts of osteoid material without appropriate mineralization, though is less frequently observed in elderly CKD patients.

Extraskeletal calcification including soft tissue and vascular calcification is a disorder of CKD-MBD and aging. Vascular calcification in particular is tightly associated with all-cause mortality by way of early onset of cardiovascular disease and diabetes.

The various bone disorders seen in CKD-MBD are summarized in the following table (Table 11.2).

Management Strategies

Consistent monitoring of serum calcium, phosphate, PTH, and vitamin D is necessary for older adults with CKD. Recommendations for treatment include replenishing vitamin D-deficient stores and ensuring adequate calcium intake of approximately 800–1000 mg daily. Serum calcium should be maintained in the normal range while mild hyperphosphatemia and hyperparathyroidism are permitted, <5.5 mg/dL and 150–300 pg/mL, respectively. Dietary modification to limit phosphate intake should be encouraged. Additionally, phosphate binders, calcimimetics such as cinacalcet, and/or active vitamin D can be utilized; titrated carefully to simultaneously limit excess bone turnover while avoiding the development of adynamic bone disease

Table 11.2 CKD-MBD defined by bone turnover

CKD-related bone disease	Features	Disorder	Manifestation
Osteitis fibrosa cystica	High turnover	Secondary hyperparathyroidism Tertiary hyperparathyroidism	Increased fracture risk, elevated calcium-phosphate product, extraskeletal calcification
Adynamic bone disease	Low turnover, decreased bone formation	Excessive PTH suppression. More common in peritoneal dialysis and diabetes	Increased fracture risk, elevated calcium-phosphate product, extraskeletal calcification
Osteomalacia	Low turnover, deficient mineralization	Associated with aluminum-containing phosphate binders, less common in elderly	

with these same agents. Additional fracture risk reduction strategies are discussed below.

Osteoporosis

CKD-MBD is associated with bone loss and fractures, both of which are additionally magnified by age and frailty. Thus, older adults with CKD are particularly vulnerable to the impact of osteoporosis, characterized by low bone mass, disrupted bone microarchitecture, skeletal fragility, and ultimately low trauma fractures. In fact, fracture incidence rates are more than fourfold higher and are associated with greater morbidity and mortality than the general population [2]. Therefore, fracture risk reduction in this growing population is prudent, and the management paradigm of CKD-related osteoporosis is shifting toward active monitoring and intervention.

Diagnosis of CKD-associated osteoporosis can be undertaken with a measurement of bone mineral density to assess fracture risk by dual-energy X-ray absorptiometry (DXA). Osteoporosis is diagnosed by a T-score < -2.5 on DXA, a T-score between -1.0 and -2.4 with an elevated fracture risk assessment tool (FRAX) score, or based on the clinical history of a low trauma fracture. The most recent KDIGO updates recommend measurement of bone mineral density (BMD) to assess fracture risk in patients with CKD-MBD or risk factors for fractures such as postmenopausal status, older age, use of glucocorticoids and low body mass index.

In patients with eGFR $\geq$30 mL/min without evidence of CKD-MBD, management is similar to patients without CKD. However, the management of CKD-associated osteoporosis is more complex. Regardless, management strategies should incorporate lifestyle optimization and balanced control of vitamin D deficiency, hyperphosphatemia, and hyperparathyroidism using the strategies outlined above. Beyond this, the addition of typical anti-fracture pharmacologic agents requires careful consideration as these medications are often cleared by the kidneys, can potentially increase the risk for hypocalcemia or adynamic bone disease, or simply, have not been adequately studied for benefit and safety in the CKD-MBD population. However, emerging bodies of evidence do suggest there is a role for specific anti-resorptive agents where the benefit may be greater than the risk for adynamic bone disease [14]. The aging population in which fragility fractures, reduced eGFR, and low BMD are common, may be of particular benefit.

The typical treatment approach is based on the presence or absence of CKD-MBD and specifically adynamic bone disease as employing pharmacologic agents that suppress bone turnover in a state of low bone turnover may not be beneficial. Traditionally, the gold standard for assessing bone turnover is conducted through a bone biopsy, which is limited by cost, availability, and patient comfort. Updated guidelines encourage the use of surrogates for bone biopsy to predict bone turnover in most cases. These markers include PTH and bone-specific alkaline phosphatase levels, both of which are associated with high bone turnover [15]. When the state of bone turnover remains unclear, a bone biopsy by an expert technician should be considered. A proposed algorithm published by the Clinical Journal of the American Society of Nephrology summarizes an approach for fracture risk screening and initiation of ant-fracture strategies in Fig. 11.2.

Anti-resorptive Agents

Bone resorption is mediated by the osteoclast activity. When there is normal to high turnover, pharmacologic agents that inhibit bone resorption may be helpful in preventing fracture.

Bisphosphonates

Bisphosphonates inhibit the synthesis of isoprenoid compounds essential to osteoclast function, resulting in osteoclast apoptosis or dysfunction. Given their high affinity for bone mineral, they are retained in the skeletal system for several years.

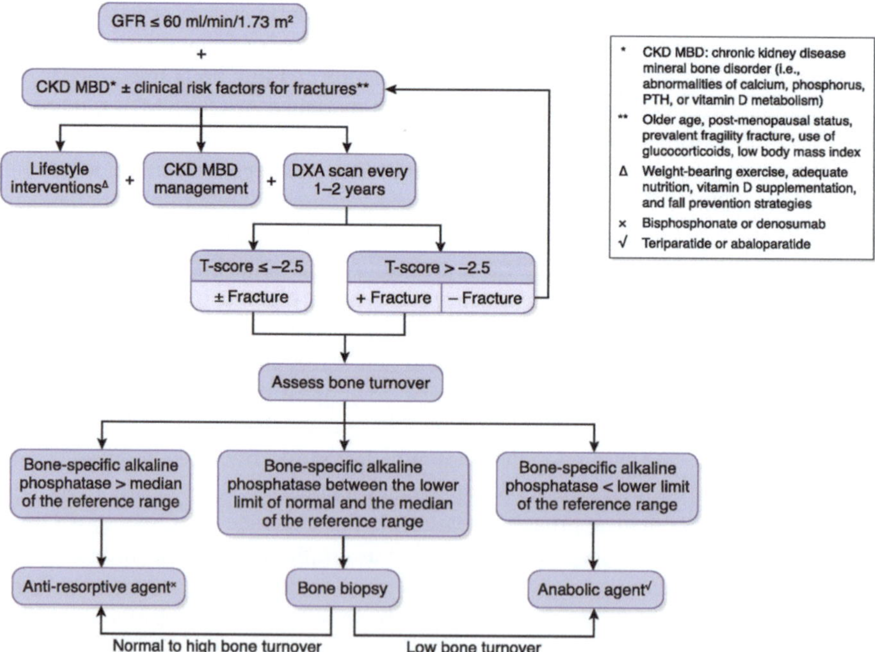

Fig. 11.2 Approach for fracture risk screening and initiation of anti-fracture risk strategies in patients with CKD. (Adapted from the Clinical Journal of the American Society of Nephrology. *CKD-MBD* CKD mineral and bone disease, *DXA* dual-energy X-ray absorptiometry, *PTH* parathyroid hormone [14])

The residual drug not taken up by bone is cleared by the kidneys. Therefore, at this time these medications are not recommended when eGFR <30 mL/min, to avoid potential oversuppression of bone turnover from drug accumulation [16]. Though more studies assessing bisphosphonate therapy specifically in the CKD-MBD population are needed, there is emerging data in post-hoc analyses that suggest improvement in lumbar BMD in patients with pre-dialysis CKD treated with bisphosphonate therapy [17–19]. Bisphosphonates are administered orally (weekly or monthly) or by annual intravenous infusion, typically for 3–5 years. Due to skeletal retention, drug holidays can be implemented without reversing the bone improvement.

Denosumab

Denosumab is a monoclonal antibody against RANK, thereby inhibiting osteoclast proliferation and development [14]. There is evidence that denosumab reduces vertebral and non-vertebral fracture risk reduction in postmenopausal women with age-related kidney function decline [20]. Because it is not cleared by the kidneys, there is less risk of oversuppression of bone remodeling and therefore unlike bisphosphonates, denosumab can be considered for lower GFR ranges. Given the potent effect of denosumab however, there is an increased risk for hypocalcemia, and thus calcium and vitamin D should be assessed prior to administration of denosumab. Hypocalcemia can be safely mitigated with adequate calcium and vitamin D supplementation. The typical course is 60 mg of denosumab administered every 6 months. Unlike bisphosphonates, denosumab is not retained for long periods of time and thus, its favorable skeletal improvements quickly reverse and place patients at risk for rebound fractures if dosing is delayed or discontinued [21]. The risk for rebound fractures increases with the duration of denosumab therapy, rendering denosumab cessation a safety concern. Therefore, patients should be encouraged to adhere to the dosing schedule, and subsequent antiresorptive treatment, often limited by kidney function, should be utilized if denosumab is discontinued.

Teriparatide and Abaloparatide

Anabolic agents such as teriparatide and abaloparatide are recombinant peptides of the PTH and PTH-rp, respectively [14]. When parathyroid hormone is administered in a pulsatile manner, it acts as an anabolic agent. As these therapeutics center on the bone formation arm of the remodeling process rather than bone turnover, there is potential utility for patients with advanced CKD and adynamic bone disease. These medications require pulsatile daily subcutaneous administration to maintain pulsatile exposure in the currently approved non-CKD-MBD population. Data for teriparatide in CKD-MBD is limited to small observational studies which showed increases in BMD at the spine and femoral including in patients with biopsy-proved adynamic bone disease [22, 23]. While abaloparatide was designed to be more purely anabolic, there is no data on its use in patients with CKD-MBD yet. Adverse

Table 11.3 Overview of available therapeutics for osteoporosis in CKD

Drug	Dosage	GFR cutoffs	Effect on mineral metabolism
Alendronate	35–70 mg per oral once weekly	eGFR ≥35 mL/min	Hypocalcemia, hypophosphatemia
Zoledronic acid	5 mg intravenous once yearly	eGFR ≥35 mL/min	Hypocalcemia, hypophosphatemia
Denosumab	60 mg subcutaneous every 6 months	Any eGFR	Hypocalcemia, hypophosphatemia
Teriparatide	20 µg subcutaneous daily	eGFR >30 mL/min	Hypercalcemia, hypercalciuria
Abaloparatide	80 µg subcutaneous daily	Any eGFR, not studied in ESRD	Hypercalcemia, hypercalciuria
Romosozumab	210 mg subcutaneous monthly	GFR >30 mL/min in trials, not studied in GFR <30 mL/min	

Adapted from Clinical Journal American Society of Nephrology with modifications

events that should be monitored if these agents are employed include hypercalcemia and hypercalciuria, which were seen more commonly in advanced CKD. These medications are administered as daily subcutaneous injections.

Romosozumab

Romosozumab is anti-sclerostin a monoclonal antibody that has both anti-resorptive and anabolic properties. Sclerostin is secreted by osteocytes and when inhibited, leads to greater bone formation than resorption. It is administered as a once-monthly subcutaneous injection in the non-CKD population. Current trials investigating Romosozumab efficacy in participants with mild to moderate CKD show benefit [24]. Studies have not yet been conducted to evaluate fracture prevention in those with more severe kidney disease.

Bone-specific pharmacology and its potential use in CKD-associated osteoporosis is summarized in Table 11.3.

Lifestyle Management

Lifestyle measures include addressing reversible risk factors and bone health optimization. These measures include adequate calcium and vitamin D intake, weight-bearing exercise, smoking cessation, limited alcohol intake, and fall prevention strategies. Implementing fall prevention strategies is particularly important in the aging population with CKD who are often frail with sarcopenia, or decreased muscle mass [25].

Case Recap

The patient presented at the beginning of the chapter is a postmenopausal older adult with multiple risk factors for osteoporosis as diagnosed by her bone density score and vertebral spinal fracture. Her risk factors include frailty, decreased mobility, infrequent calcium intake, vitamin D insufficiency, CKD, history of spinal fracture, and family history of osteoporosis. Her lab work is consistent with vitamin D insufficiency and secondary hyperparathyroidism from low vitamin D and CKD. Her serum calcium levels are reassuringly normal and do not suggest primary hyperparathyroidism. Management would begin with encouraging lifestyle changes. This would include optimizing calcium and vitamin D intake, enrolling in physical therapy for gait stability, encouraging safe weight-bearing activity, and reviewing fall precautions.

In addition, this patient would benefit from the incorporation of bone-specific therapy after adequate repletion of vitamin D and calcium. Multiple osteoporotic medication options exist and may depend on patient comfort, insurance coverage, and accessibility to consistent follow-up. Therapy could include initiating antiresorptive therapies such as an oral or IV bisphosphonate (if creatinine clearance remains above 35 mL/min) or prolia (if creatinine clearance falls below 35 mL/min). Alternatively, given her prior spinal fracture signifying more severe osteoporosis, she may be a candidate for an injectable anabolic agent such as a PTH-analog or monthly Romosozumab. Monitoring response to therapy with bone turnover markers and repeat bone density evaluation as well as routine evaluation of vitamin D, renal function and calcium status is prudent for future decision-making.

References

1. Cauley JA, Thompson DE, Ensrud KC, Scott JC, Black D. Risk of mortality following clinical fractures. Osteoporos Int. 2000;11(7):556–61. https://doi.org/10.1007/s001980070075.
2. Peacock M. Calcium metabolism in health and disease. Clin J Am Soc Nephrol. 2010;5(Suppl 1):S23–30. https://doi.org/10.2215/CJN.05910809.
3. Tejwani V, Qian Q. Calcium regulation and bone mineral metabolism in elderly patients with chronic kidney disease. Nutrients. 2013;5(6):1913–36. https://doi.org/10.3390/nu5061913.
4. Koeppen BM. Renal physiology. 5th ed. Amsterdam: Elsevier; 2012.
5. Haussler MR, Jurutka PW, Mizwicki M, Norman AW. Vitamin D receptor (VDR)-mediated actions of $1\alpha,25(OH)_2$vitamin D_3: genomic and non-genomic mechanisms. Best Pract Res Clin Endocrinol Metab. 2011;25(4):543–59. https://doi.org/10.1016/j.beem.2011.05.010.
6. Bischoff-Ferrari HA, Willett WC, Orav EJ, et al. A pooled analysis of vitamin D dose requirements for fracture prevention. N Engl J Med. 2012;367(1):40–9. https://doi.org/10.1056/NEJMoa1109617.
7. Lavi-Moshayoff V, Wasserman G, Meir T, Silver J, Naveh-Many T. PTH increases FGF23 gene expression and mediates the high-FGF23 levels of experimental kidney failure: a bone parathyroid feedback loop. Am J Physiol Renal Physiol. 2010;299(4):F882–9. https://doi.org/10.1152/ajprenal.00360.2010.

8. Shimada T, Hasegawa H, Yamazaki Y, et al. FGF-23 is a potent regulator of vitamin D metabolism and phosphate homeostasis. J Bone Miner Res. 2004;19(3):429–35. https://doi.org/10.1359/JBMR.0301264.

9. Moe S, Drüeke T, Cunningham J, et al. Definition, evaluation, and classification of renal osteodystrophy: a position statement from Kidney Disease: Improving Global Outcomes (KDIGO). Kidney Int. 2006;69(11):1945–53. https://doi.org/10.1038/sj.ki.5000414.

10. Stenvinkel P, Larsson TE. Chronic kidney disease: a clinical model of premature aging. Am J Kidney Dis. 2013;62(2):339–51. https://doi.org/10.1053/j.ajkd.2012.11.051.

11. Cannata-Andía JB, Rodriguez García M, Alonso CG. Osteoporosis and adynamic bone in chronic kidney disease. J Nephrol. 2013;26(1):73–80. https://doi.org/10.5301/jn.5000212.

12. Rodriguez Garcia M, Naves Diaz M, Cannata Andia JB. Bone metabolism, vascular calcifications and mortality: associations beyond mere coincidence. J Nephrol. 2005;18(4):458–63.

13. Naves M, Rodríguez-García M, Díaz-López JB, Gómez-Alonso C, Cannata-Andía JB. Progression of vascular calcifications is associated with greater bone loss and increased bone fractures. Osteoporos Int. 2008;19(8):1161–6. https://doi.org/10.1007/s00198-007-0539-1.

14. Khairallah P, Nickolas TL. Management of osteoporosis in CKD. Clin J Am Soc Nephrol. 2018;13(6):962–9. https://doi.org/10.2215/CJN.11031017.

15. Kidney Disease: Improving Global Outcomes (KDIGO) CKD-MBD Update Work Group. KDIGO 2017 clinical practice guideline update for the diagnosis, evaluation, prevention, and treatment of chronic kidney disease-mineral and bone disorder (CKD-MBD). Kidney Int Suppl (2011). 2017;7(1):1–59. https://doi.org/10.1016/j.kisu.2017.04.001.

16. Miller PD. The kidney and bisphosphonates. Bone. 2011;49(1):77–81. https://doi.org/10.1016/j.bone.2010.12.024.

17. Jamal SA, Bauer DC, Ensrud KE, et al. Alendronate treatment in women with normal to severely impaired renal function: an analysis of the fracture intervention trial. J Bone Miner Res. 2007;22(4):503–8. https://doi.org/10.1359/jbmr.070112.

18. Toussaint ND, Lau KK, Strauss BJ, Polkinghorne KR, Kerr PG. Effect of alendronate on vascular calcification in CKD stages 3 and 4: a pilot randomized controlled trial. Am J Kidney Dis. 2010;56(1):57–68. https://doi.org/10.1053/j.ajkd.2009.12.039.

19. Shigematsu T, Muraoka R, Sugimoto T, Nishizawa Y. Risedronate therapy in patients with mild-to-moderate chronic kidney disease with osteoporosis: post-hoc analysis of data from the risedronate phase III clinical trials. BMC Nephrol. 2017;18(1):66. https://doi.org/10.1186/s12882-017-0478-9.

20. Cummings SR, San Martin J, McClung MR, et al. Denosumab for prevention of fractures in postmenopausal women with osteoporosis. N Engl J Med. 2009;361(8):756–65. https://doi.org/10.1056/NEJMoa0809493.

21. Anastasilakis AD, Makras P, Yavropoulou MP, Tabacco G, Naciu AM, Palermo A. Denosumab discontinuation and the rebound phenomenon: a narrative review. J Clin Med. 2021;10(1):152. https://doi.org/10.3390/jcm10010152.

22. Miller PD, Schwartz EN, Chen P, Misurski DA, Krege JH. Teriparatide in postmenopausal women with osteoporosis and mild or moderate renal impairment. Osteoporos Int. 2007;18(1):59–68. https://doi.org/10.1007/s00198-006-0189-8.

23. Cejka D, Kodras K, Bader T, Haas M. Treatment of hemodialysis-associated adynamic bone disease with teriparatide (PTH1-34): a pilot study. Kidney Blood Press Res. 2010;33(3):221–6. https://doi.org/10.1159/000316708.

24. Miller PD, Adachi JD, Albergaria BH, et al. Efficacy and safety of romosozumab among postmenopausal women with osteoporosis and mild-to-moderate chronic kidney disease. J Bone Miner Res. 2022;37(8):1437–45. https://doi.org/10.1002/jbmr.4563.

25. Cruz-Jentoft AJ, Baeyens JP, Bauer JM, et al. Sarcopenia: European consensus on definition and diagnosis: Report of the European Working Group on Sarcopenia in Older People. Age Ageing. 2010;39(4):412–23. https://doi.org/10.1093/ageing/afq034.

Chapter 12
Sodium Disorders, Kidney Disease in the Elderly

Amy A. Yau and Juan Carlos Q. Velez

Introduction to Sodium Disorders

Aging increases the risk of many disease states and impacts organ function. Of these, sodium disorders are common in the elderly, and the aged kidney may play a role in their development. Hyponatremia is more common than hypernatremia in the elderly. Defined as a serum sodium level of less than 135 mmol/L, hyponatremia is commonly associated with symptoms of nausea, vomiting, and altered mentation. Despite varied age cut-offs in studies to define "elderly," various epidemiologic studies consistently show an increased prevalence of hyponatremia in patients older than 50–65 years of age compared to younger populations. Older kidneys possess an impaired ability to excrete free water, and older patients may also have underlying comorbidities or medication use which may increase their risk for hyponatremia. The aged kidney also has diluting defects, increasing the risk for hyponatremia, especially in settings of high free water intake. Hypernatremia defined by a serum sodium level of more than 145 mmol/L is less common, but it tends to develop in the elderly and infirmed population due to reduced intake of free water and increased free water excretion. The aged kidney acquires concentrating defects, which impair its ability to conserve free water, and underlying comorbidities such as dementia or neurologic deficits place patients at higher risk for reduced free water intake. Both hypernatremia and hyponatremia are associated with increased morbidity and mortality in older patients.

A. A. Yau (✉) · J. C. Q. Velez (✉)
Division of Nephrology, The Ohio State University Wexner Medical Center, Columbus, OH, USA

Department of Nephrology, Ochsner Health, New Orleans, LA, USA
e-mail: juancarlos.velez@ochsner.org

H. Kramer et al. (eds.), *Kidney Disease in the Elderly*,
https://doi.org/10.1007/978-3-031-68460-9_12

Age-Related Physiologic Changes

The aging kidney and hormonal changes prime the elderly to develop sodium disorders. Because of a reduction in glomerular filtration rate (GFR), impaired urinary dilution and concentration, and a reduction of total body water, elderly patients are primed to be susceptible to hypernatremia and hyponatremia (Fig. 12.1). Older age is associated with a reduction of total body water. Total body water is 60% of total body weight in 30–40-year-old adults and may decrease to 50% of total body weight in 75–80-year-old adults due to a loss of lean muscle mass, which corresponds to a 21% loss of plasma volume [1]. For example, a 2 kg weight loss can lead to orthostatic declines in systolic blood pressure in older but not younger patients [2, 3].

This plasma volume loss with aging increases sensitivity to volume changes, which can impact vasopressin release and free water retention.

Urinary Concentration and Dilution The classic teaching is that the range of human urine osmolality varies from 50 to 1400 mOsm/L. However, older adults have impaired dilution and concentrating defects. After receiving a water load, observational studies suggest urine can only be diluted to 92–112.8 mOsm/L in older adults while young adults dilute their urine to 52–80.9 mOsm/L [4, 5]. Older adults also have impaired concentrating defects which was first noted in the 1930s. Various studies show in response to hypertonicity or impaired access to free water (i.e., a "dry diet"), patients over 65–75 years of age have lower specific gravity compared to younger patients [6, 7]. In response to a "dry diet," one would expect the urine to concentrate to allow for free water retention. However, individuals over 65 years of age have an average urine specific gravity of 1.025 compared to their younger counterparts whose average urine specific gravity appears higher (1.029) in response to a "dry diet" [6]. Over the age of 40, concentrating ability declines by 24%, and a more abrupt reduction occurs after 65 years old [6]. In response to water deprivation, one study showed the average urine osmolality in individuals aged 68 years old was 882 mOsm/kg compared to 1109 mmol/L in younger patients aged

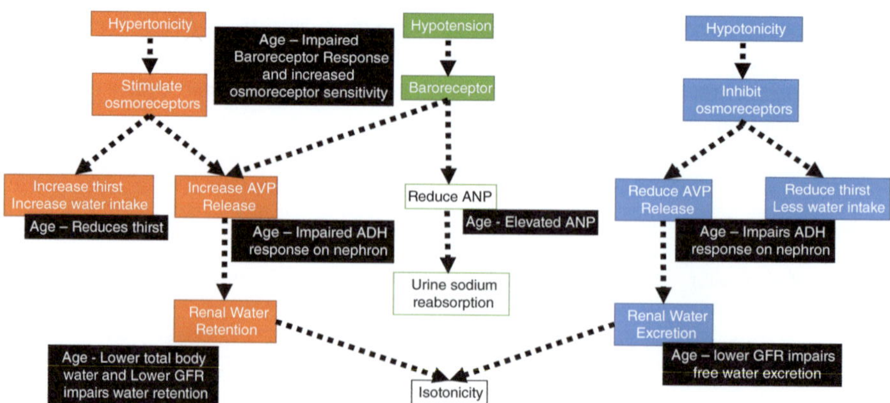

Fig. 12.1 Age related renal physiology changes

33 years old [8]. The impaired dilution predisposes the elderly to hyponatremia, whereas impaired concentration predisposes the elderly to hypernatremia.

Kidney Function The exact mechanisms are unclear, but reduced eGFR may contribute to impaired dilution and concentration in the aged kidney [7, 9]. Reduced GFR occurs likely due to loss of 20–25% of renal mass with age [10]. On average, the majority of adults will have a reduction in their glomerular filtration rate by 0.5–1 mL per minute per year after 40 years of age [11]. At 80 years old, there is a demonstrated loss of renal mass that corresponds with a reduction in GFR of 25% [11, 12]. Combined with a reduction in GFR, there is reduced renal blood flow and increased filtration fraction due to loss of cortical nephrons and preservation of juxtamedullary nephrons [13, 14]. However studies which looked at the effect of vasopressin on medullary blood flow in various kidney pathologies (pyelonephritis, hypertensive renal disease, and glomerulonephritis) demonstrated that dilution of the medullary interstitium via vasopressin contributes to reduced concentrating ability [4, 9, 10].

Role of Vasopressin Much of the ability to dilute or concentrate the urine relies on anti-diuretic hormone (ADH), which is also termed arginine vasopressin (AVP). AVP release is stimulated by decreased effective arterial blood volume through carotid baroreceptors as well as by hyperosmolality via osmoreceptors in the brain. Although it is unclear if basal AVP levels differ with age, there does appear to be a difference when attempts are made to stimulate or suppress AVP. In response to hypertonicity, AVP rose 4.5 times the baseline in older men compared to 2.5 times the baseline in younger men [5, 15]. The rise in AVP and degree of AVP release compared to baseline was faster and higher in older individuals; however, there were similar free water clearances, implying a difference in osmoreceptor sensitivity with age [5, 15]. This difference in osmoreceptor sensitivity may contribute to the risk of hyponatremia in the elderly. Despite similar free water clearances, when older men were allowed to drink water in response to a hypertonic load, AVP persisted longer than in younger men [5, 15]. However, later studies did not see this increased osmoreceptor sensitivity in older adults [5, 16]. Instead, researchers observed that older kidneys had concentrating defects as demonstrated by reduced medullary tonicity and reduced urine-to-plasma inulin ratio [4, 9, 17]. This concentrating defect necessitated higher AVP levels to achieve similar free water clearances.

AVP is also stimulated by hypotension, which may be influenced by age. After laying flat for a minimum of 8 h overnight, research subjects were asked to stand for 8 min. Older patients when standing had lower vasopressin levels compared to younger subjects, but norepinephrine levels were similar [18]. Again when the central plasma volume was increased by head-out-of-water immersion, older volunteers had an earlier and higher increase in atrial natriuretic peptide (ANP) levels compared to a young cohort [19]. The suggestion from these two studies is that the blunted AVP response seen in elderly patients is either related to a defect in the baroreceptor reflex arc or a more pronounced elevation in ANP that inhibits AVP release.

Thirst and Nutrition AVP is also affected by thirst. Thirst is the body's main defense against hypertonicity and increases once plasma osmolality is above 290–295 mOsm/kg. Thirst is satiated by the oropharyngeal mechanoreceptors even before normalization of the plasma osmolality, resulting in a step-wise reduction in plasma osmolality. In seven healthy volunteers with hypernatremia after infusion of hypertonic saline, thirst was measured on a scale. Within 5 min of drinking, plasma vasopressin and thirst were lower despite no change in plasma osmolality until 20 min [20, 21]. Elderly patients are thought to have impaired thirst sensation. In a survey of elderly individuals over 65 years old compared to middle-aged individuals, thirst was assessed with visual analog scales, which is a subjective survey where participants report relative tastes and their intensities. Elderly individuals reported less thirst and response to thirst [22]. Other studies report a higher baseline tonicity in elderly individuals to an average of 293 mOsm/L compared to 288 mOsm/L in younger individuals, and changes in perception of thirst may be partially related [5].

Older individuals are also prone to anorexia through loss of appetite and early satiety. This can be due to a host of social and physical factors, such as familiarity with different foods and products, underlying comorbidities that impact satiety, as well as loss of smell, which may impact appetite [23]. Taste and texture may also contribute to food interest and satiety. Regardless the etiology, low solute intake can predispose elderly patients to hyponatremia as a very low solute intake can impair free water excretion.

Natriuresis Impaired urinary dilution may also be a result of increased natriuresis in the elderly. When elderly men and young men were exposed to a very low sodium diet, older men required two to three times longer time to reduce urine sodium excretion in order to maintain sodium balance [4, 5, 24]. The prolonged time elderly men required to achieve sodium balance may be related to low renin levels and higher ANP levels. ANP is released by cardiac myocytes in response to stretch or increases in plasma volume. ANP inhibits renin, which reduces levels of angiotensin II and aldosterone, which are important for sodium reabsorption along the nephron. Older individuals had basal ANP levels five times higher than their younger peers, which likely explains the low renin levels seen in the elderly [1]. Older adults had lower direct renin concentrations and plasma renin activity [25]. When exposed to a low salt diet and measured supine, although levels did increase, they were significantly lower compared to the younger cohort [25]. The delayed response may be due to the delay in renin disinhibition by elevated ANP levels and places older adults at risk for hypovolemic hyponatremia.

Prostaglandins Changes in renal hemodynamics due to prostaglandins may also be important in the development of hyponatremia in the elderly, specifically in relation to thiazide-induced hyponatremia [26–28]. Through its mechanism of vasodilation of the afferent arteriole, prostaglandins increase RBF, GFR, and filtration fraction resulting in a net increase in water and sodium excretion. Prostaglandin E2 (PGE2) resulted in a net reduction of NKCC2 recycling in the thick ascending limb and aquaporin 2 (AQP2) recycling in the collecting duct [26, 27, 29, 30]. The net effect is a diuretic-like effect that leads to less sodium reabsorption and less water reabsorption, in other words, a concentrating defect. It is suggested that older individuals may have less prostaglandin levels than younger individuals, and there is some suggestion that elderly women have lower urinary excretion of prostaglandin E2 compared to younger women [28].

In individuals with thiazide-induced hyponatremia, when compared to individuals on thiazides but who were normonatremic, urine PGE2 and its metabolite were much higher [27]. When a genome-wide association study was completed for individuals with thiazide-induced hyponatremia, there was a high percentage of a gene polymorphism which impacts prostaglandin transporters in the distal nephron, and these individuals have significantly higher levels of urinary PGE2 and its metabolite [27]. Although the mechanism is not completely clear, it does suggest a role of prostaglandins in sodium balance, and may be an important factor for thiazide-induced hyponatremia, especially in response to a water load.

Hyponatremia

Case Presentation

A 73-year-old female with a past medical history of hypertension, hyperlipidemia, and history of depression presents to the hospital after a fall at home. She tried to get up from the sofa but felt weak, and fell to the floor. After standing up, she felt dizzy and lightheaded and decided to come to the hospital. She complained of watery diarrhea at least once a day for the past week without associated abdominal pain or hematochezia. She denies having fevers or chills. She admits to some nausea without vomiting, but poor oral intake. Medications include amlodipine 5 mg once a day and citalopram 40 mg once a day.

On evaluation, she has a temperature of 98.2 °F, heart rate of 85 beats per minute, and blood pressure of 122/58 mmHg. Her oxygen saturation is 98% on room air. Her examination is significant for obesity and dry mucous membranes. She has no peripheral edema, and her pulmonary and cardiac exams were otherwise unremarkable. Her laboratory evaluation on admission revealed serum chemistry significant for a sodium level of 103 mEq/L, potassium of 3.4 mEq/L, chloride of 73 mEq/L, bicarbonate of 21 mEq/L, blood urea nitrogen of 7 mg/dL and creatinine of 0.52 mg/dL. Her serum glucose was normal.

Epidemiology of Hyponatremia

The overall incidence and prevalence of hyponatremia are reported to be anywhere from 15% to 53% of hospitalized patients [31–33]. Many epidemiologic studies are single-center evaluations with different cut-offs for hyponatremia as well as for age.

A thorough review of the literature suggests the incidence of hyponatremia in elderly patients can be up to 53%. This is much higher compared to the 6% in non-geriatric wards [31, 32, 34, 35]. Hyponatremia is 2.4–2.8 times more likely to occur in elderly patients compared to younger patients in the hospital [36]. In specific study populations, the prevalence of hyponatremia may be higher or lower than in the general ward patient. For example, geriatric patients admitted with community-acquired pneumonia, spontaneous intracranial hemorrhage, and chronic obstructive pulmonary disease exacerbation had a prevalence of hyponatremia of 8%, 16%, and 16% respectively, whereas geriatric patients with cancer had a prevalence of hyponatremia of 38% [37–40].

A distinction should be made between patients who are found to have hyponatremia on outpatient laboratory evaluation, patients who present to an acute care facility with hyponatremia (i.e. community-acquired hyponatremia), and patients who develop hyponatremia during their hospitalization (i.e. hospital-acquired hyponatremia). This distinction is also important when discussing the mortality associated with hyponatremia. In community-dwelling individuals who are otherwise asymptomatic, the incidence of hyponatremia is lower, closer to 7–11% [41–44]. This percentage increases significantly in long-term care facilities where it can increase up to 22–28% [32, 35, 45].

All degrees of hyponatremia severity are seen in the elderly. In a population of patients over 80 years of age, the prevalence of mild, moderate, and severe hyponatremia was 16.3%, 23.8%, and 10.2%, respectively [31]. Severe hyponatremia defined as levels less than 125 mmol/L was more likely to occur in the elderly patient (2–5%) compared to the non-geriatric population (0.3–1%) [32, 46]. Overall, there is no consistent trend that the severity of hyponatremia is associated with increasing age [47–49].

Symptoms of Hyponatremia

Many patients with hyponatremia are asymptomatic. Up to 18.9% of patients will be asymptomatic, especially if their hyponatremia is mild [33]. Those who are symptomatic may complain of vague symptoms (Table 12.1). In two Swiss academic centers, among patients with an average age of 71 years old and sodium levels less than 125 mmol/L, the majority complained of nausea, vomiting, weakness, and fatigue [50]. Other common manifestations included neuromuscular symptoms such as confusion, mental "cloudiness," and gait disturbances [33, 47]. Many individuals have symptoms an average of 7–8 days prior to their presentation with the most prevalent symptom being nausea and vomiting [51]. As many as 9.4% of patients with hyponatremia admitted to having a fall in the previous 14 days prior to presentation [51].

The association of risk of falls and fractures to hyponatremia may be due to neuromuscular weakness or hypovolemia due to nausea and vomiting. Neuromuscular weakness is not related to strength per se versus nerve reaction time. Looking at hospitalized patients in a psychiatric ward with mild hyponatremia less than

Table 12.1 Symptoms of hyponatremia

Confusion, altered mental status
Coma
Seizures
Irritability
Nausea, vomiting
Gait unsteadiness
Headache
Weakness
Fatigue

133 mmol/L compared to a normonatremic control group and another control group (healthy non-hospitalized individuals), the individuals with hyponatremia in the psychiatric ward had a 128.73 ms slower reaction time compared to both control groups [52]. Clinically, hospitalized patients with hyponatremia due to syndrome of inappropriate antidiuresis (SIAD) had a significant improvement in their Timed Up and Go test by around 2.5 s when normonatremia was achieved, and nerve conduction velocities increased by 14.3% [53]. The delayed nerve response in the setting of hyponatremia likely contributes to the fall risk. Cross-sectional observational studies show in a population of over 75 years of age, the fall prevalence was 27.9% with an increased odds ratio of 3.02 [54] For every 5 mmol/L drop in serum sodium, the risk of falling increased by 32% [55]. Of a population of patients with hyponatremia, fractures were reported in 4% of the study population [50]. In a retrospective database in Taiwan, those patients on a thiazide who developed hyponatremia had a higher fracture rate compared to individuals on a thiazide without hyponatremia at 3 years [56]. The majority of these individuals were over 60 years of age, and the risk of fracture included increased risk of vertebral as well as hip fractures [56]. The risk of fractures beyond the initial fall may be due to intrinsic weakness of the bones due to leakage of sodium. Cell studies from rats indicate prolonged hyponatremia, not hypo-osmolality, increases osteoclastogenesis, and impacts gene expression which are responsible for osteoclast growth, differentiation, and migration [57, 58]. Bones are a reservoir for total body sodium accounting for up to 40% of total body sodium stores, which is exchangeable with circulating sodium, and prolonged sodium leak from bone may contribute to osteopenia or osteoporosis [59].

Morbidity Associated with Hyponatremia

Hyponatremia is associated with increased length of hospital stay and greater risk of hospital readmission. In a prospective observational review of all hospitalized patients with hyponatremia, the mean increase in length of stay was an average of 1.9 days [33]. In cancer patients, the length of stay increased from an average of 8.2 to 17.6 days in the setting of hyponatremia [40]. More severe hyponatremia had longer lengths of stay compared to mild hyponatremia [40]. In heart failure patients, the length of stay increased by an average of 3 days in hyponatremic patients [49].

The increase in length may be related to the type, degree, and management of hyponatremia. Older patients had later treatment of their hyponatremia during their hospitalization (9.8 days vs. 1 day) and slower correction rates compared to younger patients [33, 60]. In fact 19–51% of patients with hyponatremia during hospitalization were discharged with persistent hyponatremia [60–63]. Regarding readmission risk, up to 56.2% of individuals who presented to the emergency department with hyponatremia were readmitted at least once within the following 12 months [44]. Forty-three percent of these patients had recurrent hyponatremia [44]. Hyponatremia less than 130 mmol/L was associated with an increased readmission rate at 3 and 12 months (34.2% and 51.8%, respectively) with mortality as high as 17.4%, specifically in the hypovolemic hyponatremic cohort [51]. Increased length of stay and readmission risk may have further downstream effects of deconditioning, and weakness, and may further affect mental health which adversely affects the overall health of the geriatric population.

The risk of short- and long-term mortality is also increased in patients with hyponatremia. Patients over 65 years old have a nearly twofold increased relative risk of death (4.34 compared to 2.14) compared to younger patients and an increased odds ratio of 1.43 for death at 1 year [44, 61, 64]. When comparing mortality risk to younger patients, a large prospective observational study found younger patients had increased mortality compared to older patients with hyponatremia less than 130 mmol/L, but both elderly and younger individuals had increased risk of death [64]. In patients with SIAD, elderly patients had increased mortality compared to younger patients; however, the relative risk of death was higher in younger patients (4.34 vs. 2.14) [61, 64]. Even in patients who may have competing comorbidities for death, such as those with cancer and end-stage renal disease, patients with hyponatremia had increased mortality compared to normonatremic peers. Cancer patients with hyponatremia less than 130 mmol/L were at 4.28 times more risk of death [65]. Another study found an increased risk of mortality at 90 days for cancer patients with hyponatremia with a hazard ratio of 2.04–4.74 depending on the severity of hyponatremia [66]. Patients on peritoneal dialysis with hyponatremia and peritonitis had increased in-hospital mortality compared to their normonatremic peers [67]. Hyponatremia was an independent predictor of in-hospital mortality in this cohort [67].

This mortality risk of hyponatremia may be related more to underlying disease states, either acute or chronic, rather than due to the hyponatremia itself. Mortality risk of hyponatremia in patients on peritoneal dialysis with peritonitis correlated to low serum albumin levels and low serum phosphorus levels, suggesting a baseline malnourished state [67]. Indeed, hospitalized patients with hyponatremia and heart failure had lower serum albumin levels and higher morbidity and mortality rates [49]. In patients with malignancy, many patients with hyponatremia and SIAD had high mortality if their hyponatremia was related to malignancy or infection compared to other causes with a survival [63, 68]. Patients with SIAD due to malignancy had an overall survival of 6.1% compared to 34.5% in patients with cancer and non-malignancy-associated SIAD [63]. Although some studies note an increased risk of death with metastatic disease, others do not [40, 63].

Because of the relationship of hyponatremia to underlying disease states, there is no strong data that the resolution of hyponatremia impacts overall morbidity and mortality. Prospective studies looking at the impact of hyponatremia resolution on neurocognitive and neuromuscular outcomes showed that hyponatremic patients were indeed lower scoring on neurocognitive tests but after 14 days of treatment all symptoms there was an improvement in gait analysis of those with moderate chronic hyponatremia despite significant changes in neuromuscular function, but this may be due to prolonged bed rest and deconditioning while hospitalized [69]. On average, these patients were 60.8 years old with an increase in Na by 4.7 mmol/L and average Na of 128.8 mmol/L. Resolution of hyponatremia did improve activities of daily living (ADL) and the Mini-Mental State Examination (MMSE) mental assessment tool specifically patients with euvolemic hyponatremia with an increase in serum sodium by 5 mmol/L [70]. But, it is possible that fixing hyponatremia may help reduce fracture risk in elderly patients through osteoblast function [71]. In patients with neurologic abnormalities, specifically aneurysmal subarachnoid hemorrhage, hyponatremia was not correlated with poor neurologic outcome or change in mortality [72, 73]. In patients admitted with hyponatremia in the setting of spontaneous intracerebral hemorrhage, correction of hyponatremia apparently had no effect on mortality [38]. When looking at subtypes of hyponatremia and mortality as differentiated by volume, hypervolemic hyponatremia has the highest relative risk of mortality presumed due to the comorbidities which lend themselves to hypervolemia, such as heart failure and liver disease [49, 61]. In heart failure patients, the use of tolvaptan to assist with diuresis did improve hyponatremia, but did not have an all-cause mortality benefit [74, 75]. However when patients with heart failure and reduced ejection fraction with more significant hyponatremia below 130 mmol/dL, use of tolvaptan did have a small but significant reduction of cardiovascular mortality and hospitalizations (HR 0.6) [76].

But conflicting data in patients with malignancy suggest that hyponatremia may be a modifiable risk factor. Cancer patients with SIAD not associated with their malignancy were more likely to achieve normal serum sodium levels and showed lower mortality [63]. Normalizing sodium did seem to improve survival in patients with small cell and non-small cell lung cancer but it is unclear if this is related to the resolution of their malignancy or not. In certain populations, achieving normal serum sodium levels may help to improve quality of life through reduced hospitalizations regardless if they are symptomatic or not.

Causes of Hyponatremia

The causes of hyponatremia in the elderly are the same as in the general population, and evaluation should proceed similarly. Classically hyponatremia causes are organized based on volume status, but a newer approach recommends evaluating for the presence of inappropriate AVP activity to help evaluate causes [77]. Elderly patients in particular may be prone to low solute hyponatremia as discussed earlier, which can impair free water excretion.

Of the various causes of hyponatremia, the majority of causes are euvolemic, specifically due to the syndrome of inappropriate anti-diuretic hormone (ADH). Different epidemiologic studies point to the prevalence of SIAD as a cause of hyponatremia to be 25.5–50% [33, 47, 50, 51, 61, 70]. SIAD may be due to a variety of causes including respiratory infections, neurologic disease, and/or tumors (Table 12.2). In a retrospective review of patients over 80 years old, SIAD was related mostly to respiratory causes, followed by malignancy, and neurologic complications [31]. Another series revealed that tumor-related SIAD was mostly attributed to small cell lung cancer (11–15%) and head-eye-ear-nose-throat (3%) malignancies unrelated to metastasis including metastasis to the lung and/or brain [63, 78]. SIAD is a diagnosis of exclusion, and endocrinopathy should be ruled out. Pituitary disorders lead to hyponatremia through multiple mechanisms including a reduction in plasma volume, elevated ADH levels due to reduced cortisol-mediated AVP inhibition, or increased aquaporin 2 upregulation in cortisol deficiency [79–81]. In studies evaluating idiopathic SIAD in the elderly, only 29% of patients had adrenal function testing completed and were admitted 1–4 times before their hypopituitarism was diagnosed. In 80.7% of patients with hypopituitarism, hyponatremia was the key to their diagnosis, and hypopituitary-related hyponatremia was more often seen in elderly patients over 60 years old than young patients [82, 83].

Table 12.2 Major causes of syndrome of inappropriate antidiuresis (SIAD)

Nausea
Pain
Cancer
  Lung
  Head and neck
  Gastrointestinal, genitourinary, thymoma, lymphomas, sarcomas
Pulmonary
  Cancer
  Pneumonia
  Empyema
  Bronchiectasis
  Cavitary lesions
Central nervous system
  Meningitis, encephalitis
  Intracranial bleeding
  Cerebrovascular accident
  Spinal disorders
Drugs
  Selective serotonin reuptake inhibitors (SSRI)
  Tricyclic antidepressants
  Carbamazepine, oxcarbazepine
  Vincristine
  Antipsychotic medications
  Cyclophosphamide
  Non-steroidal anti-inflammatory drugs (NSAIDs)
Hereditary gain of function mutation of V2 receptor

However, in the elderly, the majority of cases of hyponatremia are multifactorial. Anywhere from 33% to 62% of cases of hyponatremia in the elderly are multifactorial, and severe hyponatremia is more likely to be multifactorial [33, 47, 51]. In a population of patients over 65 years old with hyponatremia, the severity of hyponatremia shows strong correlation with the number and severity of comorbidities [49, 84]. A common comorbidity among elderly patients with hyponatremia is hypertension [33, 43, 50, 60, 85, 86]. It is not clear if this is related to the use of antihypertensive therapy, specifically thiazides, or another mechanism. Polypharmacy is also a risk factor for hyponatremia. A review of a database of elderly patients over 65 years old found that hyponatremia in the community setting is associated with increased drug consumption (sevenfold higher with six or more chronic drugs), and use of antidepressants, diuretics, renin angiotensin aldosterone system (RAAS) inhibitors, antiarrhythmics, and antibiotics [41, 85]. Higher diuretic doses of furosemide, spironolactone, and thiazides have all been associated with increased rates of hyponatremia [87, 88]. Looking at thiazide-induced hyponatremia specifically, the majority of patients are over 50 years old [89]. Elderly patients on a thiazide are almost four times more likely to develop hyponatremia compared to patients younger than 70 years old [47, 88].

Diagnostic Evaluation and Management of Hyponatremia

The evaluation and management of hyponatremia in the aged adult is similar to that in the general population [77, 90]. A thorough history and physical examination should include an evaluation of the onset of symptoms, new medications or dose changes, and volume status. Laboratory assessment should include urine studies and serum studies to assess for possible pseudohyponatremia related to hyperglycemia or hypertriglyceridemia. Urine electrolytes (Fig. 12.2) can help to determine the degree to which AVP is contributing to free water retention and aldosterone to sodium retention and this should be utilized to determine the urine changes are appropriate based on the patient's history and examination. Twenty-four hour urine collections to assess osmolar excretion may be helpful to identify cases of low solute intake-induced hyponatremia.

Regardless of the etiology of hyponatremia, if patients have significant symptoms of hyponatremia including seizure, altered mental status that compromises the airway or poses a danger to the patient, they should be treated with hypertonic saline to increase the serum sodium by 4–6 mmol/L. After the patient is stabilized, acute hyponatremia can be increased by a rate of 8–12 mmol/L in a 24-h period, whereas chronic hyponatremia should be increased by a slower rate, closer to 8 mmol/L in a 24-h period. The recommended rates of correction exist to reduce the risk of osmotic demyelination. In patients with serum sodium of 120 mEq/dL or higher, the risk of osmotic demyelination is lower, so re-lowering of sodium levels which are corrected quicker than desired is not necessary [90]. The risk of osmotic demyelination is highest in individuals with a serum sodium concentration less than or equal to 105 mEq/L, hypokalemia, alcoholism, malnutrition, and advanced liver disease.

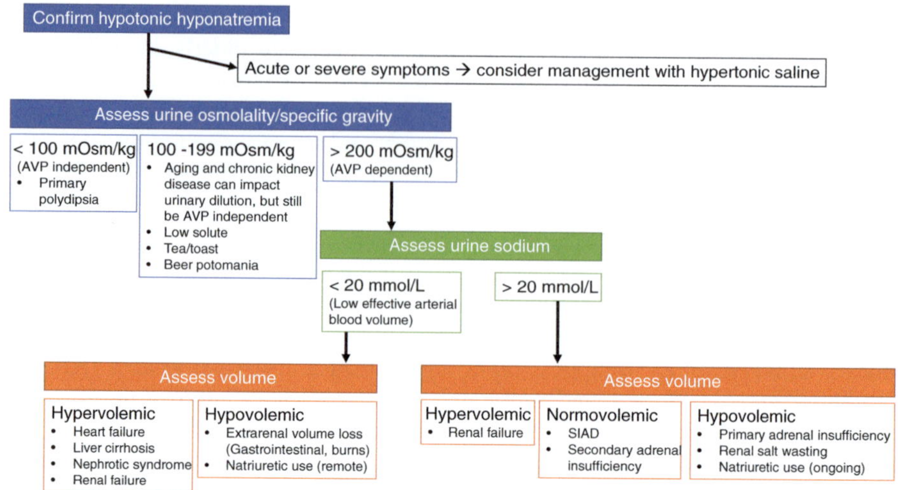

Fig. 12.2 Evaluation and causes of hyponatremia

Management should focus on ways to reduce free water intake and enhance free water excretion. Patients who have excessive free water intake such as in the case of primary polydipsia should be encouraged to reduce their intake, and other patients should be encouraged to reduce their intake to a manageable level. Free water clearance can be estimated by the Fürst eq. (Eq. 12.1). A value less than 0.5 indicates fluid restriction may be helpful if restricted to 1000 mL per day. A value of 0.5–1.0 indicates fluid restriction may be helpful if restricted to 500 mL per day. If the value is more than 1.0, then fluid restriction is unlikely to be beneficial, and other therapies should be considered

$$\text{Urine to Plasma Electrolyte Ratio} = \frac{\text{Urine}\left[\text{Na}\right] + \text{Urine}\left[\text{K}\right]}{\text{Serum}\left[\text{Na}\right]} \quad (12.1)$$

In the setting of hyponatremia, urine osmolality should be low, defined as less than 100 mOsm/L, which indicates a lack of AVP activity. Typical causes include low solute, tea and toast hyponatremia, and beer potomania. The introduction of solute by way of protein supplementation, salt tablets, or urea can help allow free water loss.

In instances of hyponatremia where urine osmolality is elevated, this indicates AVP activity is high. In the setting of hypovolemia, this response is appropriate, and management would be volume resuscitation with isotonic intravenous fluids or oral rehydration salts and other means for blood pressure support with vasopressors and alpha agonists. In patients who are hypervolemic on an exam, AVP is responding to a low effective arterial blood volume, and diuretics are utilized to help with free water loss. There is some interest in stimulating osmotic diuresis in hypervolemic patients through the use of SGLT2 inhibitors or possibly urea or salt tablets;

however, in hypervolemic patients, salt tablets may lead to further fluid retention. Others recommend the use of vaptans in the setting of hypervolemic hyponatremia to stimulate aquaresis [69, 91, 92].

When urine osmolality is elevated in the setting of hyponatremia without urinary sodium retention, endocrinopathies and occult diuretics should be evaluated and if these issues are ruled out then SIAD should be considered. Causes of SIAD should be addressed (Table 12.2) in conjunction with attempts to enhance free water excretion. Although excessive free water intake should be limited, a more strict free water restriction may be no better than a placebo and difficult to maintain outside of the hospital [93]. Protein supplements, urea, and salt tablets help to generate solute diuresis, which contributes to free water loss. Low-dose diuretics and vaptans can also be utilized to reduce free water retention depending on the degree of AVP activity [92]. The use of vaptans in severe hyponatremia should be used cautiously to avoid over-correction, especially in cases of SIAD with higher AVP activity (i.e., higher urine osmolalities). In patients with impaired access to free water or impaired mobility or cognition, vaptans should be avoided unless under close monitoring.

In the outpatient setting, patients started on diuretics, specifically, thiazides, should have frequent electrolyte checks, especially on higher doses. The incidence of hydrochlorothiazide-induced hyponatremia was 10% for patients on a 12.5 mg daily dose compared to 44% for patients on a 50 mg daily dose [94]. Alternative thiazide agents such as indapamide may have lower rates of hyponatremia [95, 96]. In patients on multiple medications of which an antidepressant or anxiolytic is to be started, one could consider initiation of buproprion rather than a selective serotonin reuptake inhibitor (SSRI) or serotonin-norepinephrine reuptake inhibitor (SNRI) [97]. Patients should be advised to drink to thirst and not encouraged to push excessive fluid intake [98]. Although many claim older individuals have impaired thirst mechanisms, there is no age-related difference between thirst and increasing plasma osmolality [5]. In the hospitalized setting, avoid administering hypotonic fluids and act on changes in sodium earlier and more aggressively during their hospitalization [60, 97].

Case Follow Up

Our patient's clinical presentation is typical of patients who present with hyponatremia. She complains of nausea and weakness associated with falls. Further history reveals that a few months ago, her citalopram dosage was increased from 20 to 40 mg once a day due to persistent depressive symptoms. On evaluation, using Fig. 12.2 as a guide, her serum osmolality was 218 mOsm/kg, confirming hypotonic hyponatremia. Although she is symptomatic, she can provide a thorough history with no evidence of seizure-like activity, so hypertonic saline can be forgone. Urine studies were obtained significantly for a random urine osmolality of 503 mmol/kg. As we discussed, the range of normal urine osmolality can decrease with age due to a host of factors (Fig. 12.1), but her urine osmolality above 200 mOsm/kg is indicative of an AVP-dependent process. Her random urine sodium of 52 mEq/L confirms that despite a desire to retain free water, her kidneys are not retaining sodium. Her examination demonstrates dry mucous membranes, which could indicate hypovolemia; however, physical exam findings are not very sensitive or specific for volume measurements. Meanwhile, her vital signs are stable, and when checking orthostatic vitals, her vitals are stable. She has no evidence of hypervolemia on exam.

On arrival at the hospital, after urine and blood samples were obtained, she was given 1 L of normal saline with stable serum and urine values. Further evaluation with a random cortisol level of 21 µg/dL effectively ruled out adrenal insufficiency. She is not on any diuretics, and knowing by history that her citalopram dose was increased, she was diagnosed with SIAD due to SSRI. Because there was no significant impact on her depressive symptoms with citalopram, she was discontinued off the medication. Management of her hyponatremia during her hospitalization included free water restriction, and potassium supplementation to normalize her serum potassium, and urea.

Hypernatremia

Case Presentation

A 70-year-old male with a past medical history of dementia and hypertension is admitted with sepsis from pneumonia. He lives in an assisted care facility, and the nurse aide states he has had a productive cough for the past 2 days. His temperature at the facility today was 100.4 °F. Due to weakness, poor oral intake, and worsening mentation, he was brought to the hospital for evaluation and management. The nurse aide states he is usually able to dress and feed himself with minor assistance, but he has been unable to do so today. He admits to feeling weak and ill, but he is not able to provide much history.

On examination, he had dry mucous membranes and skin tenting. He was minimally interactive with the exam without any peripheral edema. His serum sodium was 158 mEq/L, and his serum creatinine was 1.8 mg/dL. His serum glucose was normal. His serum creatinine was 1.1 mg/dL a month ago on a routine check. Chest X-ray was significant for a left lower lobe opacity. He was not started on any additional fluids, but given intravenous antibiotics and a dose of solu-medrol. His urine output over his first hospital day was 600 mL.

Epidemiology of Hypernatremia

The overall incidence and prevalence of hypernatremia are much lower than hyponatremia. Community-associated hypernatremia occurred in 0.2–0.4% whereas hospital-acquired hyponatremia occurred in 0.6–1% of hospitalized patients [99,

100]. Most concerning is the high incidence of hospital-acquired hypernatremia (82.5%) compared to incident hypernatremia (17.5%) in a cohort of patients with hypernatremia more than 150 mmol/L [99]. When restricted to an intensive care unit (ICU) population, 2% of patients had hypernatremia upon arrival to the unit, but 7% developed hypernatremia during their intensive care unit stay [101]. In nursing home residents, the incidence of community-associated hypernatremia rose to more than 30–60% [1, 99].

Symptoms of Hypernatremia

Patients with mild hypernatremia may present with altered mental status and complain of thirst. Severe hypernatremia is associated with seizures and coma. In a systematic review of patients with acute hypernatremia with a mean sodium of 180 mmol/L, 44% had seizures and 39% were comatose on presentation [102]. Hypernatremia is associated with intraventricular brain hemorrhage, specifically in low birth weight and premature infants with sodium levels more than 150 mmol/L, but this association has not been well defined in adults [103–105]. Hypernatremia may also impact cardiac contractility negatively and increase peripheral insulin resistance which may further contribute to the mortality risk seen in hypernatremia [101, 106, 107].

Morbidity Associated with Hypernatremia

The mortality of patients with hypernatremia is more than 40% and is higher in geriatric patients compared to non-geriatric patients [108]. In a prospective cohort study of 103 patients with hypernatremia of more than 150 mmol/L, /dL, overall mortality was 41%, but hypernatremia was determined to be the underlying cause of death in only 16% [99]. This led the authors to conclude that it is not the hypernatremia per se that is leading to death, but it may be a symptom of the patient's underlying health condition and medical comorbidities [99]. Hypernatremia appears to increase mortality by 40% and length of stay by 38% in an ICU population [109, 110]. Hospital-acquired hypernatremia is associated with a higher mortality rate of 52% compared to community-acquired hypernatremia of 29% and increased length of stay (5 days compared to 3 days) [99, 100]. Among patients with community-acquired hypernatremia, patients more than 65 years old had a higher mortality rate (64%) compared to their younger peers (47.3%) despite similar sodium levels on admission [108].

Causes of Hypernatremia

The causes of hypernatremia are related to reduced free water intake due to infirmary or altered mentation and/or increased free water excretion either from insensible volume losses, urinary losses related to water or solute diuresis, or gastrointestinal free water losses (Table 12.3) [100, 111, 112]. Medications can lead to urinary free water loss through the development of central or nephrogenic diabetes insipidus or through the result of increased free water loss through use of diuretics.

The key is that despite urinary or gastrointestinal free water loss, if a patient has ability to take in free water, hypernatremia will not develop. It is important to note that 86% of patients with hypernatremia during hospital stays lacked access to free water, and 46.1% of nursing home residents admitted with hypernatremia had Alzheimer's disease [99, 108]. Other risk factors for hypernatremia on admission included females, age over 85 years old (odds ratio 2.2), having four or more chronic conditions (odds ratio 4.0), or being bedridden (odds ratio 2.9) [113].

Table 12.3 Causes of hypernatremia

Decreased water intake
Infirmary
Dementia
Altered mental status
Increased water losses with decreased water intake
Fever
Diarrhea
Burns
Central diabetes insipidus
Nephrogenic diabetes insipidus
– Demeclocycline
– Amphotericin B
– Lithium
– Cisplatin
– Urinary obstruction
– Hypercalcemia
– Hypokalemia
– Acute tubular necrosis (ATN)
Loop diuretics
Solute diuresis
– Elevated BUN
– Steroid administration due to elevated urea
– Parenteral or enteral protein feeding
– Recovery of ATN
– Mannitol administration
– Hyperglycemia
Excessive sodium intake
Massive oral sodium intake
Hypertonic solution administration

Other causes of hypernatremia can be related to high salt intake through saline administration or salt ingestion/poisoning, and these patients are typically hypervolemic [100, 102]. A review of ICU patients with hypernatremia showed that almost all patients with hospital-acquired hypervolemic hyponatremia had evidence of edema or weight gain of more than 9 kg average attributed to saline administration, free water losses through solute diuresis due to urea, and post-acute tubular necrosis diuresis [114].

Evaluation and Management of Hypernatremia

Hypernatremia is due to impaired free water intake and may be exacerbated by renal and extrarenal water losses. Urine studies are important in the evaluation of hypernatremia (Fig. 12.3). In the setting of hypernatremia, a urine osmolality of less than 250 mOsm/kg is consistent with a water diuresis. Dilute urine is inappropriate in the setting of hypernatremia and confirms the diagnosis of diabetes insipidus. Work up to determine the completeness and type of diabetes insipidus includes the use of water deprivation or copeptin testing [115, 116]. In the setting of hypernatremia, urine osmolality more than plasma osmolality indicates the kidney's desire to preserve free water. Ergo, the main driver of hypernatremia is either due to impaired free water intake or extrarenal water losses. The ratio of electrolytes to free water in the urine can be calculated by the electrolyte-free water clearance (Eq. 12.2).

$$\text{Electrolyte Free Water Clearance} = \text{Urine Volume}\,(\text{L}) \times \left(1 - \left(\frac{\text{Urine}[\text{Na}] - \text{Urine}[\text{K}]}{\text{Serum Sodium}}\right)\right) \quad (12.2)$$

A negative electrolyte-free water clearance confirms extrarenal water loss as a main contributor to hypernatremia. A positive electrolyte-free water clearance confirms renal water losses, but depending on the total urine output, this may or may not be a significant driver of hypernatremia. Renal water losses can be due to a

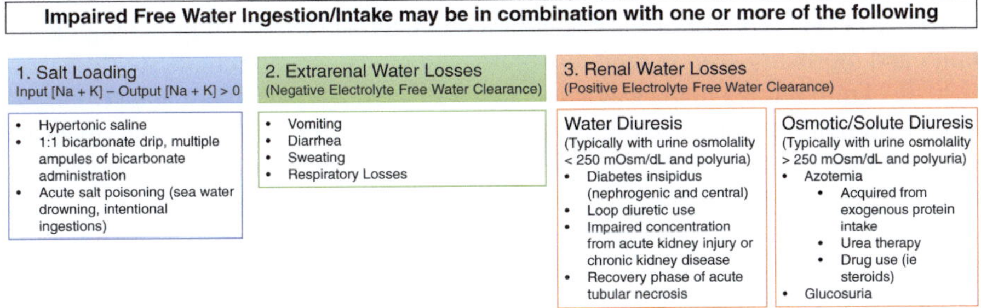

Fig. 12.3 Causes of hypernatremia

water diuresis, as described earlier, or a solute diuresis. Solute diuresis can be confirmed by calculating excreted osmoles by multiplying urine volume by urine osmolality. Given that the average adult daily solute intake is 800–900 mOsm per day, an osmolar excretion of more than that suggests solute diuresis. Hyperglycemia, azotemia, and high protein tube feeds can all lead to solute diuresis [116].

Patients with solute diuresis may also have a water diuresis that is being masked. This can be elucidated by monitoring urine osmolality relative to serum sodium in the setting of hypotonic fluid administration. If at any point of therapy, the urine osmolality decreases to less than 250 mOsm/kg in the setting of yet unresolved hypernatremia, this can indicate the addition of an underlying partial diabetes insipidus.

Management includes the administration of free water and the reduction of free water losses. For patients with renal water losses due to solute diuresis, removing or reducing the offending solute can help. The current free water deficit (Eq. 12.3) can be calculated along with an estimation of ongoing free water losses in order to improve hypernatremia. Ongoing free water losses include insensible volume losses from respiration, and sweat, as well as electrolyte-free water clearance (Eq. 12.2)

$$\text{Free Water Deficit} = \text{Percent Body Water} \times \text{Mass} \left(\text{kg} \right) \times \left(\frac{\text{Current Serum}\left[\text{Na}\right] - \text{Goal Serum}\left[\text{Na}\right]}{\text{Goal Serum}\left[\text{Na}\right]} \right) \quad (12.3)$$

For example, in the hypervolemic hypernatremic patient requiring diuresis, the amount of free water given should include the current deficit along with the urinary water clearance. In the hypovolemic patient, it would be reasonable to forgo free water administration for isotonic saline for resuscitation, then once hemodynamically stable, proceed with free water administration. In the acutely seizing or severely altered patient, a rapid reduction of serum sodium until asymptomatic is advised with boluses of free water.

Initiating free water repletion based on current and ongoing water losses helps to ensure that the hypernatremia will improve with therapy. In a retrospective study of patients admitted with hypernatremia, by hospital day three, 42% had worse or no change in their sodium level, only 32% of patients normalized their sodium levels, and patients with no sodium improvement had a significantly higher risk of death (HR 3.12) [117]. The persistent hypernatremia may be the culprit to the high mortality and morbidity seen in hypernatremic patients. Slow correction rate (less than 0.20–0.25 mmol/L per hour) was associated with increased mortality, and prolonged hypernatremia can lead to cell shrinkage [117, 118]. In patients where sodium levels were normalized after 1, 2, 3, or 3+ days, encephalopathy ratios were highest for those who corrected after 72 h (45.5%) compared to correction less than 48 h (6.9–8.8%) [108]. As described above, hypernatremia even mild (average 150 mmol/L) is a negative inotrope [106]. Empiric antibiotics may be considered given the association with sepsis and high mortality associated with hypernatremia and sepsis compared to normonatremia and sepsis [111].

A more acute reduction in sodium can be employed to reduce serum sodium by 6–8 mmol/L in the first few hours [112, 119]. In a systematic review of case reports of hyperacute hypernatremia of less than 12 h duration, treatment began within 12 h of onset with a mean max correction rate of 7.6 mmol/L per in patients who lived compared to a mean correction rate of 4.9 mmol/L per hour in patients who died [102].

For chronic hypernatremia, there is no recommended correction rate or guideline. Some studies advise a slow correction rate of no more than 0.5–1.0 mmol/L per hour with a maximum change in 24 h less than 10 mmol/L. However, this rate was suggested due to the risk of cerebral edema with resolution of hypertonicity, specifically in children admitted with diabetic ketoacidosis [120]. Most of the data concerning cerebral edema and seizures with hypernatremia correction come from pediatrics and infants [121–123]. Newer data supports the lack of side effects to include neurologic effects when the serum sodium is adjusted by a rate of correction of more than 12 mmol/L per day despite a higher peak serum sodium level [124, 125]. Slow correction may be considered in patients with cerebral dehydration seen on imaging, existing cerebral edema, and those with an alternative osmotic agent which is also being addressed (i.e., high blood urea nitrogen, hyperglycemia).

Case Follow Up

Our patient is at high risk for developing hypernatremia. He has baseline dementia and lives in an assisted living facility. Now in the setting of his acute illness, his inability to communicate well and eat and drink on his own can lead to hypernatremia. It is unclear whether he has impaired thirst mechanism, but it is clear he has impaired intake of free water due to his hypernatremia on presentation. His current free water deficit, using a weight of 70 kg and total body water in an elderly individual of 50% of weight, is 2.9 L.

Again, hypernatremia can occur either due to salt loading or renal water loss or extrarenal water loss. There is no evidence of salt loading in this case. Insensible volume losses through respiration, sweat, and stool total on average around 800 mL per day in a normal human. In a patient with a fever, the insensible volume losses may be higher than on average. To estimate renal water loss, urine studies are necessary. His urine studies revealed urine osmolality of 520 mOsm/kg, urine sodium of 18 mEq/dL, and urine potassium of 10 mEq/dL without glucosuria. His urine osmolality is elevated above his serum osmolality, thus confirming there is not a pure water diuresis (i.e., diabetes insipidus). His electrolyte-free water clearance is 569 mL, indicating he has only 569 mL of water loss. Plus the lack of polyuria is consistent with the lack of water or solute diuresis.

Knowing that his free water deficit is 2.9 L, the main driver of this patient's hypernatremia is impaired free water intake, as ingestion of around 1.4 L a day of water would have prevented the development of hypernatremia in this patient.

Conclusion

Sodium disorders are common in the elderly and arise from dilution and concentrating defects which may be age-related or related to underlying comorbidities or medications. The incidence of hyponatremia is more common in the elderly compared to young adults, and hypernatremia is quite common in the elderly. Herein, we attempt to summarize how these physiologic changes (Table 12.4) lead to the development of hyponatremia and hypernatremia in the elderly, which are exacerbated in the setting of a water load, water deprivation, and solute intake. Evaluation of the etiology of dysnatremia depends on the assessment of urine constituents, if their response is appropriate or inappropriate in the clinical setting. Management of dysnatremias will depend on the presence of symptoms, chronicity of sodium disorder, and underlying precipitant.

Table 12.4 Urine concentration and dilution in the elderly and implications in susceptibility to dysnatremias

Theoretical framework of aging-induced reduction in diluting capacity of the kidneys, the influence of solute intake in water-handling, and the risk for hyponatremia			
Maximal dilution capacity: U Osm **50** mOsm/kg	Normal daily osmolar intake 10 mOsm/kg (65 kg) = **650** mOsm	Maximum urine volume: (650) (1 L)/ (50) = **13** L	Maximum water intake before development of hyponatremia = **13** L
Aging-induced impairment in maximal dilution U Osm **150** mOsm/kg	Normal daily osmolar intake 10 mOsm/kg (70 kg) = **650** mOsm	Maximum urine volume: (650) (1 L)/ (150) = **4.3** L	Maximum water intake before development of hyponatremia = **4.3** L
Aging-induced impairment in maximal dilution U Osm **150** mOsm/kg	Fall in daily osmolar intake by half 5 mOsm/kg (65 kg) = **325** mOsm	Maximum urine volume: (325) (1 L)/ (150) = **2.17** L	Maximum water intake before development of hyponatremia = **2.17** L
E.g.: If an elderly individual keeps a daily water intake of 2.8 L per day, an excess of 0.63 L of water will be retained each day. Some of it may be eliminated through insensible losses. Nevertheless, this impaired water-handling physiology makes elderly individuals more vulnerable to hyponatremia in response to any additional insult (e.g., hypovolemia, SIAD, etc.). Impairment in diluting capacity due to aging can be exacerbated by concomitant reduction in kidney function (nephron mass)			
Theoretical framework of aging-induced reduction in concentrating capacity of the kidneys and the associated risk for hypernatremia			
Maximal concentrating capacity: U Osm **1300** mOsm/kg	Normal daily osmolar intake 10 mOsm/kg (65 kg) = **650** mOsm	Minimum urine volume: (650) (1 L)/ (1300) = **0.5** L	Obligatory renal volume loss in the context of dehydration = **0.5** L
Aging-induced impairment in maximal concentration U Osm **650** mOsm/kg	Normal daily osmolar intake 10 mOsm/kg (65 kg) = **650** mOsm	Minimum urine volume: (650) (1 L)/ (650) = **1.0** L	Obligatory renal volume loss in the context of dehydration = **1.0** L
E.g.: If an elderly individual becomes dehydrated, the renal response to retain water is suboptimal. This impaired water-handling physiology makes elderly individuals more vulnerable to hypernatremia if they have limited access to water intake. Impairment in concentrating capacity due to aging can be exacerbated by concomitant reduction in kidney function (nephron mass)			

References

1. Beck LH. Changes in renal function with aging. Clin Geriatr Med. 1998;14(2):199–209.
2. Fülöp T, Wórum I, Csongor J, Fóris G, Leövey A. Body composition in elderly people. I. Determination of body composition by multiisotope method and the elimination kinetics of these isotopes in healthy elderly subjects. Gerontology. 1985;31(1):6–14. https://doi.org/10.1159/000212676.
3. Shannon RP, Wei JY, Rosa RM, Epstein FH, Rowe JW. The effect of age and sodium depletion on cardiovascular response to orthostasis. Hypertension. 1986;8(5):438–43. https://doi.org/10.1161/01.hyp.8.5.438.
4. Lindeman RD, Lee TD, Yiengst MJ, Shock NW. Influence of age, renal disease, hypertension, diuretics, and calcium on the antidiuretic responses to suboptimal infusions of vasopressin. J Lab Clin Med. 1966;68(2):206–23.
5. Davies I, O'Neill PA, Mclean KA, Catania J, Bennett D. Age-associated alterations in thirst and arginine vasopressin in response to a water or sodium load. Age Ageing. 1995;24(2):151–9. https://doi.org/10.1093/ageing/24.2.151.
6. Lewis WH, Alving AS. Changes with age in the renal function in adult men: I. Clearance of urea. II. Amount of urea nitrogen in the blood. III. Concentrating ability of the kidneys. Am J Physiol Legacy Content. 1938;123(2):500–15. https://doi.org/10.1152/ajplegacy.1938.123.2.500.
7. Mack GW, Weseman CA, Langhans GW, Scherzer H, Gillen CM, Nadel ER. Body fluid balance in dehydrated healthy older men: thirst and renal osmoregulation. J Appl Physiol. 1994;76(4):1615–23. https://doi.org/10.1152/jappl.1994.76.4.1615.
8. Rowe JW, Shock NW, DeFronzo RA. The influence of age on the renal response to water deprivation in man. Nephron. 1976;17(4):270–8. https://doi.org/10.1159/000180731.
9. Lindeman RD. Overview: renal physiology and pathophysiology of aging. Am J Kidney Dis. 1990;16(4):275–82. https://doi.org/10.1016/S0272-6386(12)80002-3.
10. McLachlan M, Wasserman P. Changes in sizes and distensibility of the aging kidney. Br J Radiol. 1981;54(642):488–91. https://doi.org/10.1259/0007-1285-54-642-488.
11. Lindeman RD, Tobin J, Shock NW. Longitudinal studies on the rate of decline in renal function with age. J Am Geriatr Soc. 1985;33(4):278–85. https://doi.org/10.1111/j.1532-5415.1985.tb07117.x.
12. Rowe JW, Andres R, Tobin JD, Norris AH, Shock NW. The effect of age on creatinine clearance in men: a cross-sectional and longitudinal study. J Gerontol. 1976;31(2):155–63. https://doi.org/10.1093/geronj/31.2.155.
13. Fliser D, Nowack R, Ritz E. Renal functional reserve in healthy elderly subjects. J Am Soc Nephrol. 1993;3(7):1371–7.
14. Lindeman RD, Goldman R. Anatomic and physiologic age changes in the kidney. Exp Gerontol. 1986;21(4–5):379–406. https://doi.org/10.1016/0531-5565(86)90044-6.
15. Helderman JH, Vestal RE, Rowe JW, Tobin JD, Andres R, Robertson GL. The response of arginine vasopressin to intravenous ethanol and hypertonic saline in man: the impact of aging. J Gerontol. 1978;33(1):39–47. https://doi.org/10.1093/geronj/33.1.39.
16. Phillips PA, Bretherton M, Johnston CI, Gray L. Reduced osmotic thirst in healthy elderly men. Am J Phys Regul Integr Comp Phys. 1991;261(1):R166–71. https://doi.org/10.1152/ajpregu.1991.261.1.R166.
17. Miller JH, Shock NW. Age differences in the renal tubular response to antidiuretic hormone. J Gerontol. 1953;8(4):446–50. https://doi.org/10.1093/geronj/8.4.446.
18. Rowe JW, Minaker KL, Sparrow D, Robertson GL. Age-related failure of volume-pressure-mediated vasopressin release. J Clin Endocrinol Metab. 1982;54(3):661–4. https://doi.org/10.1210/jcem-54-3-661.
19. Stachenfeld NS, DiPietro L, Nadel ER, Mack GW. Mechanism of attenuated thirst in aging: role of central volume receptors. Am J Phys. 1997;272(1 Pt 2):R148–57. https://doi.org/10.1152/ajpregu.1997.272.1.R148.

20. Thompson CJ, Burd JM, Baylis PH. Acute suppression of plasma vasopressin and thirst after drinking in hypernatremic humans. Am J Phys Regul Integr Comp Phys. 1987;252(6):R1138–42. https://doi.org/10.1152/ajpregu.1987.252.6.R1138.
21. Seckl JR, Williams TD, Lightman SL. Oral hypertonic saline causes transient fall of vasopressin in humans. Am J Phys Regul Integr Comp Phys. 1986;251(2):R214–7. https://doi.org/10.1152/ajpregu.1986.251.2.R214.
22. Hendi K, Leshem M. Salt appetite in the elderly. Br J Nutr. 2014;112(10):1621–7. https://doi.org/10.1017/S0007114514002803.
23. Rolls BJ. Appetite, hunger, and satiety in the elderly. Crit Rev Food Sci Nutr. 1993;33(1):39–44. https://doi.org/10.1080/10408399309527610.
24. Epstein M, Hollenberg NK. Age as a determinant of renal sodium conservation in normal man. J Lab Clin Med. 1976;87(3):411–7.
25. Weidmann P, De Myttenaere-Bursztein S, Maxwell MH, de Lima J. Effect on aging on plasma renin and aldosterone in normal man. Kidney Int. 1975;8(5):325–33. https://doi.org/10.1038/ki.1975.120.
26. César KR, Magaldi AJ. Thiazide induces water absorption in the inner medullary collecting duct of normal and Brattleboro rats. Am J Physiol Renal Physiol. 1999;277(5):F756–60. https://doi.org/10.1152/ajprenal.1999.277.5.F756.
27. Ware JS, Wain LV, Channavajjhala SK, et al. Phenotypic and pharmacogenetic evaluation of patients with thiazide-induced hyponatremia. J Clin Invest. 2017;127(9):3367–74. https://doi.org/10.1172/JCI89812.
28. Clark BA, Shannon RP, Rosa RM, Epstein FH. Increased susceptibility to thiazide-induced hyponatremia in the elderly. J Am Soc Nephrol. 1994;5(4):1106–11. https://doi.org/10.1681/ASN.V541106.
29. Olesen ETB, Fenton RA. Is there a role for PGE2 in urinary concentration? J Am Soc Nephrol. 2013;24(2):169–78. https://doi.org/10.1681/ASN.2012020217.
30. Kokko JP. Effect of prostaglandins on renal epithelial electrolyte transport. Kidney Int. 1981;19(6):791–6. https://doi.org/10.1038/ki.1981.82.
31. Zhang X, Li XY. Prevalence of hyponatremia among older inpatients in a general hospital. Eur Geriatr Med. 2020;11(4):685–92. https://doi.org/10.1007/s41999-020-00320-3.
32. Miller M, Morley JE, Rubenstein LZ. Hyponatremia in a nursing home population. J Am Geriatr Soc. 1995;43(12):1410–3. https://doi.org/10.1111/j.1532-5415.1995.tb06623.x.
33. Dash SC, Sundaray NK, Rajesh B, Pagad T. Hyponatremia in elderly in-patients. JCDR. 2019;13(2):OC01–4. https://doi.org/10.7860/JCDR/2019/39957.12554.
34. Upadhyay A, Jaber BL, Madias NE. Incidence and prevalence of hyponatremia. Am J Med. 2006;119(7 Suppl 1):S30–5. https://doi.org/10.1016/j.amjmed.2006.05.005.
35. Naka T, Kohagura K, Kochi M, Ohya Y. Hyponatremia and mortality among very elderly residents in a geriatric health service facility. Clin Exp Nephrol. 2018;22(6):1404–10. https://doi.org/10.1007/s10157-018-1607-x.
36. Siregar P. The risk of hyponatremia in the elderly compared with younger in the hospital inpatient and outpatient. Acta Med Indones. 2011;43(3):158–61.
37. Cuesta M, Slattery D, Goulden EL, et al. Hyponatraemia in patients with community-acquired pneumonia; prevalence and aetiology, and natural history of SIAD. Clin Endocrinol. 2019;90(5):744–52. https://doi.org/10.1111/cen.13937.
38. Kuramatsu JB, Bobinger T, Volbers B, et al. Hyponatremia is an independent predictor of in-hospital mortality in spontaneous intracerebral hemorrhage. Stroke. 2014;45(5):1285–91. https://doi.org/10.1161/STROKEAHA.113.004136.
39. Chalela R, González-García JG, Chillarón JJ, et al. Impact of hyponatremia on mortality and morbidity in patients with COPD exacerbations. Respir Med. 2016;117:237–42. https://doi.org/10.1016/j.rmed.2016.05.003.
40. Berardi R, Caramanti M, Castagnani M, et al. Hyponatremia is a predictor of hospital length and cost of stay and outcome in cancer patients. Support Care Cancer. 2015;23(10):3095–101. https://doi.org/10.1007/s00520-015-2683-z.

41. Grattagliano I, Mastronuzzi T, D'Ambrosio G. Hyponatremia associated with long-term medication use in the elderly: an analysis in general practice. J Prim Health Care. 2018;10(2):167. https://doi.org/10.1071/HC17084.
42. Tay CL, Myint PK, Mohazmi M, Soiza RL, Tan MP. Prevalence and documented causes of hyponatraemia among geriatric patients attending a primary care clinic. Med J Malaysia. 2019;74(2):121–7.
43. Heybeli C, Smith L, Soysal P. Associations between mild hyponatremia and geriatric syndromes in outpatient settings. Int Urol Nephrol. 2021;53(10):2089–98. https://doi.org/10.1007/s11255-021-02789-8.
44. Winzeler B, Jeanloz N, Nigro N, et al. Long-term outcome of profound hyponatremia: a prospective 12 months follow-up study. Eur J Endocrinol. 2016;175(6):499–507. https://doi.org/10.1530/EJE-16-0500.
45. Kleinfeld M, Casimir M, Borra S. Hyponatremia as observed in a chronic disease facility. J Am Geriatr Soc. 1979;27(4):156–61. https://doi.org/10.1111/j.1532-5415.1979.tb06439.x.
46. Imai N, Osako K, Kaneshiro N, Shibagaki Y. Seasonal prevalence of hyponatremia in the emergency department: impact of age. BMC Emerg Med. 2018;18(1):41. https://doi.org/10.1186/s12873-018-0182-5.
47. Shapiro DS, Sonnenblick M, Galperin I, Melkonyan L, Munter G. Severe hyponatraemia in elderly hospitalized patients: prevalence, aetiology and outcome: severe hyponatraemia in elderly patients. Intern Med J. 2010;40(8):574–80. https://doi.org/10.1111/j.1445-5994.2010.02217.x.
48. Reddy PS, Katragadda H. A clinical study on hyponatremia in elderly, hospitalized patients. AJM. 2019;2(2):141–3. https://doi.org/10.21276/ajm.2019.2.2.36.
49. Saepudin S, Ball PA, Morrissey H. Hyponatremia during hospitalization and in-hospital mortality in patients hospitalized from heart failure. BMC Cardiovasc Disord. 2015;15(1):88. https://doi.org/10.1186/s12872-015-0082-5.
50. Nigro N, Winzeler B, Suter-Widmer I, et al. Symptoms and characteristics of individuals with profound hyponatremia: a prospective multicenter observational study. J Am Geriatr Soc. 2015;63(3):470–5. https://doi.org/10.1111/jgs.13325.
51. Ioannou P, Panagiotakis S, Tsagkaraki E, et al. Increased mortality in elderly patients admitted with hyponatremia: a prospective cohort study. JCM. 2021;10(14):3059. https://doi.org/10.3390/jcm10143059.
52. Filmyer DM, Finkel G, Plasay M, Shaughnessy RA, Josiassen RC. A comparison of simple reaction times in psychotic inpatients with and without hyponatremia. Schizophr Res. 2019;208:449–50. https://doi.org/10.1016/j.schres.2019.04.001.
53. Vandergheynst F, Gombeir Y, Bellante F, et al. Impact of hyponatremia on nerve conduction and muscle strength. Eur J Clin Investig. 2016;46(4):328–33. https://doi.org/10.1111/eci.12597.
54. Boyer S, Gayot C, Bimou C, et al. Prevalence of mild hyponatremia and its association with falls in older adults admitted to an emergency geriatric medicine unit (the MUPA unit). BMC Geriatr. 2019;19(1):265. https://doi.org/10.1186/s12877-019-1282-0.
55. Gunathilake R, Oldmeadow C, McEvoy M, et al. Mild hyponatremia is associated with impaired cognition and falls in community-dwelling older persons. J Am Geriatr Soc. 2013;61(10):1838–9. https://doi.org/10.1111/jgs.12468.
56. Yang LJ, Wu PH, Huang TH, Lin MY, Tsai JC. Thiazide-associated hyponatremia attenuates the fracture-protective effect of thiazide: a population-based study. PLoS One. 2018;13(12):e0208712. https://doi.org/10.1371/journal.pone.0208712.
57. Barsony J, Sugimura Y, Verbalis JG. Osteoclast response to low extracellular sodium and the mechanism of hyponatremia-induced bone loss. J Biol Chem. 2011;286(12):10864–75. https://doi.org/10.1074/jbc.M110.155002.
58. Barsony J, Xu Q, Verbalis JG. Hyponatremia elicits gene expression changes driving osteoclast differentiation and functions. Mol Cell Endocrinol. 2022;554:111724. https://doi.org/10.1016/j.mce.2022.111724.

59. Hannon MJ, Verbalis JG. Sodium homeostasis and bone. Curr Opin Nephrol Hypertens. 2014;23(4):370–6. https://doi.org/10.1097/01.mnh.0000447022.51722.f4.

60. Hoorn EJ, Lindemans J, Zietse R. Development of severe hyponatraemia in hospitalized patients: treatment-related risk factors and inadequate management. Nephrol Dial Transplant. 2006;21(1):70–6. https://doi.org/10.1093/ndt/gfi082.

61. Thorpe O, Cuesta M, Fitzgerald C, et al. Active management of hyponatraemia and mortality in older hospitalised patients compared with younger patients: results of a prospective cohort study. Age Ageing. 2021;50(4):1144–50. https://doi.org/10.1093/ageing/afaa248.

62. Chewcharat A, Thongprayoon C, Cheungpasitporn W, Mao MA, Thirunavukkarasu S, Kashani KB. Trajectories of serum sodium on in-hospital and 1-year survival among hospitalized patients. Clin J Am Soc Nephrol. 2020;15(5):600–7. https://doi.org/10.2215/CJN.12281019.

63. Goldvaser H, Rozen-Zvi B, Yerushalmi R, Gafter-Gvili A, Lahav M, Shepshelovich D. Malignancy associated SIADH: characterization and clinical implications. Acta Oncol. 2016;55(9–10):1190–5. https://doi.org/10.3109/0284186X.2016.1170198.

64. Al Mawed S, Pankratz VS, Chong K, Sandoval M, Roumelioti ME, Unruh M. Low serum sodium levels at hospital admission: outcomes among 2.3 million hospitalized patients. PLoS One. 2018;13(3):e0194379. https://doi.org/10.1371/journal.pone.0194379.

65. Abu Zeinah GF, Al-Kindi SG, Hassan AA, Allam A. Hyponatraemia in cancer: association with type of cancer and mortality. Eur J Cancer Care (Engl). 2015;24(2):224–31. https://doi.org/10.1111/ecc.12187.

66. Doshi SM, Shah P, Lei X, Lahoti A, Salahudeen AK. Hyponatremia in hospitalized cancer patients and its impact on clinical outcomes. Am J Kidney Dis. 2012;59(2):222–8. https://doi.org/10.1053/j.ajkd.2011.08.029.

67. Tseng MH, Cheng CJ, Sung CC, et al. Hyponatremia is a surrogate marker of poor outcome in peritoneal dialysis-related peritonitis. BMC Nephrol. 2014;15(1):113. https://doi.org/10.1186/1471-2369-15-113.

68. Basu A, Ryder REJ. The syndrome of inappropriate antidiuresis is associated with excess long-term mortality: a retrospective cohort analyses. J Clin Pathol. 2014;67(9):802–6. https://doi.org/10.1136/jclinpath-2014-202243.

69. Refardt J, Kling B, Krausert K, et al. Impact of chronic hyponatremia on neurocognitive and neuromuscular function. Eur J Clin Investig. 2018;48(11):e13022. https://doi.org/10.1111/eci.13022.

70. Brinkkoetter PT, Grundmann F, Ghassabeh PJ, et al. Impact of resolution of hyponatremia on neurocognitive and motor performance in geriatric patients. Sci Rep. 2019;9(1):12526. https://doi.org/10.1038/s41598-019-49054-8.

71. Potasso L, Refardt J, Meier C, Christ-Crain M. Effect of hyponatremia normalization on osteoblast function in patients with SIAD. Eur J Endocrinol. 2022;186(1):1–8. https://doi.org/10.1530/EJE-21-0604.

72. Zheng B, Qiu Y, Jin H, et al. A predictive value of hyponatremia for poor outcome and cerebral infarction in high-grade aneurysmal subarachnoid haemorrhage patients. J Neurol Neurosurg Psychiatry. 2011;82(2):213–7. https://doi.org/10.1136/jnnp.2009.180349.

73. Kieninger M, Kerscher C, Bründl E, et al. Acute hyponatremia after aneurysmal subarachnoid hemorrhage: frequency, treatment, and outcome. J Clin Neurosci. 2021;88:237–42. https://doi.org/10.1016/j.jocn.2021.04.004.

74. Wang J, Zhou W, Yin X. Improvement of hyponatremia is associated with lower mortality risk in patients with acute decompensated heart failure: a meta-analysis of cohort studies. Heart Fail Rev. 2019;24(2):209–17. https://doi.org/10.1007/s10741-018-9753-5.

75. Konstam MA. Effects of oral tolvaptan in patients hospitalized for worsening heart failurethe EVEREST outcome trial. JAMA. 2007;297(12):1319. https://doi.org/10.1001/jama.297.12.1319.

76. Hauptman PJ, Burnett J, Gheorghiade M, et al. Clinical course of patients with hyponatremia and decompensated systolic heart failure and the effect of vasopressin receptor antagonism with tolvaptan. J Card Fail. 2013;19(6):390–7. https://doi.org/10.1016/j.cardfail.2013.04.001.

77. Spasovski G, Vanholder R, Allolio B, et al. Clinical practice guideline on diagnosis and treatment of hyponatraemia. Nephrol Dial Transplant. 2014;29(Suppl 2):i1–i39. https://doi.org/10.1093/ndt/gfu040.

78. Gill G, Huda B, Boyd A, et al. Characteristics and mortality of severe hyponatraemia—a hospital-based study. Clin Endocrinol. 2006;65(2):246–9. https://doi.org/10.1111/j.1365-2265.2006.02583.x.

79. Ishikawa SE, Saito T, Fukagawa A, et al. Close association of urinary excretion of aquaporin-2 with appropriate and inappropriate arginine vasopressin-dependent antidiuresis in hyponatremia in elderly subjects. J Clin Endocrinol Metab. 2001;86(4):1665–71.

80. Saito T, Ishikawa SE, Ando F, Higashiyama M, Nagasaka S, Sasaki S. Vasopressin-dependent upregulation of aquaporin-2 gene expression in glucocorticoid-deficient rats. Am J Physiol Renal Physiol. 2000;279(3):F502–8. https://doi.org/10.1152/ajprenal.2000.279.3.F502.

81. Yatagai T, Kusaka I, Nakamura T, et al. Close association of severe hyponatremia with exaggerated release of arginine vasopressin in elderly subjects with secondary adrenal insufficiency. Eur J Endocrinol. 2003;148(2):221–6. https://doi.org/10.1530/eje.0.1480221.

82. Diker-Cohen T, Rozen-Zvi B, Yelin D, et al. Endocrinopathy-induced euvolemic hyponatremia. Intern Emerg Med. 2018;13(5):679–88. https://doi.org/10.1007/s11739-018-1872-4.

83. Miljic D, Doknic M, Stojanovic M, et al. Impact of etiology, age and gender on onset and severity of hyponatremia in patients with hypopituitarism: retrospective analysis in a specialised endocrine unit. Endocrine. 2017;58(2):312–9. https://doi.org/10.1007/s12020-017-1415-1.

84. Kayar NB, Kayar Y, Ekinci I, Erdem ED, Sit D. Relation between severity of hyponatremia and comorbidity in elderly patients who develop hyponatremia. Biomed Res. 2016;27(3):5.

85. Grover S, Shouan A, Mehra A, Chakrabarti S, Avasthi A. Antidepressant-associated hyponatremia among the elderly: a retrospective study. J Geriatr Ment Health. 2018;5(2):115. https://doi.org/10.4103/jgmh.jgmh_28_18.

86. Manu P, Ray K, Rein JL, De Hert M, Kane JM, Correll CU. Medical outcome of psychiatric inpatients with admission hyponatremia. Psychiatry Res. 2012;198(1):24–7. https://doi.org/10.1016/j.psychres.2012.01.022.

87. Velat I, Bušić Ž, Jurić Paić M, Čulić V. Furosemide and spironolactone doses and hyponatremia in patients with heart failure. BMC Pharmacol Toxicol. 2020;21(1):57. https://doi.org/10.1186/s40360-020-00431-4.

88. Clayton JA, Rodgers S, Blakey J, Avery A, Hall IP. Thiazide diuretic prescription and electrolyte abnormalities in primary care. Br J Clin Pharmacol. 2006;61(1):87–95. https://doi.org/10.1111/j.1365-2125.2005.02531.x.

89. Fichman MP, Vorherr H, Kleeman CR, Telfer N. Diuretic-induced hyponatremia. Ann Intern Med. 1971;75(6):853–63. https://doi.org/10.7326/0003-4819-75-6-853.

90. Verbalis JG, Goldsmith SR, Greenberg A, et al. Diagnosis, evaluation, and treatment of hyponatremia: expert panel recommendations. Am J Med. 2013;126(10):S1–S42. https://doi.org/10.1016/j.amjmed.2013.07.006.

91. Bălăceanu A. New approaches of the hyponatremia treatment in the elderly—an update. Farmacia. 2020;68(3):406–18. https://doi.org/10.31925/farmacia.2020.3.5.

92. Harbeck B, Lindner U, Haas CS. Low-dose tolvaptan for the treatment of hyponatremia in the syndrome of inappropriate ADH secretion (SIADH). Endocrine. 2016;53(3):872–3. https://doi.org/10.1007/s12020-016-0912-y.

93. Krisanapan P, Vongsanim S, Pin-On P, Ruengorn C, Noppakun K. Efficacy of furosemide, oral sodium chloride, and fluid restriction for treatment of syndrome of inappropriate antidiuresis (SIAD): an open-label randomized controlled study (the EFFUSE-FLUID trial). Am J Kidney Dis. 2020;76(2):203–12. https://doi.org/10.1053/j.ajkd.2019.11.012.

94. Sharabi Y, Illan R, Kamari Y, et al. Diuretic induced hyponatraemia in elderly hypertensive women. J Hum Hypertens. 2002;16(9):631–5. https://doi.org/10.1038/sj.jhh.1001458.

95. Roush GC, Ernst ME, Kostis JB, Tandon S, Sica DA. Head-to-head comparisons of hydrochlorothiazide with indapamide and chlorthalidone: antihypertensive and metabolic effects. Hypertension. 2015;65(5):1041–6. https://doi.org/10.1161/HYPERTENSIONAHA.114.05021.

96. Plante GE, Dessurault DL. Hypertension in elderly patients. A comparative study between indapamide and hydrochlorothiazide. Am J Med. 1988;84(1B):98–103.

97. Filippatos TD, Makri A, Elisaf MS, Liamis G. Hyponatremia in the elderly: challenges and solutions. CIA. 2017;12:1957–65. https://doi.org/10.2147/CIA.S138535.

98. Lindeman RD, Romero LJ, Liang HC, Baumgartner RN, Koehler KM, Garry PJ. Do elderly persons need to be encouraged to drink more fluids? J Gerontol A Biol Sci Med Sci. 2000;55(7):M361–5. https://doi.org/10.1093/gerona/55.7.m361.

99. Palevsky PM, Bhagrath R, Greenberg A. Hypernatremia in hospitalized patients. Ann Intern Med. 1996;124(2):197–203.

100. Snyder NA, Feigal DW, Arieff AI. Hypernatremia in elderly patients. A heterogeneous, morbid, and iatrogenic entity. Ann Intern Med. 1987;107(3):309–19. https://doi.org/10.7326/0003-4819-107-2-309.

101. Lindner G, Funk GC, Schwarz C, et al. Hypernatremia in the critically ill is an independent risk factor for mortality. Am J Kidney Dis. 2007;50(6):952–7. https://doi.org/10.1053/j.ajkd.2007.08.016.

102. Goshima T, Terasawa T, Iwata M, Matsushima A, Hattori T, Sasano H. Intracranial hemorrhage caused by acute-onset severe hypernatremia. J Community Hosp Intern Med Perspect. 2022;12(5):124–5. https://doi.org/10.55729/2000-9666.1089.

103. Simmons MA, Adcock EW, Bard H, Battaglia FC. Hypernatremia and intracranial hemorrhage in neonates. N Engl J Med. 1974;291(1):6–10. https://doi.org/10.1056/NEJM197407042910102.

104. Barnette AR, Myers BJ, Berg CS, Inder TE. Sodium intake and intraventricular hemorrhage in the preterm infant. Ann Neurol. 2010;67(6):817–23. https://doi.org/10.1002/ana.21986.

105. Lim WH, Lien R, Chiang MC, et al. Hypernatremia and grade III/IV intraventricular hemorrhage among extremely low birth weight infants. J Perinatol. 2011;31(3):193–8. https://doi.org/10.1038/jp.2010.86.

106. Kozeny GA, Murdock DK, Euler DE, et al. In vivo effects of acute changes in osmolality and sodium concentration on myocardial contractility. Am Heart J. 1985;109(2):290–6. https://doi.org/10.1016/0002-8703(85)90596-4.

107. Bratusch-Marrain PR, DeFronzo RA. Impairment of insulin-mediated glucose metabolism by hyperosmolality in man. Diabetes. 1983;32(11):1028–34. https://doi.org/10.2337/diab.32.11.1028.

108. Turgutalp K, Özhan O, Gök Oğuz E, et al. Community-acquired hypernatremia in elderly and very elderly patients admitted to the hospital: clinical characteristics and outcomes. Med Sci Monit. 2012;18(12):CR729–34. https://doi.org/10.12659/msm.883600.

109. Ni HB, Hu XX, Huang XF, et al. Risk factors and outcomes in patients with hypernatremia and sepsis. Am J Med Sci. 2016;351(6):601–5. https://doi.org/10.1016/j.amjms.2016.01.027.

110. Waite MD, Fuhrman SA, Badawi O, Zuckerman IH, Franey CS. Intensive care unit-acquired hypernatremia is an independent predictor of increased mortality and length of stay. J Crit Care. 2013;28(4):405–12. https://doi.org/10.1016/j.jcrc.2012.11.013.

111. Mahowald JM, Himmelstein DU. Hypernatremia in the elderly: relation to infection and mortality. J Am Geriatr Soc. 1981;29(4):177–80. https://doi.org/10.1111/j.1532-5415.1981.tb01761.x.

112. Liamis G, Filippatos TD, Elisaf MS. Evaluation and treatment of hypernatremia: a practical guide for physicians. Postgrad Med. 2016;128(3):299–306. https://doi.org/10.1080/00325481.2016.1147322.

113. Lavizzo-Mourey R, Johnson J, Stolley P. Risk factors for dehydration among elderly nursing home residents. J Am Geriatr Soc. 1988;36(3):213–8. https://doi.org/10.1111/j.1532-5415.1988.tb01803.x.

114. Sarahian S, Pouria MM, Ing TS, Sam R. Hypervolemic hypernatremia is the most common type of hypernatremia in the intensive care unit. Int Urol Nephrol. 2015;47(11):1817–21. https://doi.org/10.1007/s11255-015-1103-0.

115. Refardt J, Winzeler B, Christ-Crain M. Copeptin and its role in the diagnosis of diabetes insipidus and the syndrome of inappropriate antidiuresis. Clin Endocrinol. 2019;91(1):22–32. https://doi.org/10.1111/cen.13991.
116. Rose BD, Post TW. Clinical physiology of acid-base and electrolyte disorders. 5th ed. New York: McGraw-Hill; 2001.
117. Bataille S, Baralla C, Torro D, et al. Undercorrection of hypernatremia is frequent and associated with mortality. BMC Nephrol. 2014;15(1):37. https://doi.org/10.1186/1471-2369-15-37.
118. Alshayeb HM, Showkat A, Babar F, Mangold T, Wall BM. Severe hypernatremia correction rate and mortality in hospitalized patients. Am J Med Sci. 2011;341(5):356–60. https://doi.org/10.1097/MAJ.0b013e31820a3a90.
119. Sterns RH. Disorders of plasma sodium — causes, consequences, and correction. N Engl J Med. 2015;372(1):55–65. https://doi.org/10.1056/NEJMra1404489.
120. Fang C, Mao J, Dai Y, et al. Fluid management of hypernatraemic dehydration to prevent cerebral oedema: a retrospective case control study of 97 children in China. J Paediatr Child Health. 2010;46(6):301–3. https://doi.org/10.1111/j.1440-1754.2010.01712.x.
121. Bruck E, Abal G, Aceto T. Therapy of infants with hypertonic dehydration due to diarrhea. A controlled study of clinical, chemical, and pathophysiological response to two types of therapeutic fluid regimen, with evaluation of late sequelae. Am J Dis Child. 1968;115(3):281–301. https://doi.org/10.1001/archpedi.1968.02100010283001.
122. Bolat F, Oflaz MB, Güven AS, et al. What is the safe approach for neonatal hypernatremic dehydration? A retrospective study from a neonatal intensive care unit. Pediatr Emerg Care. 2013;29(7):808–13. https://doi.org/10.1097/PEC.0b013e3182983bac.
123. Kahn A, Brachet E, Blum D. Controlled fall in natremia and risk of seizures in hypertonic dehydration. Intensive Care Med. 1979;5(1):27–31. https://doi.org/10.1007/BF01738999.
124. Chauhan K, Pattharanitima P, Patel N, et al. Rate of correction of hypernatremia and health outcomes in critically ill patients. Clin J Am Soc Nephrol. 2019;14(5):656–63. https://doi.org/10.2215/CJN.10640918.
125. Didsbury M, See EJ, Cheng DR, Kausman J, Quinlan C. Correcting hypernatremia in children. Clin J Am Soc Nephrol. 2023;18(3):306–14. https://doi.org/10.2215/CJN.0000000000000077.

Chapter 13
Acute Kidney Injury in Older Adults

Matteo Floris, Antonello Pani, and Mitchell H. Rosner

Take Home Points
- Advanced age is associated with increased AKI risk.
- Molecular, cellular, structural, and functional changes associated with aging may contribute to kidney injury.
- The most common causes of AKI in older adults include postrenal obstructive disease, ischemic ATN, and hemodynamically-mediated AKI.
- The kidney insult is often multifactorial.
- Diagnostic and therapeutic issues in AKI for older patients are comparable to those observed in the general population.
- Once established, AKI is associated with a higher risk of CKD, kidney failure, and mortality.
- Due to the increased risk for frailty with advancing age, treatment strategies for AKI should be individualized and include shared decision-making.

M. Floris (✉)
Nephrology, Dialysis and Transplantation Unit, ARNAS Brotzu, Cagliari, Italy
e-mail: matteo.floris@aob.it

A. Pani
Nephrology, Dialysis and Transplantation Unit, ARNAS Brotzu, Cagliari, Italy

Department of Medical Sciences and Public Health, University of Cagliari, Cagliari, Italy

M. H. Rosner
Division of Nephrology, University of Virginia Health System, Charlottesville, VA, USA
e-mail: mhr9r@hscmail.mcc.virginia.edu

H. Kramer et al. (eds.), *Kidney Disease in the Elderly*,
https://doi.org/10.1007/978-3-031-68460-9_13

Introduction

The number of patients in the hospital including the intensive care unit (ICU) who are aged 65 years and older is rising [1–3]. Older adults show a heightened risk for the development of acute kidney injury (AKI) as defined by the KDIGO stages 1–3 [4, 5]. The development of AKI in ICU and hospitalized patients is associated with increased mortality, increased days in the ICU, increased ventilator days, higher costs, and long-term morbidity and mortality [6–10]. Avoiding AKI is likely to improve outcomes. Despite the critical need to prevent AKI and associated morbidity, clinical trials have failed to discover effective pharmacological therapies for AKI [3]. Thus, prevention of AKI remains one of the most effective strategies that could improve outcomes. In order to prevent AKI, it is important to understand the risk factors (both intrinsic and extrinsic to the patients), predisposing factors, and specific settings in which AKI may occur. Knowing these factors, patients can be monitored, and preventive strategies can be developed, studied, and implemented to decrease AKI incidence and improve outcomes, especially for the most vulnerable patients.

Case Report

An 86-year-old female with moderate to severe dementia who resides in a nursing home is brought to the emergency department with worsening confusion and a fever of 38.9 °C. She has a history of hypertension, stage 3a chronic kidney disease (CKD) (estimated glomerular filtration rate (eGFR) of 49 mL/min/1.73 m^2) and urinary retention. On admission, her blood pressure was initially 83/40 mmHg, her pulse was 124 per minute and irregular and she was arousable only to painful stimuli. Respiratory rate was 28 per minute and oxygen saturation on room air was 82%. Physical examination was notable for bibasilar rales and peripheral edema. Laboratory work was notable for a serum sodium of 132 meq/L, potassium of 5.8 meq/L, bicarbonate of 14 meq/L, and creatinine of 4.8 mg/dL. White blood cell count was 23,000/mm^3. The patient was administered intravenous fluids and broad-spectrum antibiotics but despite this, her condition deteriorated leading to respiratory failure requiring mechanical ventilation and the need for vasopressor agents to support her blood pressure. On hospital day 2, her urine output fell to <10 mL/h and a discussion was started regarding the need for kidney replacement therapy with continuous modalities. The nephrology team met with the patient's family to explain AKI, its potential treatment with KRT and its prognosis. The family expressed concerns about the patient's limited functional ability prior to this hospital admission. After a discussion between the nephrologist and the patient's family, the decision was made to treat the AKI without KRT and to move toward comfort care measures only.

Epidemiology: Older ICU Patients and the Development of AKI

Older patients (>age 65 years) represent the largest segment of patients admitted to the ICU and 55% of all American ICU bed-days are occupied by this group of patients [11]. In a multicenter study of 120,123 adult ICU admissions of more than 24 h duration, Australian New Zealand Intensive Care Society Adult Patient (ANCIZS) database researchers determined that 13% were aged >80 years and that the admission rate for this age group increased by 5.6% per year during the period between 2000 and 2005 [12]. In a more recent study, patients aged >65 years represented 45.7% of ICU admissions and these patients had a higher prevalence of heart failure (25.9–40.3%), cardiac arrhythmia (24.6–43.5%), and valvular heart disease (7.5–15.8%) [13]. Interestingly, among the very old (>85 years old), one study found that ICU admissions actually fell as compared to younger groups, suggesting that some of the oldest patients may opt for less aggressive care [14]. Choosing more conservative routes is not surprising given the reported ICU mortality exceeding 80% among hospitalized adults aged >85 years [15]. The factors independently associated with a higher rate of mortality include the acute physiology and chronic health evaluation (APACHE) II score, the need for mechanical ventilation (MV), or inotropic support, and the presence of coronary artery disease (CAD) or chronic kidney disease (CKD). Despite numerous studies, uncertainty remains whether ICU admission in this population confers any short- or long-term benefit to patients.

Almost one in four older adults in the ICU will develop AKI and a substantial number of these AKI cases will be severe [16]. A prospective multicenter study on 29,269 critically ill patients with a median age of 67 years, determined that 5.7% of the patients developed severe AKI [4]. Moreover, in a prospective cohort study on risk factors and outcomes of AKI in the ICU as evaluated by the sequential organ failure assessment (SOFA) score, 24.7% of 1411 patients developed AKI. The median age was significantly higher in the AKI group, and age >65 years was an independent risk factor for the development of AKI [5]. In a longitudinal cohort analysis of 381 critically ill octogenarians, 40% of patients admitted after 1996 developed AKI, as compared to 4% of this age group in the time period before 1978 [17]. Differences in AKI by time period could be attributed to increased awareness and better diagnosis but higher numbers of co-morbidities such as obesity and diabetes could also be operative. In their recent study comparing the RIFLE and AKIN classifications, Joannidis et al. analyzed 16,784 patients during the initial 48 h of their ICU stay and determined that the incidence of AKI ranged from 28.5% to 35.5%. The mean age of the patients was 63 years, with 25% aged >75 years [18]. An analysis showed that the incidence of AKI increases stepwise from 24.9 (75–79 years) to 34.2 (80–84 years) to 46.9 episodes (85 years and older) per 1000 patient-years, respectively [19]. In a more recent study among older men in China, there was a high rate of AKI in patients admitted to the ICU (39.0%) [6]. The median age was 87 years and the 28-day mortality rate was 25.7%. The AKI etiologies were infections (39.6%), hypovolemia (23.8%), cardiovascular events (15.9%), nephrotoxicity (12.0%), and surgery (7.1%). Multiple organ dysfunction syndrome (46.4%) and pulmonary infection (22.5%) were the principal causes of death. Not surprisingly, more severe AKI stages (stage 2: hazard ratio (HR) = 3.709; 95% CI 1.926–7.141; P <0.001 and stage 3: HR = 5.660; 95% CI 2.990–10.717; P <0.001) were independent risk factors for 28-day mortality. Identification of risk factors might lead to more intensive monitoring and opportunities for early prevention of AKI.

Recently, a study reported that 46% of COVID-19 adult patients hospitalized in in a New York City health system had AKI, and the median age of patients with AKI was significantly higher than those without non-AKI (71 vs. 63 years, P <0.001) [20]. Thus, the data consistently show a rising incidence of AKI with aging and significant AKI-associated complications and mortality.

Factors Contributing to AKI

As part of the aging process, the kidney undergoes age-dependent structural and functional alterations: a significant decrease in kidney mass, functioning nephron numbers, and baseline kidney function (Fig. 13.1) [21]. In a study of autopsy samples, a decline in kidney weight was noted in 19% of men and 9% in women aged 70–79 years compared with men and women aged 20–29 years, respectively [22]. The loss of kidney mass with aging is primarily cortical, with relative sparing of the medulla [23]. These autopsy data have been confirmed in a large population study

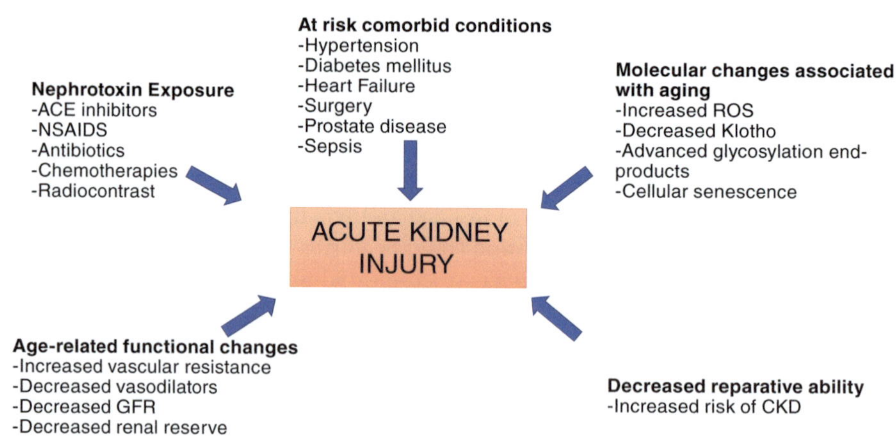

Fig. 13.1 Factors associated with development of AKI in the older patient. Older adults are predisposed to AKI due to convergence of factors such as intrinsic functional, structural, and molecular cellular changes associated with aging, increased number of comorbidities, and increased likelihood of nephrotoxin exposure. ACE (angiotensin-converting enzyme), NSAIDs (nonsteroidal anti-inflammatory drugs), ROS (reactive oxygen species), GFR (glomerular filtration rate), CKD (chronic kidney disease)

which included 3097 Sardinian individuals, 12.9% of whom were older than 70 years [24]. Among the healthy adults, kidney volume and length increased up to the fifth decade of life and then progressively decreased in men; in women, the decrease in kidney size is slower and less pronounced [24]. Independent predictors of lower kidney volume (<2.5 percentile for age and sex) include male sex, low body mass index, short height, reduced waist/hip ratio, and high serum creatinine levels (SCr) [24]. The incidence of sclerotic glomeruli rises with advancing age, increasing from less than 5% of the total glomeruli at the age of 40 years to 10–30% by the eighth decade of life [25, 26]. With kidney senescence, there is a variable decrease in glomerular filtration rate (GFR). However, the rate of decline varies according to measurement criteria, gender, race, genetic influence, and, most importantly, the presence of interacting medical conditions that can impact kidney function [27–29]. Classic studies demonstrated a highly significant reduction in creatinine clearance (CrCl) with age. Beginning at age 34 years and accelerating after age 65 years, CrCl decreased by approximately 1 mL/min per 1.73 m^2 per year after age 50 years [28, 29]. However, a decline in kidney function with aging is neither predictable nor an inevitable consequence of aging because 35% of older adults showed a stable CrCl over a 20-year period [29].

Effective renal blood flow (RBF) decreases up to 10% per decade of life [30]. Research has demonstrated that the increase in RBF in older individuals in response to provocative maneuvers such as amino acid infusion, was markedly impaired, with a higher renal vascular resistance [31]. The rise in renal vascular resistance may in part be related to reduced nitric oxide production in older individuals. Thus, GFR may be preserved to some extent through an increased filtration fraction and renal vasoconstriction. Renal sympathetic-mediated vasoconstriction appears to be exaggerated in the aging kidney while the response to vasodilatory mediators, such as atrial natriuretic peptide and prostacyclin, is poor [31, 32]. Furthermore, the aging renal vasculature appears to exhibit exaggerated angiotensin-II-mediated vasoconstriction [31, 32]. These changes may lead to a loss in functional reserve, a key measure that allows the kidney to adapt to stress and prevent AKI.

Changes in renal hemodynamics could potentiate the risk for developing AKI. For example, in combination with dehydration, a disturbance in autoregulatory defense mechanisms that would normally preserve GFR and RBF (such as increased renal vascular resistance) can lead to ischemia and AKI due to drastic falls in RBF in the older kidney [33]. In fact, changes in tubular sodium handling with aging result in impairment of urine concentrating ability and increase the risk of volume depletion in older individuals [34]. In states of stress, this impairment may lead to more rapid decreases in organ perfusion and a greater propensity for prerenal AKI.

The exact role of these molecular changes that result in the structural and functional changes in the aging kidney remains speculative and these pathways are attractive targets for therapies to prevent AKI or hasten repair after injury. Some of the molecular changes in the aging kidney that have been identified include: decreases in the anti-aging protein Klotho [35] in the tubular epithelium, activation of the Wnt/ β-Catenin pathway that may mediate the progression of CKD after AKI

[36], greater activation of the complement cascade [37] and increased production of damaging reactive oxygen species [38]. More studies on the exact role of these pathways regarding the risk of developing AKI are needed.

In addition to the structural and molecular changes that occur with aging, patients are more susceptible to AKI as they age due to the accumulation of comorbid conditions such as prostatic disease with the risk of obstructive AKI, diabetes mellitus, systolic or diastolic heart failure and the presence of underlying CKD and impaired kidney function [39]. Along with comorbidities comes the risk of polypharmacy and drug-induced AKI. Lean body mass decreases in older individuals with respect to adipose tissue, causing alterations in the volume of distribution [40]. Water-soluble drugs, such as aminoglycosides, therefore attain higher blood concentrations [40]. A decreased GFR often goes unnoticed when clinicians are focused on only looking at serum creatinine values, which in older individuals may result in an overestimate of the GFR and, ultimately, overdosage of potentially nephrotoxic medications. An example of the overlapping pathway to AKI that can be seen in older individuals is nephrotoxicity due to non-steroidal anti-inflammatory drugs (NSAIDs) where the higher predisposition of older patients for volume depletion can interact with the inhibition of renal vasodilatory prostaglandins, which exacerbates the imbalance between vasoconstrictors and vasodilators leading to AKI [41]. All of these factors may increase the risk of AKI when patients are exposed to kidney stresses such as radiocontrast agents, surgery, or sepsis (occurrences that are more common with aging) [40].

Finally, repair of kidney injury may also be impaired in the aging kidney leading to delay in resolution of AKI and more severe injury. A recent systematic review and meta-analysis of recovery of kidney function after AKI in older individuals has shown that recovery after AKI is approximately 28% less likely to occur when the patient is older than 65 years [42]. Whether these results are caused by the effects of advanced age on the kidney itself or the increased number of comorbidities (including baseline CKD) in older individuals is not certain. Long-term recovery is also less likely and it is believed that AKI in older individuals more often results in CKD [42]. The lower likelihood of kidney recovery in older individuals may be due to the effects of aging to impair the capacity for kidney repair [42]. The capacity for renal epithelial cell proliferation declines with aging as does the function of progenitor and stem cells that are critical for tubular repair [42]. The burst of cellular proliferation usually seen in response to acute damage seems to decline with age [42]. Moreover, basal rates of cellular apoptosis increase with age, both under baseline conditions as well as in response to injury. Changes in potential progenitor and immune cell functions are also seen [42]. Growth factors play a critical role in regulating cellular proliferation, migration, and apoptosis, and their expression is upregulated in response to injury. The expression of many of these growth factors decreases with aging, and their respective receptor transduction pathways are often downregulated [43]. In aggregate, healing may be impaired which may significantly alter the course of AKI leading to more prolonged episodes and incomplete healing.

Causes of AKI

Acute kidney injury in older individuals shares the same causes that afflict the general population, with some differences in terms of incidence, presentation and evolution. Since the number of kidney biopsies performed in older patients is low, information about the causes of kidney dysfunction is often obtained from clinical reports [44]. These data show that AKI occurring in older adults is often multifactorial with a predominance of iatrogenic insults, which are often drug-related, and obstructive injuries occurring in patients with greater kidney frailty compared to younger counterparts [44]. In a recent analysis involving 480 patients hospitalized for severe AKI in a tertiary center and stratified into three age groups (<65 y/o; 65–75 y/o and >75 y/o), a higher burden of comorbidities and AKI risk was noted in patients aged 75+ years. In this group, AKI was due to obstruction in 23%, sepsis in 20%, and hypovolemia in 20% [45]. On the other hand, some studies suggest that a high proportion of prerenal and ischemic causes account for at least half of the AKI episodes in older patients [46]. Once established, AKI in older individuals is associated with a worse prognosis, including poor recovery after kidney replacement therapy (KRT) initiation, prolonged hospitalization, increased CKD, and progression to kidney failure [47].

Prerenal AKI

Prerenal AKI is estimated to make up a significant proportion of AKI cases [48] and is mainly responsible for decreased kidney perfusion that may exert dangerous effects in older individuals due to stimulation of sympathetic nervous system-mediated vasoconstriction, thus ultimately reducing renal blood flow. The causes of kidney hypoperfusion include reduced cardiac output (acute and chronic cardiorenal syndromes), reduced effective circulating volume (sepsis, cirrhosis, and nephrotic syndrome), and hypovolemic issues (blood loss and dehydration). Older adults have an increased risk of dehydration due to decreased thirst response, reduced kidney function, and a higher burden of medications such as diuretics and laxatives or drugs that may decrease appetite or level of consciousness [7]. The increased risk of developing intense and prolonged febrile illnesses, which is particularly important during the SARS-Cov-2 pandemic, may increase the clinical impact of dehydration on kidney function [20, 49]. A considerable number of prerenal AKI cases may be completely or partially reversed with appropriate fluid replacement. However, a higher percentage of older patients progress to acute tubular necrosis (ATN) and show slower recovery compared to younger subjects, especially in cases of severe and prolonged insults [50]. The diagnosis of prerenal AKI is often complicated by the poor reliability of clinical signs of dehydration. Furthermore, the urinary indices, such as the fractional excretion of sodium, that are traditionally used to discriminate between prerenal and renal AKI, may better reflect both alterations of tubular sodium handling and the effects of diuretic treatments than the degree of the kidney insult itself. For these reasons, short-term administration of intravenous fluids is often the first clinical choice following careful evaluation of diuresis and changes in laboratory parameters. Foley catheter placement is warranted due to the higher percentage of urinary incontinence and the need to periodically evaluate urine output.

Renal AKI

Ischemic AKI, when prolonged, can lead to acute tubular necrosis and may occur in a wide range of settings. Some etiologies for ischemic AKI are more common in older versus younger adults and are highlighted below.

Renovascular Diseases

Due to the burden of severe atherosclerotic disease, older adults have a high risk of AKI related to acute obstruction of the renal vasculature. Other than advanced age, risk factors for renal vasculature obstruction include smoking, male sex, diabetes, hypercholesterolemia, and hypertension [51]. A cause of AKI in older adults is atheroembolic disease, a severe and systemic condition caused by dislodged cholesterol plaques from a major artery and the dissemination of micro-emboli throughout the vascular bed [51]. These emboli can lead to an inflammatory response that contributes to vascular injury and AKI [51]. This condition mainly occurs after invasive arterial procedures, although spontaneous occurrence has been reported, especially in at-risk patients [52].

Hemodynamically-Mediated AKI

Older patients are at increased risk for hemodynamically-mediated AKI due to the combination of hypoperfusion of the kidneys and administration of drugs that may reduce intraglomerular pressure. Particularly, NSAIDs may reduce the activity of vasodilatory prostaglandin on the afferent artery, while angiotensin-converting enzyme inhibitors (ACEis) and angiotensin II Receptor Blockers (ARBs) predominantly decrease the angiotensin II-mediated resistance of the efferent artery. According to a large population study among patients older than 65 years of age, NSAID administration increases the risk of developing AKI by about 40% and hyperkalemia by 50% [53]. In this population, NSAID use accounts for 25% of all AKI causes as compared to 15% among the general population [54]. Besides old age, well-known risk factors include atherosclerotic disease, pre-existing CKD, and renal hypoperfusion [55]. Due to their well-known effects on hypertension and proteinuria, renin-angiotensin system (RAS) blockers are frequently prescribed to patients with CKD, thus slowing CKD progression [56]. However, when administered together with NSAIDs, RAS blockers carry significant risk of AKI, especially in the presence of dehydration and/or sepsis [56]. In older adults with CKD, administering RAS blockers almost doubles the risk of AKI, which may occur in up to 42% of patients [57, 58]. Of note, many ACEis are cleared by the kidney and can accumulate in the setting of low GFR, thus inducing more severe RAS inhibition that may contribute to acute declines in kidney function, especially in the presence of other conditions such as dehydration and/or renovascular diseases [59].

Acute Tubular Necrosis

Acute tubular necrosis is likely the most frequent cause of AKI in older adults, with a prevalence ranging between 25% and 87% depending on the study population [60]. The insults leading to this condition are mainly ischemic, but can also be due to drug or contrast media exposure or pigment-induced (nephrotoxic ATN). Ischemic ATN in older individuals often occurs as a consequence of cardiac surgery (aortic aneurysm repair, bypass surgery), and involves multiple mechanisms including hemodynamic and inflammatory factors such as ischemia-reperfusion injury and oxidative stress, microembolization (associated or not with cardio-pulmonary bypass) and neurohormonal activation that can exert greater damage on frail kidneys [61]. These mechanisms may act synergistically, often in association with toxic exposure. Older adults are more prone to develop systemic infections that can lead to sepsis and multiorgan failure. At least half of older adults with sepsis develop AKI [62–64].

Drug toxicity represents one of the leading causes of ATN in older individuals. Commonly involved drugs include antibiotics (particularly aminoglycosides, vancomycin, and piperacillin/tazobactam), immunosuppressive agents (cyclosporine and tacrolimus), contrast medium and antineoplastic drugs. The most common risk factors, besides advanced age, include CKD and other pre-existing chronic medical conditions, hypoperfusion status, and polypharmacy [65].

Older adults are susceptible to developing AKI after iodinated contrast administration. This entity, named contrast-associated nephropathy (CAN), has been called into question but seems to be most prevalent in high-risk patients exposed to large volumes of iodinated contrast in the setting of hemodynamic instability [66]. Risk factors for CAN include: advanced age, undergoing percutaneous coronary intervention, baseline eGFR below 60 mL/min, left ventricular ejection fraction less than 45%, and poorly controlled diabetes [67]. Prevention strategies include administering periprocedural fluids and, when possible, reducing the impact of concomitant risk factors such as anemia, dehydration/hypotension, and high-dose contrast medium administration.

Older patients may develop rhabdomyolysis and consequent myoglobin-induced ATN due to falls, other trauma and/or immobilization (more than half of AKI causes), sepsis, and seizures, often in the context of cerebrovascular accidents, electrolyte disorders and hyperosmolar states [68].

Acute Interstitial Nephritis

Acute interstitial nephritis (AIN) is an important cause of AKI in older individuals. Compared to younger individuals, older patients have a significantly higher risk of developing drug-induced AIN mainly due to penicillin and omeprazole administration, although a number of substances including herbal remedies may be involved. Autoimmune or systemic causes of AIN are less common in comparison to the occurrence in younger patients (7% vs. 27%) [69]. Proton pump inhibitor-related AIN exerts less severe but more prolonged kidney damage compared to AIN caused by other drugs. Once established, AIN among older adults tends to be more severe and more often leads to KRT initiation compared to younger patients regardless of the cause; nevertheless, more than 85% of older patients show partial or complete recovery within 6 months after AIN diagnosis [69]. Prompt initiation of corticosteroid therapy is positively associated with quick and sustained recovery of kidney function in many cases.

Glomerulonephritis

Older adults have an increased incidence of glomerulonephritis with a rate of 30.8 per million population (pmp) compared to the general population (25.7 pmp). Clinicians should consider presence of glomerulonephritis when patients have urinary abnormalities (particularly microhematuria and inflammatory urinary casts along with proteinuria) and GFR reduction higher than expected based on age (around 1.7 mL/min per year in the absence of severe comorbidities) [70]. Rapidly progressive glomerulonephritis, often associated with ANCA-associated vasculitis (AAV) (particularly granulomatosis with polyangiitis (GPA) and microscopic polyangiitis) is more common among older adults In patients aged ≥ 80 years undergoing renal biopsy for rapidly progressive glomerulonephritis, AAV is the histological diagnosis in 19% of cases overall and in 33% when RPGN is the indication for histological evaluation [71]. Although advanced age is often associated with poor kidney survival and increased risk of adverse events, the percentage of older patients who show response to therapy is similar to the percentage of younger patients. Initiation of immunosuppressive (corticosteroids and cyclophosphamide or rituximab) therapy is associated with a fivefold higher relative risk of death compared to the younger population. Nevertheless, it was also associated with a 73% reduction in ESKD risk and a 67% reduction in death risk compared to a control group of untreated patients [72]. In order to provide adequate treatment while preventing the risk of excessive immunosuppression, careful dosing and monitoring of immunosuppressive agents in consultation with a pharmacist is strongly advised [73].

Post-renal AKI

Post-renal causes account for 9% of AKI in patients aged over 70 years old and depend on extrinsic or intrinsic obstruction that may occur in any part of the urinary tract [74]. Prostate enlargement secondary to benign hypertrophy or carcinoma is the primary cause of urinary tract obstruction in males, while the second is urethral strictures that may occur secondary to trauma, infection and after treatment for prostate cancer. Up to 8.4% of patients undergoing either radical prostatectomy or non-surgical therapy for prostate cancer develop urethral strictures [75]. The most common post-renal AKI in females is ureteral obstruction caused by pelvic malignancy, usually invasive carcinoma of the cervix or ovarian neoplasms. Ultrasonography at the time of admission is part of the diagnostic work-up in any AKI case and is especially relevant in older individuals for whom urinary catheterization is warranted. Clinically relevant obstruction is associated with hydronephrosis in 95% of cases [76]. False-negative ultrasonography may be observed in patients with retroperitoneal fibrosis and in cases of severe volume depletion and early obstruction [77].

Laboratory Evaluation

Prompt diagnosis of AKI is crucial in order to limit the progression of the insult and the related clinical consequences. Although numerous biomarkers have been developed and tested over the years, the diagnosis of AKI still relies on serum creatinine and urine output according to KDIGO guidelines. The criteria of increasing serum creatinine and decreasing urine output do not differ by age group, although age is one of the variables that most significantly confounds the association of serum creatinine with true GFR, which makes the detection of AKI in older adults challenging [78].

To address the low sensitivity for detecting AKI, especially in older adults, ongoing research continues to focus on the identification of new biomarkers for early AKI risk and prognosis. Currently, the most important biomarkers are neutrophil gelatinase-associated lipocalin (NGAL), kidney injury molecule 1 (KIM-1), interleukin 18 (IL-18), cystatin C and the product of urinary tissue inhibitor metalloproteinase 2 (TIMP-2), and insulin-like growth factor binding protein 7 (IGFBP7). Although none of these biomarkers are recommended for clinical use, these biomarkers may be most useful in older adults. Urinary NGAL showed diagnostic power for AKI in patients with sepsis and advanced age [79], while cystatin C detects reduced GFR in older adults and appears to be a strong predictor of death and cardiovascular events in this population [80]. Urinary TIMP-2 and IGFBP7 (either alone or combined) are able to predict the need for KRT and 30-day mortality after elective cardiac surgery [81]. However, although the new biomarkers show some diagnostic utility for AKI, no biomarker has been adopted for widespread assessment.

Once AKI is diagnosed, the laboratory evaluation follows the diagnostic classification that is aided by a careful history and physical examination as well as a review of recent clinical events and potential nephrotoxin exposure (prerenal, renal, and post-renal causes). Urinary sediment analysis is of particular importance since it facilitates the differential diagnosis between prerenal and renal AKI causes. In fact, urinary sediment in patients affected by prerenal AKI is usually bland or contains some hyaline casts. However, in ATN renal tubular epithelial (RTE) cells and RTE cell casts are frequent, as are granular casts or mixed cellular casts [82]. Furthermore, when combined with urinalysis or urine dipstick, urinary sediment analysis may provide information about the renal compartment involved. Urinary acanthocytes and red blood cell casts, along with albuminuria are indicative of glomerular injury, while culture-negative leukocyturia with RTE cells, white blood cell casts and granular casts may point to acute or chronic tubulointerstitial disease [83]. Since the incidence of kidney biopsy complications does not differ with regard to age groups, prompt histological evaluation, unless clinically contraindicated, should be offered to all patients in whom AKI diagnosis is not clear.

Recovery of Kidney Function and Prognosis of AKI in Older Adults

CKD and ESRD After AKI in Older Adults

Acute kidney injury is no longer considered a completely reversible condition and with the exception of prerenal AKI, the repair process after AKI is often incomplete. As a consequence, the functional outcome after acute AKI may range from a subclinical condition, characterized by reduced kidney function reserve, to CKD that may be progressive [84–86]. The recovery of kidney function after AKI in older individuals is substantially impaired and estimated to be approximately 28% less likely to occur when patients are older than 65 years of age [87], while the risk of developing CKD can be up to 20 times higher compared to younger patients [88]. These effects may depend on intrinsic characteristics of the aged kidney (see Fig. 13.1), and on the substantial burden of comorbidities in an older population. Little is known about the effects of management of age-related comorbidities in hampering the incidence of reduced kidney recovery from AKI in older populations [89]. Given the risk of CKD after AKI, it is recommended that close follow-up by a nephrologist should be part of any follow-up plan for these patients.

Mortality After AKI in Older Patients

Acute kidney injury in older patients is associated with increased short- and long-term mortality. Short-term mortality, defined as the time between the onset of AKI and 90 days from diagnosis, ranges from 20% to 45% depending on the cohort analyzed [48]; in fact, compared to community-acquired AKI, hospital-acquired AKI is characterized by higher mortality [90]. Furthermore, the worst outcomes have been observed when renal AKI occurs, compared to prerenal [90] and when oliguria or anuria is present [91–94].

The mortality of patients with AKI in the ICU has been variously reported between 31% and 80% reflective of differences in age definition, treatment intensity and characteristics, severity of diseases, and length of follow-up [39]. Although some studies report that advanced age is an independent risk factor for death in older patients, other reports did not find this association. Conversely, these studies identified mortality risk that was related to higher KDIGO AKI stage, the presence of multi-organ dysfunction, and patient frailty.

Long-term mortality, defined as death occurring after 3 months from AKI diagnosis, has been evaluated in a few studies in older patients. One study from Brazil reported that up to 66% of older patients with AKI requiring dialysis die within 12 months [95]. A retrospective study on older patients requiring continuous kidney replacement therapy (CKRT) showed that age above 75 years was associated with increased short- and long-term mortality [96]. It is important to note that these observational studies may be confounded by the multiple interacting co-morbidities found in older patients.

Quality of Life After AKI in Older Patients

Health-related Quality of life (HRQoL) is rarely evaluated in older patients after AKI. The Prolonged Outcomes Study of the Randomized Evaluation of Normal versus Augmented Level Replacement Therapy (POST-RENAL) study highlighted that AKI survivors (median follow-up of 3.5 years) have lower physical and mental components of HRQoL compared with the general population. Statistically significant variables for low HRQoL after AKI episodes were advanced age and poor kidney function at follow-up [62]. In other reports, the impact of age in driving worse HRQoL outcomes in older patients is less clear, while the overall burden of comorbidities seems to be more significant [97, 98].

Prevention of AKI in the Older Patient

Unfortunately, many risk factors for AKI in older patients are not modifiable. Besides advanced age, AKI risk factors include male sex as well as presence of multiple chronic conditions such as heart failure, diabetes, hypertension, obesity and CKD. As a consequence, the first step toward preventing AKI is to assess the individual risk of developing this condition. Numerous risk assessment models have been developed and validated in multiple clinical settings when the timing of primary insult is known (i.e., surgery, percutaneous coronary interventions, and contrast medium administration). These models usually include the most important clinical variables in a logistic regression model which determines the total AKI risk. Estimating the AKI risk before a procedure that could cause kidney injury may provide substantial advantages. First, estimating AKI risk would allow clinicians to apply all available strategies to minimize the risk of the procedure (i.e., early application of KDIGO bundle for AKI prevention that includes maximizing kidney perfusion and minimizing nephrotoxin exposure). The KDIGO bundle includes the following elements: discontinuation of nephrotoxic agents when possible, ensuring volume status and perfusion pressure, employing hemodynamic monitoring when feasible, close monitoring of serum creatinine and urine output, avoidance of hyperglycemia, considering alternatives to radiocontrast studies and ensuring appropriate drug dosing in the setting of AKI. Second, knowing the risk of AKI could improve informed consent acquisition by giving patients more information prior to the intervention. Lastly, it might be used to assess quality improvement programs by analyzing the difference between real versus expected AKI events secondary to a known exposure [99–101].

The main elements in any prevention strategy include maintaining appropriate kidney perfusion pressure and avoiding or limiting the administration of any known nephrotoxic substance [46]. Regarding patients in the ICU, available guidelines suggest preserving kidney hemodynamics by prompt resuscitation of the circulation to ensure adequate hydration, using vasopressors to maintain adequate blood pressure, and administering saline infusion before and after contrast media administration.

In older adults at risk for AKI, careful treatment review is warranted and should be focused on limiting the action of drugs that may impair renal hemodynamics, such as RAS blockers, diuretics, and laxatives. When possible, nephrotoxic drug levels must be measured in order to prevent overdosage (Table 13.1).

Treatment of AKI in Older Patients

The general principles of AKI treatment in the older patients are the same as those applied to the general population. Since older patients may show increased vulnerability to uremic complications as well as reduced tolerance to fluid overload, early

Table 13.1 Prevention strategies

Limitation of loss of function of aged kidney
• Blood pressure control, promotion of healthy lifestyle (diet and exercise), control of weight, glucose, and lipids • RAASi, SGLT2i, vitamin D replacement therapy
Prevention of AKI
Avoidance of nephrotoxin-mediated AKI • Identification of potential nephrotoxic agents, high risk patients and clinical settings • Avoidance of exposure to multiple nephrotoxins • Use of lowest dose and for shortest time possible • Frequent monitoring of drug dose and renal function • Pharmacovigilance
Maintain adequate renal perfusion • Avoid agents that impair renal blood flow autoregulation (NSAIDs, RAASi) • Maintain euvolemia (crystalloids)
Minimization of nosocomial infection
Use of computer surveillance systems • Identify high-risk patients and medications • Application of risk prevention bundles • Determine the correct dose for GFR
Special conditions
Rhabdomyolysis • Intravenous hydration/urine alkalinization
Contrast media exposure • Intravenous hydration (normal saline) • Vitamin C • Iso-osmolar contrast
Tumor lysis syndrome • Allopurinol/rasburicase • Intravenous hydration/urine alkalinization
Aminoglycoside antibiotics • Once-daily dose • Monitoring of drug levels
Methotrexate • Intravenous hydration/urine alkalinization
Acyclovir • Intravenous hydration

RAASi (renin angiotensin aldosterone system inhibitors); SGLT2i (sodium-glucose cotransporter 2 inhibitors); AKI (acute kidney injury); NSAIDs (non-steroidal anti-inflammatory drugs); GFR (glomerular filtration rate)

interventions may be considered in order to minimize treatment-related complications. Furthermore, it is critical to carefully dose medications, to avoid further nephrotoxic exposure, to maintain hemodynamic stability in order to provide adequate kidney perfusion, and to guarantee appropriate nutritional support. In order to provide all of these elements, prolonged intermittent renal replacement therapy (PIRRT) or CRRT may offer substantial advantages compared to intermitted RRT [102].

There are no studies specifically in older patients that compare outcomes of various KRT modalities and thus these decisions should be individualized.

Ethical Perspectives

Clinicians are often faced with difficult decisions regarding the provision of aggressive care for patients with advanced age and critical illness. For nephrologists, this generally means the provision of some form of KRT for patients with KDIGO stage 3 AKI. A recent review on mortality in patients with advanced age in the ICU concluded that, after adjustment for disease severity, mortality rates are higher in older patients than in younger populations [103]. However, their long-term prognosis depends mostly on functional status, not on initial disease severity [103, 104]. In fact, a prospective study of previously healthy older patients in the ICU documented a high mortality rate which increased with age and was mostly related to pre-morbid quality of life [105]. Clearly, chronological age alone is unable to measure the ability of individuals to benefit from a treatment, and should not be the sole criterion used when deciding upon starting dialysis. The decision to start KRT in an older and critically ill patient must therefore be approached in a case-by-case manner. End-of-life wishes are difficult to predict, vary greatly between patients, and can change during the course of an illness. A shared-decision making model that accounts for the risks and benefits of dialysis along with clear goal-setting and expectations for recovery should be instituted. Frequent reassessments of the patient trajectory are also warranted. In some cases, a trial of dialysis can be offered but if no improvement occurs, then consideration of withdrawal of this support may be appropriate. In some cases, consultation with a specialist in ethics and palliative care can be helpful, especially when there may be disagreements between the care team and family or caregivers.

Conclusions

AKI represents a major health problem, especially among critically ill individuals. ATN and urinary tract obstruction are frequent clinical causes of AKI in older adults. AKI onset in the older population may be insidious thus leading to delayed diagnosis, and high risk of complications, and poor outcomes including progression to CKD, kidney failure, and heightened mortality risk. The preservation of kidney perfusion and prevention of further nephrotoxic insults are the main preventive strategies. Since advancing age increases the likelihood of poor outcomes, decisions regarding care for AKI should be individualized and based on the patient's functional status and wishes.

References

1. Lieberman D, Nachshon L, Miloslavsky O, Dvorkin V, Shimoni A, Lieberman D. How do older ventilated patients fare? A survival/functional analysis of 641 ventilations. J Crit Care. 2009;24(3):340–6.
2. Shahidi S, Schroeder TV, Carstensen M, Sillesen H. Outcome and survival of patients aged 75 years and older compared to younger patients after ruptured abdominal aortic aneurysm repair: do the results justify the effort? Ann Vasc Surg. 2009;23(4):469–77.
3. Foerch C, Kessler KR, Steckel DA, Steinmetz H, Sitzer M. Survival and quality of life outcome after mechanical ventilation in elderly stroke patients. J Neurol Neurosurg Psychiatry. 2004;75(7):988–93.
4. Uchino S, Kellum JA, Bellomo R, Doig GS, Morimatsu H, Morgera S, et al. Acute renal failure in critically ill patients: a multinational, multicenter study. JAMA. 2005;294(7):813–8.
5. de Mendonca A, Vincent JL, Suter PM, Moreno R, Dearden NM, Antonelli M, et al. Acute renal failure in the ICU: risk factors and outcome evaluated by the SOFA score. Intensive Care Med. 2000;26(7):915–21.
6. Li Q, Zhao M, Zhou F. Hospital-acquired acute kidney injury in very elderly men: clinical characteristics and short-term outcomes. Aging Clin Exp Res. 2020;32(6):1121–8.
7. Chronopoulos A, Cruz DN, Ronco C. Hospital-acquired acute kidney injury in the elderly. Nat Rev Nephrol. 2010;6(3):141–9.
8. Li Q, Zhao M, Wang X. The impact of transient and persistent acute kidney injury on short-term outcomes in very elderly patients. Clin Interv Aging. 2017;12:1013–20.
9. Li Q, Mao Z, Hu P, Kang H, Zhou F. Analysis of the short-term prognosis and risk factors of elderly acute kidney injury patients in different KDIGO diagnostic windows. Aging Clin Exp Res. 2020;32(5):851–60.
10. Rewa O, Bagshaw SM. Acute kidney injury-epidemiology, outcomes and economics. Nat Rev Nephrol. 2014;10(4):193–207.
11. Angus DC, Barnato AE, Linde-Zwirble WT, Weissfeld LA, Watson RS, Rickert T, et al. Use of intensive care at the end of life in the United States: an epidemiologic study. Crit Care Med. 2004;32(3):638–43.
12. Bagshaw SM, Webb SA, Delaney A, George C, Pilcher D, Hart GK, et al. Very old patients admitted to intensive care in Australia and New Zealand: a multi-centre cohort analysis. Crit Care. 2009;13(2):R45.
13. Fuchs L, Chronaki CE, Park S, Novack V, Baumfeld Y, Scott D, et al. ICU admission characteristics and mortality rates among elderly and very elderly patients. Intensive Care Med. 2012;38(10):1654–61.
14. Yu W, Ash AS, Levinsky NG, Moskowitz MA. Intensive care unit use and mortality in the elderly. J Gen Intern Med. 2000;15(2):97–102.
15. Miniksar OH, Ozdemir M. Clinical features and outcomes of very elderly patients admitted to the intensive care unit: a retrospective and observational study. Indian J Crit Care Med. 2021;25(6):629–34.
16. Kellum JA, Angus DC. Patients are dying of acute renal failure. Crit Care Med. 2002;30(9):2156–7.
17. Akposso K, Hertig A, Couprie R, Flahaut A, Alberti C, Karras GA, et al. Acute renal failure in patients over 80 years old: 25-years' experience. Intensive Care Med. 2000;26(4):400–6.
18. Joannidis M, Metnitz B, Bauer P, Schusterschitz N, Moreno R, Druml W, et al. Acute kidney injury in critically ill patients classified by AKIN versus RIFLE using the SAPS 3 database. Intensive Care Med. 2009;35(10):1692–702.
19. Collins AJ, Foley RN, Herzog C, Chavers B, Gilbertson D, Herzog C, et al. US Renal Data System 2012 Annual Data Report. Am J Kidney Dis. 2013;61(1 Suppl 1):A7, e1–476.
20. Chan L, Chaudhary K, Saha A, Chauhan K, Vaid A, Zhao S, et al. AKI in hospitalized patients with COVID-19. J Am Soc Nephrol. 2021;32(1):151–60.

21. Choudhury D, Levi M. Kidney aging—inevitable or preventable? Nat Rev Nephrol. 2011;7(12):706–17.

22. Wald H. The weight of normal adult human kidneys and its variability. Arch Pathol Lab Med. 1937;23:493–500.

23. Tauchi H, Tsuboi K, Okutomi J. Age changes in the human kidney of the different races. Gerontologia. 1971;17(2):87–97.

24. Piras D, Masala M, Delitala A, Urru SAM, Curreli N, Balaci L, et al. Kidney size in relation to ageing, gender, renal function, birthweight and chronic kidney disease risk factors in a general population. Nephrol Dial Transplant. 2020;35(4):640–7.

25. Goyal VK. Changes with age in the human kidney. Exp Gerontol. 1982;17(5):321–31.

26. Kappel B, Olsen S. Cortical interstitial tissue and sclerosed glomeruli in the normal human kidney, related to age and sex. A quantitative study. Virchows Arch A Pathol Anat Histol. 1980;387(3):271–7.

27. Epstein M. Aging and the kidney. J Am Soc Nephrol. 1996;7(8):1106–22.

28. Lindeman RD, Tobin J, Shock NW. Longitudinal studies on the rate of decline in renal function with age. J Am Geriatr Soc. 1985;33(4):278–85.

29. Rowe JW, Andres R, Tobin JD, Norris AH, Shock NW. The effect of age on creatinine clearance in men: a cross-sectional and longitudinal study. J Gerontol. 1976;31(2):155–63.

30. Fliser D, Zeier M, Nowack R, Ritz E. Renal functional reserve in healthy elderly subjects. J Am Soc Nephrol. 1993;3(7):1371–7.

31. Lakatta EG. Cardiovascular regulatory mechanisms in advanced age. Physiol Rev. 1993;73(2):413–67.

32. Zhang XZ, Qiu C, Baylis C. Sensitivity of the segmental renal arterioles to angiotensin II in the aging rat. Mech Ageing Dev. 1997;97(2):183–92.

33. Davies DF, Shock NW. Age changes in glomerular filtration rate, effective renal plasma flow, and tubular excretory capacity in adult males. J Clin Invest. 1950;29(5):496–507.

34. Epstein M, Hollenberg NK. Age as a determinant of renal sodium conservation in normal man. J Lab Clin Med. 1976;87(3):411–7.

35. Xu Y, Sun Z. Molecular basis of Klotho: from gene to function in aging. Endocr Rev. 2015;36(2):174–93.

36. Wang Y, Zhou CJ, Liu Y. Wnt signaling in kidney development and disease. Prog Mol Biol Transl Sci. 2018;153:181–207.

37. Gaya da Costa M, Poppelaars F, van Kooten C, Mollnes TE, Tedesco F, Wurzner R, et al. Age and sex-associated changes of complement activity and complement levels in a healthy Caucasian population. Front Immunol. 2018;9:2664.

38. Vlassara H, Torreggiani M, Post JB, Zheng F, Uribarri J, Striker GE. Role of oxidants/inflammation in declining renal function in chronic kidney disease and normal aging. Kidney Int Suppl. 2009;114:S3–11.

39. Chronopoulos A, Rosner MH, Cruz DN, Ronco C. Acute kidney injury in elderly intensive care patients: a review. Intensive Care Med. 2010;36(9):1454–64.

40. Aymanns C, Keller F, Maus S, Hartmann B, Czock D. Review on pharmacokinetics and pharmacodynamics and the aging kidney. Clin J Am Soc Nephrol. 2010;5(2):314–27.

41. Jerkic M, Vojvodic S, Lopez-Novoa JM. The mechanism of increased renal susceptibility to toxic substances in the elderly. Part I. The role of increased vasoconstriction. Int Urol Nephrol. 2001;32(4):539–47.

42. Schmitt R, Cantley LG. The impact of aging on kidney repair. Am J Physiol Renal Physiol. 2008;294(6):F1265–72.

43. Tran KT, Rusu SD, Satish L, Wells A. Aging-related attenuation of EGF receptor signaling is mediated in part by increased protein tyrosine phosphatase activity. Exp Cell Res. 2003;289(2):359–67.

44. Waikar SS, Wald R, Chertow GM, Curhan GC, Winkelmayer WC, Liangos O, et al. Validity of international classification of diseases, ninth revision, clinical modification codes for acute renal failure. J Am Soc Nephrol. 2006;17(6):1688–94.

45. Cardinale A, Messikh Z, Antoine V, Aglae C, Reboul P, Cariou S, et al. Specificity of severe AKI aetiology and care in the elderly. The IRACIBLE prospective cohort study. J Nephrol. 2022;35:2097.
46. Cheung CM, Ponnusamy A, Anderton JG. Management of acute renal failure in the elderly patient: a clinician's guide. Drugs Aging. 2008;25(6):455–76.
47. Chao C-T, Tsai H-B, Lin Y-F, Ko W-J. Acute kidney injury in the elderly: only the tip of the iceberg. J Clin Gerontol Geriatr. 2013;5(1):7–12.
48. Pascual J, Liano F. Causes and prognosis of acute renal failure in the very old. Madrid Acute Renal Failure Study Group. J Am Geriatr Soc. 1998;46(6):721–5.
49. Xu H, Garcia-Ptacek S, Annetorp M, Bruchfeld A, Cederholm T, Johnson P, et al. Acute kidney injury and mortality risk in older adults with COVID-19. J Nephrol. 2021;34(2):295–304.
50. Rosner MH. Acute kidney injury in the elderly. Clin Geriatr Med. 2013;29(3):565–78.
51. Bourgault M, Grimbert P, Verret C, Pourrat J, Herody M, Halimi JM, et al. Acute renal infarction: a case series. Clin J Am Soc Nephrol. 2013;8(3):392–8.
52. Mesiano P, Rollino C, Beltrame G, Ferro M, Quattrocchio G, Fenoglio R, et al. Acute renal infarction: a single center experience. J Nephrol. 2017;30(1):103–7.
53. Nash DM, Markle-Reid M, Brimble KS, McArthur E, Roshanov PS, Fink JC, et al. Nonsteroidal anti-inflammatory drug use and risk of acute kidney injury and hyperkalemia in older adults: a population-based study. Nephrol Dial Transplant. 2019;34(7):1145–54.
54. Kleinknecht D, Landais P, Goldfarb B. Pathophysiology and clinical aspects of drug-induced tubular necrosis in man. Contrib Nephrol. 1987;55:145–58.
55. Blackshear JL, Davidman M, Stillman MT. Identification of risk for renal insufficiency from nonsteroidal anti-inflammatory drugs. Arch Intern Med. 1983;143(6):1130–4.
56. Abuelo JG. Normotensive ischemic acute renal failure. N Engl J Med. 2007;357(8):797–805.
57. Zeren G, Avci II, Sungur MA, Simsek B, Sungur A, Can F, et al. Effects of RAAS blocker use on AKI in elderly hypertensive STEMI patients with propensity score weighed method. Clin Exp Hypertens. 2022;44(5):487–94.
58. Coca SG, Garg AX, Swaminathan M, Garwood S, Hong K, Thiessen-Philbrook H, et al. Preoperative angiotensin-converting enzyme inhibitors and angiotensin receptor blocker use and acute kidney injury in patients undergoing cardiac surgery. Nephrol Dial Transplant. 2013;28(11):2787–99.
59. Chaumont M, Pourcelet A, van Nuffelen M, Racape J, Leeman M, Hougardy JM. Acute kidney injury in elderly patients with chronic kidney disease: do angiotensin-converting enzyme inhibitors carry a risk? J Clin Hypertens (Greenwich). 2016;18(6):514–21.
60. Lameire N, Verspeelt J, Vanholder R. A review of the pathophysiology, causes and prognosis of acute renal failure in the elderly. Geriatr Nephrol Urol. 1991;1:77–91.
61. Vives M, Hernandez A, Parramon F, Estanyol N, Pardina B, Munoz A, et al. Acute kidney injury after cardiac surgery: prevalence, impact and management challenges. Int J Nephrol Renovasc Dis. 2019;12:153–66.
62. Wang J, Li J, Wang Y. [Clinical characteristics and prognosis of acute kidney injury in elderly patients with sepsis]. Zhonghua Wei Zhong Bing Ji Jiu Yi Xue. 2019;31(7):837–41.
63. Wardle EN. Acute renal failure and multiorgan failure. Nephrol Dial Transplant. 1994;9(Suppl 4):104–7.
64. Teles F, Santos RO, Lima H, Campos RP, Teixeira EC, Alves ACA, et al. The impact of dialysis on critically ill elderly patients with acute kidney injury: an analysis by propensity score matching. J Bras Nefrol. 2019;41(1):14–21.
65. Naughton CA. Drug-induced nephrotoxicity. Am Fam Physician. 2008;78(6):743–50.
66. Alsafi A, Alsafi Z, Lakhani A, Strickland NH. Changes in renal function in elderly patients following intravenous iodinated contrast administration: a retrospective study. Radiol Res Pract. 2014;2014:459583.
67. Fu N, Li X, Yang S, Chen Y, Li Q, Jin D, et al. Risk score for the prediction of contrast-induced nephropathy in elderly patients undergoing percutaneous coronary intervention. Angiology. 2013;64(3):188–94.

68. Wongrakpanich S, Kallis C, Prasad P, Rangaswami J, Rosenzweig A. The study of rhabdomyolysis in the elderly: an epidemiological study and single center experience. Aging Dis. 2018;9(1):1–7.
69. Muriithi AK, Leung N, Valeri AM, Cornell LD, Sethi S, Fidler ME, et al. Clinical characteristics, causes and outcomes of acute interstitial nephritis in the elderly. Kidney Int. 2015;87(2):458–64.
70. Hemmelgarn BR, Zhang J, Manns BJ, Tonelli M, Larsen E, Ghali WA, et al. Progression of kidney dysfunction in the community-dwelling elderly. Kidney Int. 2006;69(12):2155–61.
71. Moutzouris DA, Herlitz L, Appel GB, Markowitz GS, Freudenthal B, Radhakrishnan J, et al. Renal biopsy in the very elderly. Clin J Am Soc Nephrol. 2009;4(6):1073–82.
72. Bomback AS, Appel GB, Radhakrishnan J, Shirazian S, Herlitz LC, Stokes B, et al. ANCA-associated glomerulonephritis in the very elderly. Kidney Int. 2011;79(7):757–64.
73. Mukhtyar C, Guillevin L, Cid MC, Dasgupta B, de Groot K, Gross W, et al. EULAR recommendations for the management of primary small and medium vessel vasculitis. Ann Rheum Dis. 2009;68(3):310–7.
74. Macias-Nunez JF, Lopez-Novoa JM, Martinez-Maldonado M. Acute renal failure in the aged. Semin Nephrol. 1996;16(4):330–8.
75. Elliott SP, Meng MV, Elkin EP, McAninch JW, Duchane J, Carroll PR, et al. Incidence of urethral stricture after primary treatment for prostate cancer: data from CaPSURE. J Urol. 2007;178(2):529–34; discussion 34.
76. Spital A, Valvo JR, Segal AJ. Nondilated obstructive uropathy. Urology. 1988;31(6):478–82.
77. Faubel S, Patel NU, Lockhart ME, Cadnapaphornchai MA. Renal relevant radiology: use of ultrasonography in patients with AKI. Clin J Am Soc Nephrol. 2014;9(2):382–94.
78. Murray PT, Devarajan P, Levey AS, Eckardt KU, Bonventre JV, Lombardi R, et al. A framework and key research questions in AKI diagnosis and staging in different environments. Clin J Am Soc Nephrol. 2008;3(3):864–8.
79. da Rocha EP, Yokota LG, Sampaio BM, Cardoso Eid KZ, Dias DB, de Freitas FM, et al. Urinary neutrophil gelatinase-associated lipocalin is excellent predictor of acute kidney injury in septic elderly patients. Aging Dis. 2018;9(2):182–91.
80. Fliser D, Ritz E. Serum cystatin C concentration as a marker of renal dysfunction in the elderly. Am J Kidney Dis. 2001;37(1):79–83.
81. Esmeijer K, Schoe A, Ruhaak LR, Hoogeveen EK, Soonawala D, Romijn F, et al. The predictive value of TIMP-2 and IGFBP7 for kidney failure and 30-day mortality after elective cardiac surgery. Sci Rep. 2021;11(1):1071.
82. Perazella MA, Coca SG, Hall IE, Iyanam U, Koraishy M, Parikh CR. Urine microscopy is associated with severity and worsening of acute kidney injury in hospitalized patients. Clin J Am Soc Nephrol. 2010;5(3):402–8.
83. Perazella MA. The urine sediment as a biomarker of kidney disease. Am J Kidney Dis. 2015;66(5):748–55.
84. Bhandari S, Turney JH. Survivors of acute renal failure who do not recover renal function. QJM. 1996;89(6):415–21.
85. Schiffl H. Renal recovery from acute tubular necrosis requiring renal replacement therapy: a prospective study in critically ill patients. Nephrol Dial Transplant. 2006;21(5):1248–52.
86. Liano F, Felipe C, Tenorio MT, Rivera M, Abraira V, Saez-de-Urturi JM, et al. Long-term outcome of acute tubular necrosis: a contribution to its natural history. Kidney Int. 2007;71(7):679–86.
87. Schmitt R, Coca S, Kanbay M, Tinetti ME, Cantley LG, Parikh CR. Recovery of kidney function after acute kidney injury in the elderly: a systematic review and meta-analysis. Am J Kidney Dis. 2008;52(2):262–71.
88. Parikh CR, Coca SG, Wang Y, Masoudi FA, Krumholz HM. Long-term prognosis of acute kidney injury after acute myocardial infarction. Arch Intern Med. 2008;168(9):987–95.

89. Kashani K, Shao M, Li G, Williams AW, Rule AD, Kremers WK, et al. No increase in the incidence of acute kidney injury in a population-based annual temporal trends epidemiology study. Kidney Int. 2017;92(3):721–8.
90. Yilmaz R, Erdem Y. Acute kidney injury in the elderly population. Int Urol Nephrol. 2010;42(1):259–71.
91. Oweis AO, Alshelleh SA. Incidence and outcomes of acute kidney injury in octogenarians in Jordan. BMC Res Notes. 2018;11(1):279.
92. Coca SG. Acute kidney injury in elderly persons. Am J Kidney Dis. 2010;56(1):122–31.
93. Lameire N, Matthys E, Vanholder R, De Keyser K, Pauwels W, Nachtergaele H, et al. Causes and prognosis of acute renal failure in elderly patients. Nephrol Dial Transplant. 1987;2(5):316–22.
94. Ali T, Khan I, Simpson W, Prescott G, Townend J, Smith W, et al. Incidence and outcomes in acute kidney injury: a comprehensive population-based study. J Am Soc Nephrol. 2007;18(4):1292–8.
95. Acuna K, Costa E, Grover A, Camelo A, Junior RS. [Clinical-epidemiological characteristics of adults and aged interned in an intensive care unity of the Amazon (Rio Branco, Acre)]. Rev Bras Ter Intensiva. 2007;19(3):304–9.
96. Rhee H, Jang KS, Park JM, Kang JS, Hwang NK, Kim IY, et al. Short- and long-term mortality rates of elderly acute kidney injury patients who underwent continuous renal replacement therapy. PLoS One. 2016;11(11):e0167067.
97. Landoni G, Zangrillo A, Franco A, Aletti G, Roberti A, Calabro MG, et al. Long-term outcome of patients who require renal replacement therapy after cardiac surgery. Eur J Anaesthesiol. 2006;23(1):17–22.
98. Noble JS, Simpson K, Allison ME. Long-term quality of life and hospital mortality in patients treated with intermittent or continuous hemodialysis for acute renal and respiratory failure. Ren Fail. 2006;28(4):323–30.
99. Englberger L, Suri RM, Li Z, Dearani JA, Park SJ, Sundt TM III, et al. Validation of clinical scores predicting severe acute kidney injury after cardiac surgery. Am J Kidney Dis. 2010;56(4):623–31.
100. Jorge-Monjas P, Bustamante-Munguira J, Lorenzo M, Heredia-Rodriguez M, Fierro I, Gomez-Sanchez E, et al. Predicting cardiac surgery-associated acute kidney injury: the CRATE score. J Crit Care. 2016;31(1):130–8.
101. Inohara T, Kohsaka S, Abe T, Miyata H, Numasawa Y, Ueda I, et al. Development and validation of a pre-percutaneous coronary intervention risk model of contrast-induced acute kidney injury with an integer scoring system. Am J Cardiol. 2015;115(12):1636–42.
102. Ostermann M, Joannidis M, Pani A, Floris M, De Rosa S, Kellum JA, et al. Patient selection and timing of continuous renal replacement therapy. Blood Purif. 2016;42(3):224–37.
103. Boumendil A, Somme D, Garrouste-Orgeas M, Guidet B. Should elderly patients be admitted to the intensive care unit? Intensive Care Med. 2007;33(7):1252.
104. Iribarren-Diarasarri S, Aizpuru-Barandiaran F, Munoz-Martinez T, Loma-Osorio A, Hernandez-Lopez M, Ruiz-Zorrilla JM, et al. Health-related quality of life as a prognostic factor of survival in critically ill patients. Intensive Care Med. 2009;35(5):833–9.
105. Sacanella E, Perez-Castejon JM, Nicolas JM, Masanes F, Navarro M, Castro P, et al. Mortality in healthy elderly patients after ICU admission. Intensive Care Med. 2009;35(3):550–5.

Chapter 14
Pharmacotherapeutic Considerations in Older Individuals with Kidney Disease

Sharon See and Elsen Jacob

Take Home Points
- Older adults have altered pharmacokinetics and pharmacodynamics that require medication dose adjustments and monitoring.
- Several tools and strategies are available to help clinicians reduce inappropriate prescribing.

Introduction

Thirty-eight percent of older adults have a diagnosis of chronic kidney disease (CKD) in the United States [1]. Older adults are commonly prescribed inappropriate medications that can negatively impact their care [2–4]. An interdisciplinary team and evidence-based strategies can optimize the care of older adults by addressing important topics such as polypharmacy, deprescribing, and prescribing cascades. This team should include physicians, nurses, pharmacists, social workers as well as patients, families, and caregivers [5, 6]. Older adults present with variations in pharmacokinetics and pharmacodynamics which can impact medication selection, dosing, and patient response. In older adults, especially those with reduced kidney function, regular medication assessments are critical to avoid adverse outcomes and optimize drug therapy.

S. See (✉)
Department of Clinical Health Professions, College of Pharmacy and Health Sciences, St. John's University, Queens, New York, NY, USA
e-mail: sees@stjohns.edu

E. Jacob
Field Medical, Outcomes & Analytics, Pfizer Inc., New York, NY, USA
e-mail: elsen.jacob@pfizer.com

H. Kramer et al. (eds.), *Kidney Disease in the Elderly*,
https://doi.org/10.1007/978-3-031-68460-9_14

Pharmacokinetics

Case 1

Mary is an 82-year-old woman with a past medical history of atrial fibrillation, reduced ejection fraction heart failure (HFrEF), osteoarthritis, and gastroesophageal reflux disease (GERD). She presents to the physician's office complaining of weight gain and shortness of breath. She denies chest pain, fever, nausea, vomiting, or pain. Her home medications include apixaban 5 mg po twice a day, sacubitril 49 mg-valsartan 51 mg po twice a day, metoprolol succinate 50 mg po daily, pantoprazole 40 mg po daily, and ibuprofen 400 mg po 3 times a day. Her vital signs include BP of 160/98 mmHg, HR of 79 bpm, and O_2 saturation of 96% on room air. She weighs 50 kg. What pharmacokinetic (PK) and pharmacodynamic (PD) principles should be considered in Mary?

Pharmacokinetics (PK) is commonly described as 'what the body does to a drug'. It explains the changes in drug concentration as the drug moves to different parts of the body. PK is further defined through four separate, yet related concepts: absorption (A), distribution (D), metabolism (M), and excretion (E). Older adults experience changes in pharmacokinetics related to the aging process. Thus, in caring for older adults, it is important for clinicians to recognize age-related pharmacokinetic changes, so they can tailor regimens that optimize outcomes while reducing the likelihood of adverse effects [7]. Table 14.1 provides examples of medications that are impacted by altered PK in older adults.

Table 14.1 Common medications with altered pharmacokinetics in older persons [8]

Medication	Pharmacokinetic parameter	Effect
Calcium, vitamin B12, iron	Absorption	Achlorhydria may reduce absorption
Digoxin	Distribution	Vd is decreased resulting in increased drug levels
Diazepam	Distribution	Lipophilicity leads to increased Vd which reduces plasma concentration leading to longer time to steady state; toxicity
Diazepam	Metabolism	Undergoes Phase I metabolism which is impaired in older adults; leads to toxicity
Gabapentin	Elimination	Primarily eliminated by kidney, reduced kidney function leads to toxicity including somnolence
Morphine	Metabolism and elimination	Metabolized in kidney; reduced renal function leads to toxicity
Metformin	Elimination	Primarily eliminated by kidney, reduced kidney function leads to toxicity including lactic acidosis
Phenytoin	Distribution	Highly protein bound; levels increase with hypoalbuminemia
Warfarin	Distribution	Highly protein bound; levels increase with hypoalbuminemia

Absorption

Absorption describes the process of uptake of a medication into the systemic circulation.

It is dependent on the route by which the medication is administered and on the properties of the medication. When a medication is taken enterally or transdermally, it has to pass through barriers such as the gastrointestinal tract or dermal layers before reaching systemic circulation. On the other hand, intravenous administration directly enters the systemic circulation. Absorption is not thought to be significantly affected by the aging process, but older adults do experience some alterations in medication absorption secondary to drug interactions, and changes in gut motility, acidity in the stomach, and skin composition [7, 8].

As older adults are more likely to be prescribed a larger number of medications, clinically relevant drug interactions that impact absorption are more common. Older adults may be more likely to experience alterations in gut motility which can lead to changes in medication absorption. Gut motility can be slowed by medications like stimulant laxatives or medical conditions like short bowel syndrome. These conditions can reduce medication transit time through the enteral tract resulting in reduced medication absorption. Opioids can delay gut motility and increase medication absorption. The acidity of the stomach can also impact medication absorption. For example, acid-lowering medications, such as proton pump inhibitors or H2-antagonists can reduce the absorption of ketoconazole because it requires an acidic environment for absorption. Changes in skin composition such as atrophy or hyperproliferation can also impact the absorption of topically administered medications such as patches, creams, and ointments, leading to reduced or enhanced absorption of medications [7–9].

Distribution

Distribution addresses the passage of medication to various compartments in the body. Older adults typically experience increased body fat, decreased total body water, and reduced protein. These changes lead to alterations in volumes of distribution (Vd) and plasma concentration of medications. Hydrophilic medications have reduced volumes of distribution which can lead to increased medication concentrations in the plasma, while lipophilic medications have larger volumes of distribution resulting in reduced concentration in the plasma. The larger volumes of distribution of lipophilic medications such as diazepam can lead to increased time to arrive at steady-state concentrations and accumulation of medication in older adults. Reduced protein in older adults can impact the distribution of highly protein-bound medications such as warfarin. This is clinically meaningful as only the free or unbound medication is active. Increased concentrations of free medication, can increase distribution which can lead to a higher likelihood of adverse effects [7, 8, 10, 11].

Metabolism

Metabolism, sometimes referred to as biotransformation, describes the process by which medications become altered to prepare for excretion from the body. The liver is responsible for the metabolism of most medications, although the skin, kidneys, and intestines play a secondary role. Medication metabolism is primarily conducted through phase I and phase II reactions, which are described below [7, 11–14].

Phase I reactions typically transform medications into inactive metabolites through hydroxylation, oxidation, dealkylation, and reduction. Cytochrome P450 isoenzymes are primarily responsible for these reactions. Phase II reactions transform medications through conjugation, glucuronidation, and acetylation into more water-soluble inactive metabolites. Older adults have decreased phase I reactions while phase II reactions are unaffected by aging [7, 11, 13, 14].

Physiological changes associated with the aging process result in reduced hepatic blood flow and liver size and can impact the metabolism of medications. In first-pass metabolism, enterally administered medications enter the hepatic portal system and then the liver, leading to a reduced percentage of medication that reaches systemic circulation. As such, older adults are at a higher risk of adverse effects by medications that undergo first-pass such as nitrates due to higher concentrations [7, 11, 12].

Excretion

Excretion refers to medication removal from the body as a metabolite or in an unchanged form. While kidneys most commonly participate in the excretion of medications, other routes such as the biliary, fecal, sweat, and lung routes also play a role. Age-related decline in kidney function impacts many medications and can lead to an increased risk of medication accumulation and adverse effects. This is especially important in medications with narrow therapeutic windows such as lithium [9, 11].

It is critical that clinicians exercise caution and clinical judgment when evaluating the kidney excretion of medications. Clinicians must keep in mind that using serum creatinine as a marker for kidney function in older adults may be misleading and may be over-estimated in older adults who exhibit sarcopenia or age-related reduction in skeletal muscle. This chapter will explore CKD and its impact on pharmacotherapy in greater detail.

Pharmacodynamics

Pharmacodynamics is often described as "what the drug does to the body." It refers to the association between concentrations of medication and the responses elicited in individuals. In comparison to younger adults, older adults may experience changes in medication effects that are related to receptor sensitivity, changes in the number of receptors and medication affinity to receptors, and counter-regulatory mechanisms such as orthostatic changes. For example, beta blocker use in older adults can cause negative alterations in heart rate. Typically, older adults are more sensitive to the effects of beta blockers and therefore at an increased risk of adverse effects like bradycardia. Thus, slow titration of beta blockers in older adults is generally recommended to reduce the likelihood of adverse effects [7, 8, 13].

Case 1 Answer

Mary presents with weight gain and shortness of breath. Given her history of heart failure, ibuprofen is inappropriate because NSAIDs can cause fluid retention and could cause heart failure exacerbation. Pharmacodynamic changes in homeostasis mechanisms increase the risk of this medication's adverse effects. Thus, especially considering findings of likely volume overload, it would be advisable to select an alternative pain regimen [15]. The patient is also on apixaban, due to her history of atrial fibrillation. Due to changes in pharmacokinetics associated with aging, older adults are more likely to have increased exposure to apixaban, and as such there are dose adjustments to consider. As the patient is over 80 years of age and under 60 kg, the dose of apixaban should be reduced from 5 mg po BID to 2.5 mg po BID [16, 17].

Medication Management Strategies and Tools

Determining Kidney Function

This is an area of confusion for clinicians as there are many equations to calculate kidney function including Cockcroft Gault (CG), MDRD, and CKD-Epi. The choice of equation is based on institutional and clinician preferences. CG is the most commonly used equation although it has many limitations. It was studied in only 249 white males, not standardized to current serum creatinine assays, and often underestimates kidney function. PK/PD studies used CG for many years to determine drug dosing adjustments in kidney impairment and as a result, became the most commonly used estimating equation. The MDRD equation was developed in 1620 adults with CKD and is expressed as eGFR. It used standardized assays and race in the calculation and was shown to be more accurate than CG; however, it is no longer recommended [18]. More recently, CKD Epi has been shown to be a more accurate calculation and has gone through several iterations. The National Kidney Foundation and the American Society of Nephrology recommend CKD-Epi which does not include a race modifier [19]. The FDA now requires drug development to use eGFR using standardized creatinine assays. This has implications for clinicians who rely on drug company package inserts to make clinical decisions. Medication package inserts will recommend dosing reductions based on either CG (mL/min) for older medications or eGFR (mL/min/1.73 m^2) for more recent medications.

Polypharmacy

Many older individuals struggle with managing their medications due in part to having multiple chronic conditions also known as "multimorbidity" [20]. As a result, these individuals are prescribed multiple medications resulting in polypharmacy. While there is no consensus as to how many medications constitute polypharmacy, it is generally defined as five or more medications [21]. An analysis of the Center for Disease Control and Prevention's National Ambulatory Medical Care Survey revealed that out of 2 billion office visits, 65% experienced polypharmacy, and 37% qualified as major polypharmacy (5 or more medications) [22]. If a patient is prescribed a drug for which there is no indication, then that is a contributor to polypharmacy. While polypharmacy is associated with negative outcomes, it is sometimes appropriate for a patient to be on multiple medications. For example, a patient with HFrEF should be on guideline-directed therapy which often includes a loop diuretic, beta blocker, mineralocorticoid receptor antagonists (MRAs), angiotensin receptor II blocker -neprilysin inhibitor (ARNI) and sodium-glucose cotransporter-2 inhibitors (SGLT2i) [23].

Polypharmacy can lead to adverse drug reactions, drug interactions, falls, urinary incontinence, functional decline, cognitive impairment and can be costly to the patient [21]. One of the guiding principles of managing an older patient with multimorbidity is optimizing medication therapy so that it minimizes adverse effects, ensures benefit of therapies and improves quality of life [20]. Clinicians can begin to optimize therapy by identifying inappropriate or dangerous medications using screening tools and guidance documents such as START(Screening Tool to Alert to Right Treatment)/STOPP (Screening Tool of Older Persons' Prescriptions), Beer's Criteria, and the Medication Appropriateness Index [24–26]. START/STOPP and Beer's Criteria are explicit tools that provide criteria that review drug-drug interactions, duration of therapy, dosage as well as drug-disease interactions. The disadvantage of these tools is that they do not include patient preferences, life expectancy, and they need to be updated often. The Medication Appropriateness Index uses implicit criteria, which enables the clinician to use patient specific characteristics to determine appropriateness. The Medication Appropriateness Index is highly sensitive but requires an experienced clinician for use and takes time [27]. Choosing

Wisely is another excellent resource to aid in reducing polypharmacy [28]. This series is sponsored by the American Board of Internal Medicine and is endorsed by various medical organizations including the American Society of Consultant Pharmacists. This series provides evidence-based recommendations to improve patient care and addresses polypharmacy, deprescribing, and time to benefit which will be discussed below. As an example, with regard to polypharmacy, Choosing Wisely states, "Don't use three or more CNS active medications, especially in older adults" [28].

Deprescribing

Another tool to reduce inappropriate prescribing is to deprescribe. Deprescribing is the process of determining whether a medication should and can be removed from the patient's medication regimen. This is an important part of the medication evaluation process to ensure that unnecessary or harmful medications are not continued. The deprescribing process should include consideration of harms versus benefits, medications with no indications, patient values and goals and life expectancy [29]. Patients taking alendronate for osteoporosis are good candidates to consider for deprescribing. After taking alendronate for 5 years, patients are not at increased risk for non-vertebral fractures for up to 5 years off of alendronate compared to those who continued alendronate for 5 more years, thus still possessing fracture benefit even after discontinuing alendronate [30]. Given that data, deprescribing alendronate could free a patient from onerous medication administration (drinking 8 ounces of water sitting upright), high costs and adverse effects.

A helpful website for deprescribing information is www.deprescribing.org [31]. This website is open to the public, healthcare providers, and researchers and provides links to evidence-based research on deprescribing and helpful algorithms for deprescribing common medications that are often prescribed with no indication or are inappropriate for the patient.

Time to Benefit

Besides weighing harms and benefits, life expectancy/time to benefit and patient values must also be considered before deprescribing. Time to benefit is a concept that describes how long a patient needs to be on a particular medication in order to achieve the benefit or outcome [32]. Consider an 80-year-old patient who has been told by her primary care physician that because her atherosclerotic cardiovascular disease (ASCVD) risk is high, he would like to start her on atorvastatin. She has never had a cardiac event before. Her medical conditions include hypertension, chronic kidney disease and reduced ejection fraction heart failure (HFrEF). She has been admitted to the hospital multiple times this year for heart failure exacerbation and chronic kidney disease (CKD) and has a poor prognosis. Her medications include metoprolol, lisinopril, furosemide, sevelamer, and erythropoietin. The patient wants to know if atorvastatin is really necessary at this stage of her life given all of her chronic conditions and her frustration with taking so many medications. A logical first step to help in decision making is to determine her life expectancy. There is limited data on using statins in adults older than 75 years of age. Current cholesterol guidelines do suggest moderate-intensity statins in patients aged 40–75 years if they have diabetes and possibly high intensity if risk factors are present. In patients without diabetes, a risk discussion should take place about whether or not a moderate-intensity statin would be appropriate [33]. The time to benefit from an HMG CoA Reductase Inhibitor is 2–5 years to prevent a cardiac event in patients [34].

While data exists for patients younger than 80 years, there is limited data for those older than 80 years of age. A recent retrospective cohort study in veterans found that starting a statin in adults greater than 75 years of age without a history of cardiovascular disease (CVD) had a reduced risk of all-cause mortality and cardiovascular death after taking a statin for 6.8 years [35]. Given this patient's multimorbidity, it is unlikely that she would live long enough to achieve a benefit from a statin. By recommending not to start atorvastatin, the team would prevent adding another medication to complicate her medication regimen and decrease the risk of potential adverse effects and potential drug-drug interactions. In addition, the patient has expressed her desire to stop the medication. Her values and goals of care must be incorporated into the deprescribing process.

Prescribing Cascades

Polypharmacy can also result from prescribing cascades. A prescribing cascade describes a series of events that starts when a medication is prescribed and results in an adverse event. The adverse event in turn is then treated with another medication [36, 37]. In the context of multimorbidity, this cascade can continue indefinitely if an intervention is not made and a deliberate attempt to assess the appropriateness of medications in the first place does not occur. Consider a patient with knee osteoarthritis, heart failure, and chronic kidney disease. The patient is prescribed an NSAID to alleviate the pain from the osteoarthritis but it then causes a heart failure exacerbation due to fluid retention. The edema and pulmonary congestion are then treated with furosemide. The furosemide in turn causes hypokalemia which prompts the addition of potassium chloride to his regimen (Fig. 14.1) [38]. In order to avoid this prescribing cascade, it is important to evaluate the need for the NSAID in the first place. Could the osteoarthritis be treated with acetaminophen? Can other options such as topical NSAIDs or capsaicin be considered instead?

Gabapentin-induced edema is another good example of causing a prescribing cascade.

Fig. 14.1 An example of a prescribing cascade: NSAID use can cause heart failure exacerbation with edema which is treated with loop diuretics. As a result, hypokalemia may occur, requiring the need for potassium supplementation

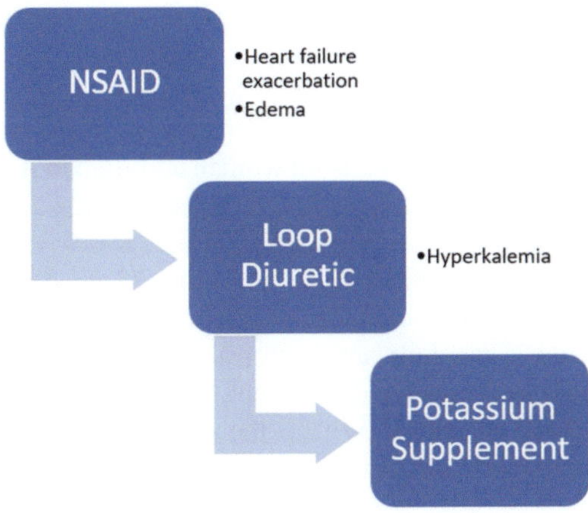

A population-based cohort study demonstrated that older individuals prescribed with gabapentin for low back pain were more likely to be prescribed a diuretic to treat gabapentin-induced edema [39]. At 90 days, patients on gabapentin had a 2.1% risk of being prescribed a diuretic compared to 1.4% in the non-gabapentinoid group (ARR 0.7%). If clinicians can identify patients who do not have an indication for gabapentin, they can deprescribe this drug to reduce risks of gabapentin including CNS depression, dizziness, abuse, and kidney impairment.

Medication Considerations in Kidney Disease

A central focus of medication management in older adults is attention to dosing due to the natural decline of kidney function as individuals age. The two main reasons for a dose reduction are either to avoid direct drug-induced nephrotoxicity or drug-related toxicity due to drug accumulation. It is important to understand that if there is a dosing recommendation with reduced kidney function in a package insert or drug monograph, it does not necessarily mean that it is because a drug is directly nephrotoxic. The provider must check the drug's pharmacokinetic parameters and determine how it is eliminated and to what extent. Useful resources for kidney dosing and PK/PD information include medication databases such as Lexi Comp and Micromedex. Both are paid subscriptions but are often provided by hospitals and academic institutions. The next section will highlight various medications that are cleared by the kidney.

Drug Related Nephrotoxicity-Accumulation

Case 2

Darlene is a 94-year-old woman admitted to the hospital after a fall at home. X-rays revealed she had a right femur fracture. It was also discovered during her exam that her glucose was 300 mg/dL, HA1C was 9% and her serum creatinine was 2.8 mg/dL with an eGFR of 25 mL/min/1.73 m^2 BSA. Her past medical history includes hypertension and type 2 diabetes. Her home medications include hydrochlorothiazide 25 mg daily and metformin 1000 mg twice daily. She reports 10 out of 10 pain. In the emergency department, she received morphine 15 mg by mouth every 4 h for a total of 4 doses. What is the appropriate management of Darlene's pain and diabetes in light of her reduced kidney function?

Diabetes

Without a dose reduction, drugs eliminated by the kidney can accumulate in patients with reduced kidney function and can accumulate and result in toxicities. There are many diabetes medications that are excreted by the kidneys including metformin, dipeptidyl peptidase 4 (DPP4) Inhibitors, and sulfonylureas. According to the manufacturer, metformin is contraindicated when eGFR is below 30 mL/min/1.73 m^2 [40]. This recommendation is not because metformin is directly nephrotoxic, but because the drug may accumulate with reduced kidney function and increase plasma lactate levels via inhibition of mitochondrial respiration in the liver. The DPP4 inhibitor sitagliptin (Januvia) is also cleared by the kidney and dosing reductions are recommended with eGFR between 30 and 45 mL/min/1.73 m^2. The manufacturer advises reducing the dose of sitagliptin to 25 mg daily when eGFR falls below 30 mL/min/1.73 m^2. Failure to reduce drug dosing of DPP4 inhibitors when kidney function is low may result in adverse effects such as dermatologic reactions, hypersensitivity reactions, and pancreatitis due to drug accumulation [41].

Glyburide has long been considered an inappropriate medication in older individuals due to the fact that it has a long half-life of 10 h and has an active metabolite that accumulates in patients with reduced kidney function [26]. As a result, older adults are at high risk for becoming hypoglycemic. If an older individual requires diabetes medication, consider other safer alternatives such as metformin or SGLT2i. Glipizide would be a safer choice if a sulfonylurea is desired.

Pain

Gabapentin was the tenth most prescribed medication in the United States in 2019 with almost half a million prescriptions reported [42]. This medication is often used to treat many off label indications including neuropathic pain despite lack of evidence. As previously stated, older adults are particularly vulnerable to the many dose-dependent adverse effects of gabapentin due to reduced kidney clearance. As such, gabapentin requires dose adjustment in patients with CrCl between 30–49, 15–29, and <15 mL/min. Adverse effects include dizziness, gait disturbance, and somnolence which can easily lead to falls in older individuals [43].

Geriatric patients often require pain medication for severe, chronic, or acute pain. When considering opioids, morphine should be avoided when CrCl <30 mL/min because of accumulation of active metabolites. Morphine is metabolized in the liver to morphine-3 (M3) and morphine-6 glucuronide (MG6) which are 70–80% eliminated by the kidney, and accumulate in patients with reduced kidney function [44, 45]. This accumulation can cause neuroallodynia, myoclonus, seizures, and respiratory depression. In addition, morphine can worsen kidney function via hypotension leading to hypoperfusion; hyperkalemia may also occur secondary to constipation and urinary retention [46]. Hydromorphone is a safer alternative to morphine in older adults with reduced kidney function.

Anticoagulation

Bleeding risk increases in patients with kidney failure which is an important monitoring parameter that should be checked prior to prescribing direct oral anticoagulants (DOACs). This is particularly relevant to older adults as many have reduced kidney function and require anticoagulation for indications such as venous thromboembolism treatment and prophylaxis and stroke prevention in atrial fibrillation. Dabigatran and rivaroxaban are cleared via the kidneys to a much greater extent than apixaban, and thereby both agents can increase the risk of bleeding in kidney failure (See Table 14.2) [47]. Dabigatran and rivaroxaban are associated with an increased risk of gastrointestinal bleeding (GIB) compared to warfarin in patients with atrial fibrillation trials. In the RE-LY trial, dabigatran 150 mg twice daily caused a significantly higher risk of GIB compared to warfarin (RR, 1.50; 95% CI, 1.19–1.89; P <0.001) [48]. In another study, the rates of major bleeding were similar between rivaroxaban and warfarin (5.5% vs. 5.4%). The major bleeds that did occur were gastrointestinal (upper, lower, and rectal) in nature [49]. Apixaban was associated with significantly less major bleeding than warfarin in the landmark trial of apixaban versus warfarin for stroke prevention in patients with atrial fibrillation (HR, 0.69; 95% CI, 0.60–0.80; P <0.001) [50]. Additionally, there was no

Table 14.2 Direct acting oral anticoagulants pharmacokinetics [54–57]

DOAC	Excretion
Dabigatran	80% kidney (excreted unchanged) after IV administration
Rivaroxaban	36% kidney (excreted unchanged)
Apixaban	27% kidney (excreted unchanged)
Edoxaban	50% kidney (primarily unchanged)

difference in the rate of GIB (HR 0.89; 95% CI, 0.70–1.15; $P = 0.37$). The rate of GIB in the apixaban group was 1.15% compared to 1.31% for warfarin [50]. While apixaban does have a low risk of GIB, the package insert does recommend a dose reduction in patients with atrial fibrillation from 5 mg twice daily to 2.5 mg twice daily in patients who fulfill 2 out of 3 of the following criteria: weight ≤60 kg, serum creatinine ≥1.5 mg/dL and age ≥80 years [17]. All DOACs have kidney dosing instructions for atrial fibrillation. Rivaroxaban, edoxaban and dabigatran are not recommended for CrCl <15 mL/min. Prescribers should refer to the package insert for each medication for dosing recommendations in the setting of reduced eGFR. Several retrospective cohort studies suggest that apixaban is safe to use in patients with CKD Stage 4 or 5 who may or may not be on dialysis [51–53].

Case 2 Answer

Because Darlene's eGFR is less than 30 mL/min/1.73 m^2 BSA, hydromorphone would be a more appropriate opioid for her femur fracture pain. Morphine has an active metabolite which can accumulate with kidney failure and lead to severe adverse effects including respiratory depression and seizures. Metformin should be discontinued, and an alternative agent such as empagliflozin can be considered because the accumulation of metformin in kidney failure can lead to toxicities such as lactic acidosis.

Conclusion

Older adults require a nuanced strategy to ensure optimal use of medications. A general understanding of PK and PD principles is essential to avoid inappropriate prescribing. This chapter offers a review of PK and PD principles, examples of consequences of drug accumulation and other medication considerations in older patients. Suggestions for evidence-based tools are provided to reduce inappropriate prescribing. A patient-centered, interdisciplinary, team-based approach is critical to the care of older adults who have complex medication therapies.

References

1. Chronic kidney disease in the United States, 2021. 2022 [cited 2022 Aug 22]. https://www.cdc.gov/kidneydisease/publications-resources/ckd-national-facts.html.
2. Khanal A, Peterson GM, Castelino RL, Jose MD. Potentially inappropriate prescribing of renally cleared drugs in elderly patients in community and aged care settings. Drugs Aging. 2015;32(5):391–400.

3. Molnar AO, Bota S, Jeyakumar N, McArthur E, Battistella M, Garg AX, et al. Potentially inappropriate prescribing in older adults with advanced chronic kidney disease. PLoS One. 2020;15(8):e0237868.
4. Chang F, O'Hare AM, Miao Y, Steinman MA. Use of renally inappropriate medications in older veterans: a national study. J Am Geriatr Soc. 2015;63(11):2290–7.
5. Partnership for Health in Aging Workgroup on Interdisciplinary Team Training in Geriatrics. Position statement on interdisciplinary team training in geriatrics: an essential component of quality health care for older adults. J Am Geriatr Soc. 2014;62(5):961–5.
6. Hung WW, Ross JS, Farber J, Siu AL. Evaluation of the mobile acute care of the elderly (MACE) service. JAMA Intern Med. 2013;173(11):990–6.
7. Bauer LA. Clinical pharmacokinetics and pharmacodynamics. In: Applied clinical pharmacokinetics. 11th ed. New York: McGraw Hill; 2020. [cited 2022 Jun 22]. https://accesspharmacy-mhmedical-com.jerome.stjohns.edu/content.aspx?sectionid=234135883&bookid=2577&Resultclick=2#1182422075.
8. Hutchison LC. Biomedical principles of aging. In: Hutchison LC, Sleeper RB, editors. Fundamentals of geriatric pharmacotherapy: an evidence-based approach. 1st ed. Bethesda, MD: American Society of Health-System Pharmacists, Inc; 2010. p. 53–70.
9. Buxton ILO. Pharmacokinetics: the dynamics of drug absorption, distribution, metabolism, and elimination. In: Hilal-Dandan R, Brunton LL, editors. Goodman and Gilman's manual of pharmacology and therapeutics. 2nd ed. New York: McGraw Hill Medical; 2014. [cited 2022 Jun 23]. https://accesspharmacy-mhmedical-com.jerome.stjohns.edu/content.aspx?sectionid=124489661&bookid=1810&Resultclick=2#1127547288.
10. Suarez S, Marroum PJ, Hughes M. Biopharmaceutic considerations in drug product design and in vitro drug product performance. In: Shargel L, Yu ABC, editors. Applied biopharmaceutics & pharmacokinetics. 7th ed. New York: McGraw Hill Medical; 2012. [cited 2022 Jun 23]. https://accesspharmacy-mhmedical-com.jerome.stjohns.edu/content.aspx?sectionid=100673007&bookid=1592#100673269.
11. Tillmann J, Reich A. Psychopharmacology and pharmacokinetics. In: Dekosky ST, Asthana S, editors. Handbook of clinical neurology, Geriatric neurology, vol. 167. Amsterdam: Elsevier; 2019. p. 37–56. [cited 2022 Jun 23]. https://www.sciencedirect.com/science/article/pii/B9780128047668000030.
12. Gonzalez FJ, Coughtrie M. Drug metabolism. In: Brunton LL, Knollman BC, editors. Goodman & Gilman's: the pharmacological basis of therapeutics. 14th ed. New York: McGraw Hill Medical; 2022. [cited 2022 Jun 23]. https://accesspharmacy-mhmedical-com.jerome.stjohns.edu/content.aspx?sectionid=266700137&bookid=3191#1191685126.
13. Donohoe KL, Price ET, Gendron TL, Slattum PW. Geriatrics: physiology of aging. In: DiPiro JT, Yee GC, Posey LM, Haines ST, Nolin TD, Ellingrod VL, editors. DiPiro: pharmacotherapy a pathophysiologic approach. 12th ed. New York: McGraw Hill; 2021.
14. Drenth-van Maanen AC, Wilting I, Jansen PAF. Prescribing medicines to older people—how to consider the impact of ageing on human organ and body functions. Br J Clin Pharmacol. 2020;86(10):1921–30.
15. Feenstra J, Heerdink ER, Grobbee DE, Stricker BHC. Association of nonsteroidal anti-inflammatory drugs with first occurrence of heart failure and with relapsing heart failure: the Rotterdam Study. Arch Intern Med. 2002;162:265–70.
16. Byon W, Garonzik S, Boyd RA, Frost CE. Apixaban: a clinical pharmacokinetic and pharmacodynamic review. Clin Pharmacokinet. 2019;58(10):1265–79.
17. Eliquis [package insert]. Princeton, NJ: Bristol-Myers Squibb; 2012.
18. GFR estimates. [cited 2023 Feb 15]. https://www.kidney.org/sites/default/files/441-8491_2202_faqs_aboutgfr_v5.pdf.
19. Delgado C, Baweja M, Crews DC, Eneanya ND, Gadegbeku CA, Inker LA, et al. A unifying approach for GFR estimation: recommendations of the NKF-ASN Task Force on reassessing the inclusion of race in diagnosing kidney disease. Am J Kidney. 2022;79(2):268–288.e1.

20. Guiding principles for the care of older adults with multimorbidity: an approach for clinicians. Guiding principles for the care of older adults with multimorbidity: an approach for clinicians: American Geriatrics Society Expert Panel on the care of older adults with multimorbidity. J Am Geriatr Soc. 2012;60(10):E1–25.
21. Maher RL, Hanlon JT, Hajjar ER. Clinical consequences of polypharmacy in elderly. Expert Opin Drug Saf. 2014;13(1):10.1517/14740338.2013.827660.
22. Young EH, Pan S, Yap AG, Reveles KR, Bhakta K. Polypharmacy prevalence in older adults seen in United States physician offices from 2009 to 2016. PLoS One. 2021;16(8):e0255642.
23. Heidenreich PA, Bozkurt B, Aguilar D, Allen LA, Byun JJ, Colvin MM, et al. 2022 AHA/ACC/HFSA guideline for the management of heart failure: executive summary: a report of the American College of Cardiology/American Heart Association Joint Committee on clinical practice guidelines. Circulation. 2022;145(18):e876–94.
24. O'Mahony D, Cherubini A, Guiteras AR, et al. STOPP/START criteria for potentially inappropriate prescribing in older people: version 3. Eur Geriatr Med. 2023;14(4):625–32. https://doi.org/10.1007/s41999-023-00777-y. Epub 2023 May 31. Erratum in: Eur Geriatr Med. 2023;14(4):633. https://doi.org/10.1007/s41999-023-00812-y. PMID: 37256475; PMCID: PMC10447584.
25. Hanlon JT, Schmader KE, Samsa GP, Weinberger M, Uttech KM, Lewis IK, et al. A method for assessing drug therapy appropriateness. J Clin Epidemiol. 1992;45(10):1045–51.
26. By the 2023 American Geriatrics Society Beers Criteria® Update Expert Panel. American Geriatrics Society 2023 updated AGS Beers Criteria® for potentially inappropriate medication use in older adults. J Am Geriatr Soc. 2023;71(7):2052–81. https://doi.org/10.1111/jgs.18372. Epub 2023 May 4. PMID: 37139824.
27. Hanlon JT, Schmader KE. The medication appropriateness index at 20: where it started, where it has been, and where it may be going. Drugs Aging. 2013;30(11):893–900.
28. Beier MT, Brodeur MR. ASCP's 2021 Choosing Wisely® Recommendations: A Proud Accomplishment. Sr Care Pharm. 2022;37(5):171–80. https://doi.org/10.4140/TCP.n.2022.171. PMID: 35450559.
29. Scott IA, Hilmer SN, Reeve E, Potter K, Le Couteur D, Rigby D, et al. Reducing inappropriate polypharmacy: the process of deprescribing. JAMA Intern Med. 2015;175(5):827–34.
30. Effects of continuing or stopping alendronate after 5 years of treatment: the fracture intervention trial long-term extension (FLEX): a randomized trial | Geriatrics | JAMA | JAMA Network. [cited 2022 Jun 15]. https://jamanetwork.com/journals/jama/fullarticle/204789.
31. Deprescribing.org—optimizing medication use. Deprescribing.org. [cited 2022 Aug 17]. https://deprescribing.org/.
32. Holmes HM, Hayley DC, Alexander GC, Sachs GA. Reconsidering medication appropriateness for patients late in life. Arch Intern Med. 2006;166(6):605–9.
33. 2018 AHA/ACC/AACVPR/AAPA/ABC/ACPM/ADA/AGS/APhA/ASPC/NLA/PCNA guideline on the management of blood cholesterol: executive summary. [cited 2022 Jun 21]. https://www.jacc.org/doi/epdf/10.1016/j.jacc.2018.11.002.
34. Lee SJ, Kim CM. Individualizing prevention for older adults. J Am Geriatr Soc. 2018;66(2):229–34.
35. Orkaby AR, Driver JA, Ho YL, Lu B, Costa L, Honerlaw J, et al. Association of statin use with all-cause and cardiovascular mortality in US veterans 75 years and older. JAMA. 2020;324(1):68–78.
36. Rochon PA, Gurwitz JH. Drug therapy. Lancet. 1995;346(8966):32–6.
37. McCarthy LM, Visentin JD, Rochon PA. Assessing the scope and appropriateness of prescribing cascades. J Am Geriatr Soc. 2019;67(5):1023–6.
38. Forman DE, Maurer MS, Boyd C, Brindis R, Salive ME, Horne FM, et al. Multimorbidity in older adults with cardiovascular disease. J Am Coll Cardiol. 2018;71(19):2149–61.
39. Read SH, Giannakeas V, Pop P, Bronskill SE, Herrmann N, Chen S, et al. Evidence of a gabapentinoid and diuretic prescribing cascade among older adults with lower back pain. J Am Geriatr Soc. 2021;69(10):2842–50.

40. DailyMed—METFORMIN tablet, extended release. [cited 2022 Jun 16]. https://dailymed. nlm.nih.gov/dailymed/lookup.cfm?setid=49a0b5c2-ebaf-4c4c-905f-dfd1962ac647.
41. DailyMed—JANUVIA—sitagliptin tablet, film coated. [cited 2022 Jun 16]. https://dailymed. nlm.nih.gov/dailymed/drugInfo.cfm?setid=f85a48d0-0407-4c50-b0fa-7673a160bf01.
42. The Top 200 of 2019. [cited 2022 Jun 21]. https://clincalc.com/DrugStats/Top200Drugs.aspx.
43. Wiffen PJ, Derry S, Bell RF, Rice AS, Tölle TR, Phillips T, et al. Gabapentin for chronic neuropathic pain in adults. Cochrane Database Syst Rev. 2017;6:CD007938. [cited 2022 Jun 21]. https://www-cochranelibrary-com.jerome.stjohns.edu/cdsr/doi/10.1002/14651858. CD007938.pub4/full.
44. Coluzzi F, Caputi FF, Billeci D, Pastore AL, Candeletti S, Rocco M, et al. Safe use of opioids in chronic kidney disease and hemodialysis patients: tips and tricks for non-pain specialists. Ther Clin Risk Manag. 2020;16:821–37.
45. Vondracek SF, Teitelbaum I, Kiser TH. Principles of kidney pharmacotherapy for the nephrologist: core curriculum 2021. Am J Kidney Dis. 2021;78(3):442–58.
46. Pham PC, et al. 2017 update on pain management in patients with chronic kidney disease. Clin Kidney J. 2017;10(5):688–97. https://academic.oup.com/ckj/article/10/5/688/4085328? login=true.
47. Benamouzig R, Guenoun M, Deutsch D, Fauchier L. Review article: gastrointestinal bleeding risk with direct oral anticoagulants. Cardiovasc Drugs Ther. 2022;36(5):973–89. https://doi. org/10.1007/s10557-021-07211-0. Epub 2021 Jun 18. PMID: 34143317.
48. Connolly SJ, Ezekowitz MD, Yusuf S, Eikelboom J, Oldgren J, Parekh A, et al. Dabigatran versus warfarin in patients with atrial fibrillation. N Engl J Med. 2009;361(12):1139–51.
49. Patel MR, Mahaffey KW, Garg J, Pan G, Singer DE, Hacke W, et al. Rivaroxaban versus warfarin in nonvalvular atrial fibrillation. N Engl J Med. 2011;365(10):883–91.
50. Granger CB, Alexander JH, McMurray JJV, Lopes RD, Hylek EM, Hanna M, et al. Apixaban versus warfarin in patients with atrial fibrillation. N Engl J Med. 2011;365(11):981–92.
51. Hanni C, Petrovitch E, Ali M, Gibson W, Giuliano C, Holzhausen J, et al. Outcomes associated with apixaban vs warfarin in patients with renal dysfunction. Blood Adv. 2020;4(11):2366–71.
52. Siontis KC, Zhang X, Eckard A, Bhave N, Schaubel DE, He K, et al. Outcomes associated with apixaban use in patients with end-stage kidney disease and atrial fibrillation in the United States. Circulation. 2018;138(15):1519–29.
53. Herndon K, Guidry TJ, Wassell K, Elliott W. Characterizing the safety profile of apixaban versus warfarin in moderate to severe chronic kidney disease at a Veterans Affairs Hospital. Ann Pharmacother. 2020;54(6):554–60.
54. DailyMed—PRADAXA—dabigatran etexilate mesylate capsule. [cited 2022 Aug 22]. https:// dailymed.nlm.nih.gov/dailymed/lookup.cfm?setid=ba74e3cd-b06f-4145-b284-5fd6b84ff3c9.
55. DailyMed—XARELTO—rivaroxaban tablet, film coated. [cited 2022 Jul 19]. https://dailymed.nlm.nih.gov/dailymed/drugInfo.cfm?setid=3e95389b-0a93-4560-98c5-02637fb2600f.
56. DailyMed—ELIQUIS—apixaban tablet, film coated. [cited 2022 Aug 22]. https://dailymed. nlm.nih.gov/dailymed/drugInfo.cfm?setid=33a9046a-41cc-46c1-becc-2ff4d7d71538.
57. DailyMed—SAVAYSA—edoxaban tosylate tablet, film coated. [cited 2022 Aug 22]. https://dailymed.nlm.nih.gov/dailymed/drugInfo.cfm?setid=e77d3400-56ad-11e3-949a-0800200c9a66.

Chapter 15
Dialysis in the Elderly

Michelle Carver and Michael Alan Kraus

Case 1

A 74-year-old Taiwanese American female who speaks little English receiving maintenance hemodialysis has a dry weight of 68 kg and for the last 12 months, her prescription has been hemodialysis thrice weekly for 3.5 h. The etiology of ESKD (end-stage kidney disease) is unknown, and past medical history includes hypertension, and heart failure with reduced left ventricular (LV) function (LVEF 30% and moderate LV hypertrophy). For the last year on hemodialysis, she has been hospitalized with symptomatic volume overload on five separate occasions. She is not eating well, and serum albumin continues to decline. She has become frailer, uses a wheelchair to leave the home, and is mostly inactive. Hemodialysis is complicated with severe hypertension pre-dialysis although adherent with five blood pressure-lowering medications. She suffers from frequent severe intradialytic hypotension.

Case 2

An 82-year-old, 80 kg male, who cares for his elderly wife who suffers from dementia has been receiving automated peritoneal dialysis (PD) for the last 6 months. He has no cognitive impairment but has mild depression. His PD prescription is 3 exchanges of 2 L over 8.5 h. Residual renal function is 5 mL/min and Kt/V >1.9. His phosphorus and blood pressure have been increasing over the last 2 months. Being

M. Carver
Fresenius Medical Care, Pickrell, NE, USA

M. A. Kraus (✉)
Fresenius Kidney Care, Waltham, MA, USA

H. Kramer et al. (eds.), *Kidney Disease in the Elderly*,
https://doi.org/10.1007/978-3-031-68460-9_15

his wife's primary caregiver remains his biggest concern because they have no family near them. At night, his wife frequently awakens confused and may get out of bed without warning. His depression is worsening and being on the APD cycler at night adversely impacts his ability to care for her. He is strongly considering going to the incenter unit so his treatment schedule can better accommodate his wife's needs.

Introduction

The mean age of patients receiving maintenance dialysis in the United States is now 63 years and almost 50% are 65 years and older. The effects of aging noted in the general population are important to consider when planning dialysis in an older patient. According to the 2022 USRDS Annual report, dialysis in an older patient (age 65 years) is not uncommon and unfortunately, data that provide guidance for the best dialysis prescription suitable for older patients remains scarce. This chapter will therefore rely on pragmatic suggestions based on the aging process and the physiology or "physiology" of dialysis.

Dialysis Results Among the Elderly

Kidney failure is a common disease among the older population; in fact, the prevalence rate of kidney failure in older adults has risen significantly from 2000 to 2020 (54.6% rise in those over 74, and 40.6% rise in adults aged 65–74 years). The prevalence rate of kidney failure is highest among the elderly with just under 7200 patients per million population in both groups. Among adults aged 65 years and older, transplant rates are much lower and home therapies remain underutilized. In 2020, among the patients 75 years or older with ESKD, only 13.6% (18,696) were transplanted. Of the remaining, 8.8% (10,447) were treated with peritoneal dialysis, 0.94% (1116) were on home hemodialysis and 90.2% (106,763) received incenter hemodialysis. Among those aged 65–74 years, 27.9% were transplanted, 10.8% were treated with PD, and 1.6% received home hemodialysis. Kidney failure is common among the older populations. While the incidence and prevalence of kidney failure varies somewhat by country, the older populations have the highest incidence and prevalence rates of kidney failure in most countries. Therefore, dialysis in older populations is indeed a global concern [1].

How dialysis is prescribed for older patients in the United States today is instructive as we consider the potential for better practices. Of patients receiving peritoneal dialysis in the United States in 2020, 86.4% were prescribed APD. This practice was similar in patients aged 65–74 years, where 86.4% also received APD versus continuous ambulatory PD (CAPD). In contrast, APD was less commonly prescribed, 84.9%, in patients 74 years and older. Home hemodialysis prescriptions based on frequency and time also have had some variance based on age. In 2020 the number of patients on five or more treatments per week decreased to 43.6% from 58.9% in 2015. Younger patients, aged 65–74 years, were more likely to receive treatment five times per week as compared to patients older than 74 years, 42% vs. 33% respectively. The total weekly duration of dialysis also decreases with advancing age. In 2020, 36.1% of patients receiving home hemodialysis (HHD) dialyzed less than 12 h per week. This shorter weekly duration is more common in older populations with 38.5% of those between 65 and 74 years of age and 44.25% of those 75 and over were prescribed less than 12 h of total dialysis per week [1]. The trends in dialysis prescriptions have moved toward less frequency and duration in all patients, but this trend is exaggerated with advancing age. We should consider if this trend is appropriate based on physiology or not.

Home Dialysis Complications with Age

As we look at infectious outcomes, peritonitis rates and dialysis access infections in home hemodialysis patients are lowest in the oldest age groups, well below the overall rates for these infections. Conversion from home, either PD or HHD, to incenter dialysis modality is also lowest in the most advanced age group. Perhaps surprisingly the rate of conversion to incenter hemodialysis from HHD is similar across age groups for the first 5 months, but after 5 months, dialysis conversion is lowest in patients aged 75 years or older [1]. These data suggest that home therapies can be safe and well tolerated in the oldest patients.

As expected, advancing age is associated with increased mortality, but survival on home therapies remains acceptable. Patients receiving PD who are 75 years and older (starting at day 61) had a 22.1% cumulative incidence of death at 1 year and 44% at 2 years. Patients aged 65–74 years experienced a 14.7% risk of death at 12 months and a 30.7% risk at 24 months. For those patients aged 75 years and older receiving HHD, the cumulative mortality was 41.9% at 12 months and 62.2% at 34 months, while mortality in the age group 65–74 years was 27.7% and 45.4% at 12 and 34 months, respectively. All-cause mortality in patients receiving any dialysis modality was 307 per 1000 patient-years in 2019 and rose to 347.6 in 2020 with COVID-19 for those 75 and older and 203.3 in 2019, 237.7 in 2020 for those 65–74 years old [1]. Renal replacement therapy is therefore a viable option for many of the elderly and in-center hemodialysis, HHD and PD may be successful options of care.

In fact, in the United States, 5-year survival among those initiating in 2016 was 22.9% for those 75+ and 35% in those aged 65–74. Canada has reported similar survival in these age groups and these survival rates improved during the 1990s. Despite increased comorbidity over the decade, the unadjusted 1-, 3-, and 5-year survival rates among patients aged 65–74 years at dialysis initiation rose from 74.4%, 44.9%, and 25.8% in 1990–1994 to 78.1%, 51.5% and 33.5% in era 1994–1999. The respective survival rates among those aged 75 years and older at dialysis initiation increased from 67.2%, 32.3%, and 14.2% in 1990–1994 to 69.0%, 36.7%, and 20.3% in 1994–1999. This survival advantage persisted after adjustment for diabetes, sex, and comorbidity in both age groups (65–74 years: hazard ratio [HR] 0.76, 95% confidence interval [CI] 0.72–0.81; 75 years or more: HR 0.86, 95% CI 0.80–0.92) [2].

Dialysis is a good option for many older people with kidney failure. An individualized approach to the dialysis prescription should be considered to improve the present outcomes. Individualizing care for the elderly patient needs to assess comorbidities carefully and understand the benefits of dialysis on morbidity and survival. Key components to consider when prescribing dialysis and modality include the social situation, cognitive function, and cardiovascular status. Cardiovascular disease and fluid overload remain the critical aspects of care and prescription for all dialysis patients today. Cognitive function is particularly important with education and selecting modality choices.

Aging and CKD, Cardiovascular Effects

Independent of CKD or ESKD, cardiovascular status, especially LVH worsens with aging. Advanced stages of CKD and ESKD are associated with higher prevalence of LVH, cardiovascular morbidity/mortality, and even sudden cardiac death. LVH remains a significant risk factor for mortality in patients receiving dialysis, especially in patients with advanced age. LVH and heart failure (HFpEF and HFrEF) worsen in the elderly even without ESRD and CKD.

In the general population with hypertension, the prevalence of LVH increases with age; notably, women with hypertension have a greater progression than men [3]. LVH is greater with hypertension, prehypertension, and diabetes [3, 4].

The Framingham study, a community cohort in Framingham Massachusetts, has shown that the prevalence of LVH increases dramatically with age and is present in 33% of men and 40% of women aged 70 years and older [5].

The heightened prevalence of LVH in older adults is an important consideration when determining optimal care for kidney failure. In 1995, Dr. Foley showed that the majority (73.9%) of patients receiving dialysis had LVH, 35.5% had LV dilatation and 14.8% had reduced systolic function. The most important predictive factors for LVH were advancing age, female gender, wide arterial pulse pressures, low blood urea, and low serum albumin [6]. The association of increasing LVH as GFR declines is consistently seen. It has been reported that LVH prevalence increases from 70% in CKD stage 3 to 85% with CKD stage 5D [7] (Table 15.1).

Dialysis appears to accelerate progression of LVH by approximately 0.50 g/m^2 per month and progression of LVH is associated with a threefold greater risk for both all-cause mortality and major adverse cardiovascular events [8]. Prescription of dialysis in the elderly should consider these cardiovascular risks and individualize treatments and modalities to modulate these risk factors when appropriate.

Table 15.1 Progression of LVH through declining GFR [7]

CKD stage	Prevalence of increased left ventricular mass (%)
CKD Stage 2	9
CKD Stage 3 GFR 30–59 mL/min/1.73 m²	70
CKD Stage 4 GFR 15–29 mL/min/1.73 m²	83
ESKD GFR <15 mL/min/1.73²	85

Aging and Cognitive Function, Depression with ESKD

Much like LVH, advancing age in the general population remains a risk factor for depression and cognitive impairment regardless of etiology [9]. Similarly, kidney failure remains a risk factor for both depression and cognitive impairment. Even in the general aging population, there is also a relationship between increased CVD risk and cognitive dysfunction. The risk factors of CVD or CVD itself affect cognition; there is a correlation between increased CVD and cognitive dysfunction [10]. Understanding cognitive impairment and depression are important aspects of the ability to educate the patient and determine the support needed to succeed in any modality of renal replacement therapy.

Cognitive dysfunction is common in older patients with CKD. It has been estimated that up to 70% of patients aged 55 years and older have moderate to severe cognitive impairment which is largely underdiagnosed. Murray noted that using a detailed 45-min neuropsychological battery, 37% of patients had severe impairment, 36% moderate and 14% had mild cognitive impairment. Surprisingly only 13% of older dialysis patients had no cognitive impairment [11]. Much like CV disease, cognitive function declines with decreasing eGFR [12].

The role dialysis plays in the worsening cognitive dysfunction is unknown, but there is significant concern that hemodialysis can worsen impairment. MRI and spectroscopy show evidence of cerebral ischemia dialysis [13]. In a study of Japanese patients receiving dialysis, 34% of cerebral infarcts occurred within 30 min of treatment initiation [14]. Cerebral function declines during dialysis with cerebral edema, decreased intra-cerebral blood pressure, velocity, and perfusion. It has been postulated that decreasing dialysis rates may help decrease these conditions as well [15]. Understanding the effects of dialysis on the CNS system and determining ways to modify therapy are likely to continue to become relevant in the future and warrant consideration today.

As cognition declines, the risk for morbidity and mortality increases. In older patients with kidney failure, dementia and depression are common, and should be elucidated to optimize the dialysis care. Prescription and modality should be individualized to protect and treat the cognitive status of the patient. Clinicians should also ensure patients and their caregivers receive the needed support and education is modified to their needs and abilities. Support needed, how to educate, suitability for dialysis modality, and even risk modification are dependent on the correct diagnosis and treatment of these underlying conditions.

Dialysis in the Elderly

All patients should have choices so they can utilize the therapy that is best for them at that particular point in time. As they age, the treatment that is best for them may change. Much like younger patients, older patients may be exposed to multiple renal replacement modalities during their ESKD life. Peritoneal dialysis (PD)—either ambulatory peritoneal dialysis with manual exchanges (CAPD) or automated peritoneal dialysis with dry days or with daytime fluid (APD, NIPD, CCPD), hemodialysis either at home (HHD) or in a center (ICHD), transplantation, and even hospice care with or without renal replacement therapy should all be offered and discussed. Each of these care paths/modalities may be used at some point in the life span of the patient.

The choice to dialyze versus conservative care at any point in the patient's course is essential to discuss and offer. Palliative care without dialysis is discussed elsewhere in this book. This is usually based on the patient's desires, beliefs, quality of life, morbidity, and perceived benefits and risks of renal replacement therapy. A trial of dialysis is sometimes chosen to see if an individual may benefit from renal replacement therapy. Multiple studies show various results as to improved quality of life in older patients with dialysis but benefits from dialysis also vary between patients depending on the comorbidities. One thing to consider is that the course of dialysis is a major determinant in morbidity and mortality [16]. If the educated and engaged patient and family agree to renal replacement therapy, in general, the medical staff should be supportive.

When the decision to proceed or continue with dialysis is made, the decision on modality and prescription is vital. Education is the cornerstone to empowering patients. Elderly patients and their support groups should be empowered to make the best decisions for them—dialysis should be a decision between the patient, family, and care team. Cornerstones of empowered care require access to care, multidisciplinary care, smooth transitions of care with continuity, involvement of family or support groups, reliable non-biased information, emotional and medical support, and respect for a patient's decisions [17].

Supporting patients as they begin dialysis may be particularly useful with older patients. Transitional care units are designed to care for incident patients with increased support, education, and care. Patients spend a 4–6 week period with the goals of medical and emotional/social support over the first 1–2 weeks with increased directed education and modality exposure over the following weeks [18, 19]. Transitional care units may be a valuable tool for assisting older patients with transitioning to end-stage kidney disease (ESKD) and assuring education and support when and as appropriate [18].

Transitional care units have been shown to improve placement of permanent access, waitlisting to transplant, and increased likelihood of home utilization [19]. Bowman also demonstrated improved mortality and hospitalization [18]. The benefits of transitional care are achieved with consistent education and include the plan of medical and emotional care to stabilize the transitioning patients and improve patient comprehension of dialysis education. While not yet specifically studied, it is reasonable to believe that the use of transitional care units is beneficial to older patients. Modality and prescription should be an integral part of education.

Cognitive function and an evaluation for depression should be undertaken to assist in the decision process. It is imperative to remember that cognition and depressive symptoms may change over time and should be reassessed as the patient's condition changes (positively or negatively). Social support is essential to evaluate as well. Are there family or friends willing to assist in the delivery of dialysis in the home? Is there family or support willing to assist in travel and care needs required for success with any modality? Can the dialysis unit or local social services provide some or all the assistance that may be required? Is there adequate access to medicine, food, medical care, housing, and other essential social determinants of health? Can access be improved?

Initial and Ongoing Evaluation

Older patients should be considered a high-risk population and may benefit from a very thorough initial evaluation. This includes the evaluation of the social determinants of health and the evaluation of the social needs a patient requires to improve overall health. Do they have access to food, medication, travel to physician appointments/dialysis, stable housing, and utilities? The level of support for the patient's needs and the best methods to deliver resources to assist in daily living and better health should be assessed. Screening older patients to find unrecognized impairments which might improve with care is warranted and will help ensure access to the support needed to be successful in any modality. There are many screens available. The Montreal Cognitive Assessment (MOCA) has been verified in patients receiving dialysis and this tool is simple to deliver [20]. For depression screening two Patient Health Questionnaire (PHQ) tools, PHQ 2 and PHQ 9, are routinely used and established as part of the conditions of coverage for dialysis entities [21].

HHD and PD in older adults may be particularly useful in clinical risk reduction but require the ability to safely perform dialysis in the home. Performing dialysis at home requires adequate cognitive function and usually, but not universally, in-house support as well. The risks of HHD and PD include the potential for social isolation, acute complications of therapy, less frequent interactions with Health care professionals, storage requirements, and the burden of therapy with burnout. These risks may be obviated if adequate social support and close attention are paid to older patients. Even in the in-center environment many of these concerns exist but more frequent face-to-face interactions may increase the ability to pick up these concerns sooner. Older patients and their partners deserve careful attention to declines in health, welfare, and mental capacity. Support needs may increase and change over the lifespan of the dialysis patient. All members of the dialysis community are responsible for ongoing evaluation, and this should not be relegated to only the social worker, although they play a critical role in going assessments and support needs. In-home therapies respite care, frequent telehealth visits, competency reviews, and discussions with care partners are all valuable tools in ensuring ongoing success and preventing negative events.

Hemodialysis (Incenter and Home)

Case 1

A 74-year-old Taiwanese American female who speaks little English.

In-center hemodialysis performed thrice weekly is the most common therapy for ESKD in the world today and has acceptable outcomes even in the older population [1]. All hemodialysis should be prescribed with the patient's needs in mind. Goal-directed therapy is essential and a frequency of 2 days per week may have merit but has not been examined in the older population specifically [22]. The advantages to in-center dialysis include the potential for increased socialization, the benefit of being evaluated by health care professionals thrice weekly, and a perception of decreased burden for caretakers However, caretaker burden is high in all modalities. In-center dialysis requires travel to and from the unit, and the schedule may be inflexible. Moving dialysis to an in-center unit may lead to a perceived loss of independence, and the symptoms associated with thrice weekly prescriptions—postdialysis fatigue, nausea, headaches, hypotension, and more may add burden to patient symptoms. Thrice-weekly dialysis may also increase cardiac and cerebral morbidity. The dialysis prescription should be written to minimize risk and complications. Ultrafiltration rate (UFR) is associated with many of the morbidities and recent data suggests that should be limited in most. Assimon and Flythe found that increasing UFR above 6 mL/h/kg was associated with increased atrial fibrillation and a 3% increased risk of death for every mL/h/kg [23–25]. More recently, the question of UFR was shown to be more significant as the mortality associated with high UFR doubled in the more obese patients. Evaluation of ultrafiltration and death increased to greater than 10% for all patients when UFR was greater than 800 mL/h regardless of weight [26, 27]. Hemodialysis in older patients should be prescribed to limit the ultrafiltration rate and increased time and or frequency may be needed.

Sudden cardiac death is also a significant risk in ESKD, and the dialysis prescription should consider such risks. Sudden cardiac death remains a leading cause of death on dialysis and continuous monitoring has shown that arrhythmias—atrial fibrillation and bradyarrhythmia occur frequently. On hemodialysis, the bradyarrhythmias are the most common life-threatening event and occur in a pattern resembling thrice weekly dialysis—with peaks generally just prior to dialysis and most prevalent around the 2-day gap [28]. Increasing frequency and reducing intradialytic volume loading may help decrease this risk of sudden death and potentially be the reason for improvement in LVH [29, 30].

Home hemodialysis offers the benefit of flexibility of prescription and becomes technically easier to prescribe increased frequency and increasing duration to minimize cardiac risk and improve LVH, hypertension, hypotension, and reduction in antihypertensives [29].

Careful and frequent evaluations and support are necessary to prevent the concerns outlined above.

Case 1 Follow-Up

The patient has significant cognitive deficits initially, a language barrier, and severe cardiac morbidity with thrice weekly in-center dialysis. Care meetings with the patient, family, and interdisciplinary team occurred, and all options of therapy were discussed. The patient's daughter would be the main support and was adamant that she would be willing to try anything to make her mother's life better and perhaps longer. A thorough discussion ensued, and the family wished to try HHD with the benefit of more frequent dialysis. A prescription of frequent dialysis was discussed and a prescription of 6 days per week with 15 h per week to ensure low ultrafiltration rates and decreased intradialytic weight gains. The hope of and evidence for decreased cardiac complications was discussed. UFR was maintained under 6 mL/h/kg (<500 mL/h) for therapy. The patient thrived and 2 years later the dialysis frequency was decreased to 5 days per week, maintaining 14–15 h per week of treatment. The patient survived 9 years with a total of only four hospitalizations in that time (none related to volume or CV morbidity). Her cognitive function improved, and her depression resolved. She became less frail and ambulatory. She traveled to Taiwan independently twice, receiving more frequent incenter therapy while traveling.

In-center dialysis should be prescribed with the same attention and care desired in the home setting. More frequent dialysis should be considered but is pragmatically limited by travel, unit capacity, and patient preferences. Attempts to maintain a weekly duration of dialysis to keep safe ultrafiltration rates remain important in-center as well. The patient's and sometimes family's desire for reducing dialysis time is significant and not all patients will allow increasing time. If dialysis is complicated with symptoms, the following prescription changes may alleviate these symptoms: Increasing time and hence decreasing ultrafiltration rates decrease hypotension, ischemia, and even post-dialysis fatigue; there may be a benefit to lower sodium dialysis to near serum sodium; dialysate cooling had some early support but may not be as useful as hoped [31].

Just like in-home therapies, ongoing evaluations should be routine to evaluate changes in health, cardiovascular issues, declines in social determinants of health, and changes in cognitive/depressive status (Fig. 15.1).

Evaluation: To be performed initially and as clinically and socially indicated (q3-6 months)

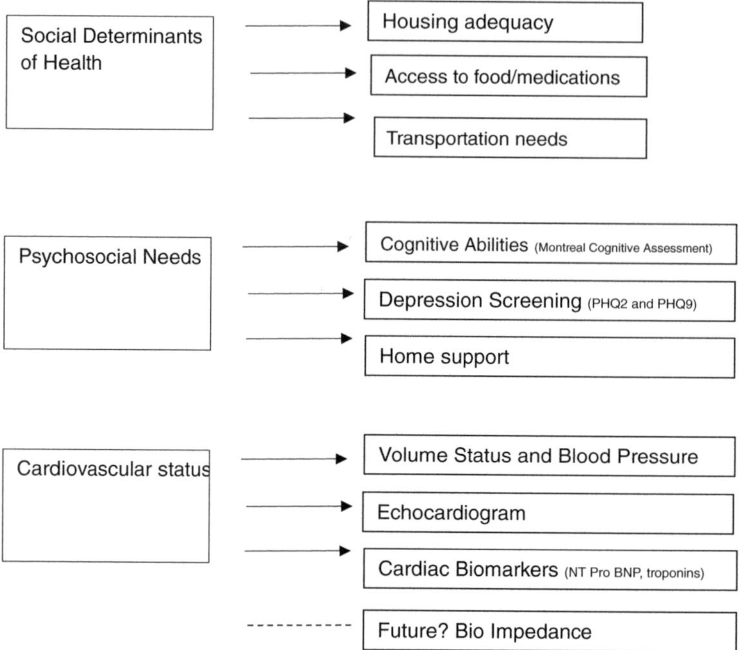

Fig. 15.1 Dialysis in the elderly—evaluation. Evaluation: to be performed initially and as clinically and socially indicated (q3-6 months)

In Europe today and perhaps in the future in the United States, hemodiafiltration (HDF) looks to be a promising addition to renal replacement therapy options. The CONVINCE trial in Europe showed a significant improvement in mortality with HDF versus conventional high flux HD. Frequency was thrice weekly and duration greater than 12 h weekly was standard in both arms. The survival benefit was clinically and statistically significant in the elderly population. Patients aged more than 65 years experienced a 32% improvement in mortality [32]. Note that hemodiafiltration in this randomized controlled study was 23 L per treatment and requires specific technology to employ.

Peritoneal Dialysis

Case 2

Eighty-two-year-old, 80 kg male, who cares for his elderly wife who suffers from dementia.

Care of the elderly with PD needs to be individualized to meet the patient's needs, reduce burden, and address cardiac status. Both CAPD and APD have potential benefits for many patients, but unfortunately in the United States CAPD use has decreased to 13.6% [1]. The true reason for the decline is unstudied, but it has not occurred elsewhere in the world. It seems reasonable to opine that healthcare providers may perceive the burden and risk of CAPD are greater than with APD. Hence patients are "educated" to choose APD. One certainly can argue that many of these perceptions may not be universally true, and individualization of therapy may require increased utilization of CAPD (Fig. 15.2).

CAPD in older patients has many obvious advantages. Longer dwell times accommodate sodium removal, phosphorus removal, and efficient urea removal [33]. It is the simplest home therapy to learn and understand as it does not require utilization and troubleshooting associated with learning a new technique and device. Since CAPD does not require transportation, water, or electricity, it is the most reliable modality for any patient during weather emergencies or even inclement weather, as transportation to and from dialysis necessitates exposure to extremes of temperature and conditions. CAPD allows for more restful nights in many, as there are no interruptions of sleep due to exchanges or machine alarms. Since CAPD is a simple therapy to learn and perform, patients with mild and perhaps even moderate cognitive dysfunction may be able to perform this independently longer. One further advantage of CAPD is smaller storage needs than CCPD. CAPD generally uses

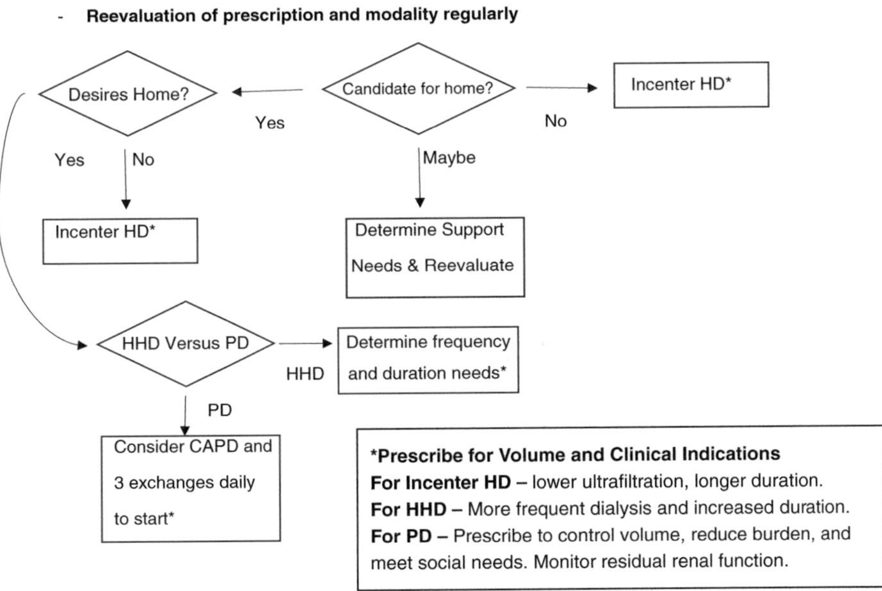

Fig. 15.2 Dialysis in the elderly—modality selection. Educate on modalities, conservative management, and hospice care. Reevaluation of prescription and modality regularly

40–50% less fluid, smaller bags, and less daily disposables than APD. This may be beneficial to elderly patients with limited living space. When necessary, supplies can be delivered more frequently so storage needs can be minimized further. Finally, CAPD may be preferred in low and low-average transport patients as studies have shown better survival in CAPD with low transporters and better sodium and phosphorus clearance in low and low-average patients [34, 35].

APD remains an excellent therapy for many patients as well. APD offers the advantage of fewer daytime interruptions but requires being connected to a device for a prolonged period. Nightly APD is best prescribed with keeping dwell times >2 h to combat the effects of sodium sieving (more rapid exchange of water than sodium occurs for the initial dwell time due to the movement of water through aquaporin channels early in the exchange, with diffusion of sodium moving greater than water movement after 1.5 h [36]). Prescriptions for APD should consider daytime dwells or even daytime dwells with an evening exchange. This improves sodium and phosphorus clearance [34]. Icodextrin can be used if there is negative ultrafiltration with longer exchanges or more ultrafiltration is required than can be achieved with nocturnal dialysis.

APD does offer a significant advantage in an elderly patient who requires assistance with connections and exchanges. This is particularly helpful if the care partner works or is away during the day, or as in many cases may not live with the patient. APD can be initiated in the evening and disconnected in the AM reducing the burden on the care provider but leaving the patient on the device for 10–12 h generally.

For both therapies incremental dialysis may be useful, but care is required to ensure residual renal function is monitored closely, as even short periods of underdialysis may lead to poor outcomes. With CAPD, three exchanges a day may be very useful. This can be done to minimize burden and still improve volume control and phosphorus removal. The exchanges can be initiated in the morning, in the evening, and at bedtime, thus minimizing the burden on the patient. This prescription provides significant dialysis clearance, but providers must monitor small solute clearance closely. Others may wish for dry nights with one or two daily exchanges; however, this provides less small solute and phosphorus clearance and declines in residual renal function may significantly impact clearances, hence there may be a need to increase therapy more often. In APD incremental dialysis can be initiated with as little as two exchanges nightly, but again this requires careful monitoring of the patient and residual renal function. With any incremental dialysis, care is needed to ensure volume is controlled, BP is controlled, and phosphorus and potassium remain controlled in addition to the usual push to maintain urea clearance.

A final consideration for PD in the elderly may be the preservation of cognitive function. Cerebral blood flow and cognitive function may decrease during hemodialysis sessions and MRI and spectroscopy demonstrate acute brain injury during dialysis. The overall impact of these repeated changes in thrice weekly dialysis has not yet been definitively demonstrated but should be considered [13, 37, 38].

These regular CNS challenges are not expected to occur with PD.

Case 2 Follow Up

Plan of care meeting ensued, and the social worker initiated the conversation about the burden of APD with this patient especially the impact on his ability to care for his wife, particularly at night. A note was made by the care team that BP, PO4, and edema were increasing concurrently to a slowly declining residual renal function. The patient was educated and decided to try CAPD before switching to hemodialysis. The patient was retrained on CAPD and initiated CAPD with three 2.5-L exchanges daily. He used a 2.5% exchange at night and either 1.5% or 2.5% exchanges during the day depending on volume needs. The patient rapidly improved. His depression and anxiety improved as he no longer had concerns about caring for his wife at night. He noted that he felt better, his BP decreased, and his meds were reduced. Phosphorus improved and binders decreased as well.

Monitoring Dialysis Therapies

Understanding that dialysis is a journey and patients may experience more than one form of modality during their life's journey. At some point, the elderly may choose PD, in-center HD, home HD, Transplant, and even hospice care. The care team's responsibility is to ensure patients are educated, empowered, and supported to meet their individual goals.

Volume status, blood pressure, adherence, and metabolic control must be assessed monthly to make sure the modality and prescription are right for the patient and readjusted as needed. In older patients, regular evaluation of social support, cognitive function, depression, and assessment of social determinants of health by an interdisciplinary team is critical for ongoing success. Finally, regular cardiac assessment is critical to ensure that the care of the heart is maintained. Cardiac biomarkers, such as NT Pro BNP (N-terminal Pro Brain Natriuretic Peptide), and regular echocardiograms to assess LVH progression, cardiac function, and volume status may be helpful in directing modification of prescription or modality [39].

Dialysis in elderly patients is a lifesaving therapy. Balancing patients' social needs, technical skills, and clinical status to deliver the best care is critical to meeting the needs of the elderly. Renal replacement therapy prescribed and performed well prolongs life and should improve quality of life as long as possible.

References

1. United States Renal Data System. Annual data report; 2022.
2. Jassal SV, Trpeski L, Zhu N, Fenton S, Hemmelgarn B. Changes in servival amoung elderly patients initiating dialysis from 1990 to 1999. Can Med Assoc J. 2007;177(9):1033–8.
3. Drazner MH. The progression of hypertensive heart disease. Circulation. 2011;123:327–34.

4. Aronow WS. Hypertension and left ventricular hypertrophy. Ann Transl Med. 2017;5(15):310.
5. Levy D, Anderson KM, Savage DD, Kannel WB, Christiansen JC, Castelli WP. Echocardiographically detected left ventricular hypertrophy: prevalence and risk factors. The Framingham Heart Study. Ann Intern Med. 1998;108(1):7–13.
6. Foley RN, Parfrey PS, Harnett JD, Kent GM, Martin CJ, Murray DC, Barre PE. Clinical and echocardiographic disease in patients starting end-stage renal disease therapy. Kidney Int. 1995;47(1):186–92.
7. Bansal N, Keane M, Delafontaine P, Dries D, Foster E, Gadegbeku CA, Go AS, Hamm LL, Kusek JW, Ojo AO, Rahman M, Tao K, Wright JT, Xie D, Hsu C-y, CRIC Study Investigators. A longitudinal study of left ventricular function and structure from CKD to ESRD: the CRIC study. Clin J Am Soc Nephrol. 2013;8(3):355–62.
8. Zoccali C, Benedetto FA, Mallamaci F, Tripepi G, Giacone G, Stancanelli B, Cataliotti A, Malatino LS. Left ventricular mass monitoring in the follow-up of dialysis patients: prognostic value of left ventricular hypertrophy progression. Kidney Int. 2004;65(4):1492–8.
9. Murman DL. The impact of age on cognition. Semin Hear. 2015;36(3):111–21.
10. Dregan A, Stewart R, Gulliford MC. Cardiovascular risk factors and cognitive decline in adults aged 50 and over: a population-based cohort study. Age Aging. 2013;42(3):338–45.
11. Murray AM. Cognitive impairment in the aging dialysis and chronic kidney disease populations: an occult burden. Adv Chronic Kidney Dis. 2008;15(2):123–32.
12. Kurella M, Chertow GM, Luan J, Yaffe K. Cognitive impairment in chronic kidney disease. J Am Geriatr Soc. 2004;52(11):1863–9.
13. Anazodo UC, Wong DY, Théberge J, Dacey M, Gomes J, Penny JD, van Ginkel M, Poirier SE, McIntyre CW. Hemodialysis-related acute brain injury demonstrated by application of intradialytic magnetic resonance imaging and spectroscopy. J Am Soc Nephrol. 2023;34(6):1090–104.
14. Toyoda K, Fujii K, Fujimi S, Kumai Y, Tsuchimochi H, Ibayashi S, Iida M. Stroke in patients on maintenance hemodialysis: a 22-year single-center study. Am J Kidney Dis. 2005;45(6):1058–66.
15. Murray AM, Pederson SL, Tupper DE, Hochhalter AK, Miller WA, Li Q, Zaun D, Collins AJ, Kane R, Foley RN. Acute variation in cognitive function in hemodialysis patients: a cohort study with repeated measures. Am J Kidney Dis. 2007;50(2):270–8.
16. O'Hare AM, Batten A, Burrows NR, Pavkov ME, Taylor L, Gupta I, Todd-Stenberg J, Maynard C, Rodriguez RA, Murtagh FEM, Larson EB, Williams DE. Trajectories of kidney function decline in the 2 years before initiation of long-term dialysis. Am J Kidney Dis. 2012;59(4):513–22.
17. Picker.org. The picker principles of person centered care; 2023.
18. Bowman BT. Transitional care units: greater than the sum of their parts. Clin J Am Soc Nephrol. 2019;14(5):765–7.
19. Blankenship DM, Usvyat L, Kraus MA, Chatoth DK, Lasky R, Turk Jr JE, Maddux FW. Assessing the impact of transitional care units on dialysis patient outcomes: a multicenter, propensity score-matched analysis. Hemodial Int. 2023;27(2):165–73.
20. Amatneeks TM, Hamdan AC. Montreal Cognitive Assessment for cognitive assessment in chronic kidney disease: a systematic review. J Bras Nefrol. 2019;41(1):112–23.
21. Kondo K, Antick JR, Ayers CK, Kansagara D, Chopra P. Depression screening tools for patients with kidney failure: a systematic review. Clin J Am Soc Nephrol. 2020;15(12):1785–95.
22. Soi V, Faber MD, Paul R. Incremental hemodialysis: what we know so far. Int J Nephrol Renovasc Dis. 2022;15:161–72.
23. Assimon MM, et al. Ultrafiltration rate and mortality in maintenance hemodialysis patients. Am J Kidney Dis. 2016;68(6):911–22.
24. Flythe JE, Liu S, Montez-Rath ME, Winkelmayer WC, Chang TI. Ultrafiltration rate and incident atrial fibrillation among older individuals initiating hemodialysis. Nephrol Dial Transplant. 2021;36(11):2084–93.
25. Flythe JE, Assimon MM, Wang L. Ultrafiltration rate scaling in hemodialysis patients. Semin Dial. 2017;30(3):282–3.

26. Mermelstein A, Raimann JG, Wang Y, Kotanko P, Daugirdas JT. Ultrafiltration rate levels in hemodialysis patients associated with weight-specific mortality risks. Clin J Am Soc Nephrol. 2023;18(6):767–76.
27. Raimann JG, Wang Y, Mermelstein A, Kotanko P, Daugirdas JT. Ultrafiltration rate thresholds associated with increased mortality risk in hemodialysis, unscaled or scaled to body size. Kidney Int Rep. 2022;7(7):1585–93.
28. Roy-Chaudhury P, Tumlin JA, Koplan BA, Costea AI, Kher V, Williamson D, Pokhariyal S, Charytan DM, MiD Investigators and Committees. Primary outcomes of the Monitoring in Dialysis Study indicate that clinically significant arrhythmias are common in hemodialysis patients and related to dialytic cycle. Kidney Int. 2018;93(4):941–51.
29. Chertow GM, Levin NW, et al. FHN Trial Group: In-center hemodialysis six times a week versus three times a week. N Engl J Med. 2010;363(24):2287–300.
30. Rocco MV, Lockridge RS, Beck GJ, et al. The effects of frequent nocturnal home hemodialysis: The Frequent Hemodialysis Network Nocturnal Trial. Kidnet Int. 2011;80(10):1080–91.
31. Committee TW. Peronalized cooler dialysate for patients receiving maintenance hemodialysis: a pragmatic, cluster-randomized trial. Lancet. 2022;400(10364):1693–703.
32. Blankestijn PJ, Vernooij RWM, Hockham C, Strippoli GFM, Canaud B, Hegbrant J, Barth C, Covic A, Cromm K, Cucui A, Davenport A, Rose M, CONVINCE Scientific Committee Investigators. Effect of hemodiafiltration or hemodialysis on mortality in kidney failure. N Engl J Med. 2023;389(20):e42.
33. Borrelli S, La Milia V, De Nicola L, Cabiddu G, Russo R, Provenzano M, Minutolo R, Conte G, Garofalo C, Study group Peritoneal Dialysis of Italian Society of Nephrology. Sodium removal by peritoneal dialysis: a systematic review and meta-analysis. J Nephrol. 2018;32(2):231–9.
34. Courivaud C, Davenport A. Phosphate removal by peritoneal dialysis: the effect of transporter status and peritoneal dialysis prescription. Perit Dial Int. 2015;36(1):85–93.
35. Johnson DW, Hawley CM, McDonald SP, Brown FG, Rosman JB, Wiggins KJ, Bannister KM, Badve SV. Superior survival of high transporters treated with automated versus continuous ambulatory peritoneal dialysis. Nephrol Dial Transplant. 2010;25(6):1973–9.
36. Heimbürger O, Waniewski J, Werynski A, Lindholm B. A quantitative description of solute and fluid transport during peritoneal dialysis. Kidney Int. 1992;41(5):1320–32.
37. Sprick JD, Nocera JR, Ihab Hajjar W, O'Neill C, Bailey J, Park J. Cerebral blood flow regulation in end-stage kidney disease. Am J Renal Physiol. 2020;319(5):F782–91.
38. Findlay MD, Dawson J, Dickie DA, Forbes KP, McGlynn D, Quinn T, Mark PB. Investigating the relationship between cerebral blood flow and cognitive function in hemodialysis patients. J Am Soc Nephrol. 2019;30(1):147–58.
39. Paniagua R, Ventura M-d-J, Avila-Díaz M, Hinojosa-Heredia H, Méndez-Durán A, Cueto-Manzano A, Cisneros A, Ramos A, Madonia-Juseino C, Belio-Caro F, García-Contreras F, Trinidad-Ramos P. NT-proBNP, fluid volume overload and dialysis modality are independent predictors of mortality in ESRD patients. Nephrol Dial Transpl. 2009;25(2):551–7.

Chapter 16
Nutrition in the Elderly Patient with CKD

Yoko Narasaki, Connie M. Rhee, and Kamyar Kalantar-Zadeh

Take Home Points
- During the nutritional assessment and dietary counseling of elderly patients with CKD, it is imperative to utilize a tailored, individualized approach that prioritizes shared-decision making.
- Dietary restrictions should be avoided among patients who are malnourished or at risk for malnutrition. Using a personalized approach that takes into consideration patients' underlying characteristics is necessary to ensure appropriate dietary intake, optimal clinical outcomes, and better quality of life.
- Elderly patients with non-dialysis dependent CKD should be informed that they have a higher risk of cardiovascular death than kidney failure which will facilitate informed decision making for better health-related quality of life.
- Dietary modification may be more challenging in older adults with long-held dietary habits, decreased appetite, lack of energy or enthusiasm to cook, loss of ability to prepare food, and inability to access groceries.

Y. Narasaki · C. M. Rhee
Harold Simmons Center for Chronic Disease Research and Epidemiology, Division of Nephrology, Hypertension and Kidney Transplantation, University of California, Irvine, Orange, CA, USA

Tibor Rubin Veterans Affairs Long Beach Healthcare System, Long Beach, CA, USA
e-mail: ynarasak@hs.uci.edu

K. Kalantar-Zadeh (✉)
Tibor Rubin Veterans Affairs Long Beach Healthcare System, Long Beach, CA, USA

Harold Simmons Center for Chronic Disease Research and Epidemiology, Division of Nephrology, Hypertension and Kidney Transplantation, University of California, Irvine Medical Center, Orange, CA, USA
e-mail: kkz@uci.edu; kkz@hs.uci.edu

H. Kramer et al. (eds.), *Kidney Disease in the Elderly*,
https://doi.org/10.1007/978-3-031-68460-9_16

Case

A 65-year-old male with a history of stage 3B chronic kidney disease (CKD) due to hypertension presents to the nephrology clinic for follow-up of his kidney disease. His baseline estimated glomerular filtration rate (eGFR) is 36 mL/min/1.73 m^2, and his urine-to-albumin creatinine ratio levels are within the normal reference range. After a recent hospitalization for non-anginal chest pain, he is very concerned about his cardiovascular and kidney health. His medical history is also notable for coronary artery disease for which he underwent a coronary artery bypass graft surgery 3 years ago, dyslipidemia, and overweight status based on his body mass index. His medications include lisinopril, metoprolol succinate, and atorvastatin for his cardiovascular health; sevelamer bicarbonate for this hyperphosphatemia; and sodium bicarbonate for his metabolic acidosis.

Since his hospitalization, he has been trying to lose weight through increased physical activity (walking 20 min several times per week) to improve his body mass index. While he has previously consumed red meat on a frequent basis, he is interested in making dietary changes to improve his health status. He is seeking guidance on an optimal heart-healthy diet that can optimize his cardiac and kidney health.

Introduction

CKD is a global public health problem that is highly prevalent in the elderly population [1]. Across the age spectrum of CKD, dietary interventions are a major cornerstone in the management of kidney disease and its ensuing sequelae. Typically, a low protein diet coupled with adjustment of dietary potassium, phosphorus, and sodium intake are the mainstays in the nutritional management of this population to reduce the risk of CKD progression and its potential complications.

Given the decline in kidney function as well as other physical functions that occur with chronic disease and aging, elderly patients with CKD are highly prone to developing poor nutritional status or protein-energy-wasting (PEW), which is a state of nutritional and metabolic derangements characterized by the loss of systemic protein and energy stores. Other factors that contribute to PEW include malnutrition, decreased physical activity, uremia-induced catabolism, acidosis, and persistent inflammation, which may exacerbate PEW-related morbidity and mortality [2–4]. Thus, in order to slow kidney function decline while also maintaining adequate energy and nitrogen balance, nutritional management in the elderly with CKD requires a multi-faceted approach. This chapter focuses on summarizing existing evidence on the nutritional abnormalities and wasting conditions in elderly patients with CKD, and the practical implementation of nutritional management in this population, including dietary protein restriction with or without supplementation in order to reduce kidney disease progression and its related complications.

Protein-Energy Wasting, Sarcopenia, and Frailty in Elderly Patients with Chronic Kidney Disease

PEW, a condition of metabolic and nutritional derangements, is common in CKD, particularly among older adults, and it is often accompanied by sarcopenia (i.e., loss of muscle mass and function) and frailty (i.e., multisystem impairment associated with increased vulnerability to stressors) [5]. The etiologies of PEW in older adults with CKD may be classified as: (1) aging, (2) advanced CKD, or (3) a combination of both conditions (Fig. 16.1). Age-related physiological changes include impaired digestive function (i.e., decrease in adaptive relaxation of the fundus of the stomach), hormonal changes (i.e., increased cholecystokinin, reduction in testosterone followed by increases in leptin), and alterations of smell, taste, and vision that may contribute to decreased appetite and post-prandial energy or nutrition utilization efficacy [6]. Moreover, depression, inability to access groceries, lack of enthusiasm or energy to cook, and loss of ability to prepare food contribute to anorexia with aging [6]. The activation of pro-inflammatory cytokines combined with a hypercatabolic state, as well as decreased consumption of protein and energy following perturbations in appetite-regulating hormones (i.e., ghrelin and leptin) that occur with CKD progression, may also heighten the risk of PEW [7–9]. Moreover, uremic toxins, including catabolic by-products of protein metabolism, may exert harmful effects ranging from oxidative stress to endothelial dysfunction, nitric oxide disarrays, renal interstitial fibrosis, sarcopenia, and worsening proteinuria and kidney function [10–12].

Dietary Protein Restriction in Elderly Patients with Chronic Kidney Disease

Dietary protein restriction (0.6–0.8 g/kg/day) has been generally recommended among patients with stages 3B-5 non-dialysis dependent (NDD) CKD for several decades (Table 16.1) because of its inhibitor effects on kidney function decline and potential to avert or delay the onset of uremic symptoms [13]. During the 1960s, Giovannetti and Maggiore showed for the first time the reno-protective effects of dietary protein restriction, such as reduction in nitrogen waste products and uremic symptoms [14]. Subsequent research has shown that dietary protein restriction decreases kidney workload by lowering intra-glomerular pressure [15]. While the primary results of the Modification of Diet in Renal Disease (MDRD) study were not conclusive with regard to the efficacy of dietary protein restriction on the progression of CKD because of a nonlinear glomerular filtration rate (GFR) decline and limited duration of follow-up [16], a subsequent re-analysis of the MDRD study as well as expert opinion/commentaries support the role of dietary protein restriction on retarding CKD progression and delaying initiation of maintenance dialysis therapy [17]. Moreover, reduced dietary protein intake has favorable effects on

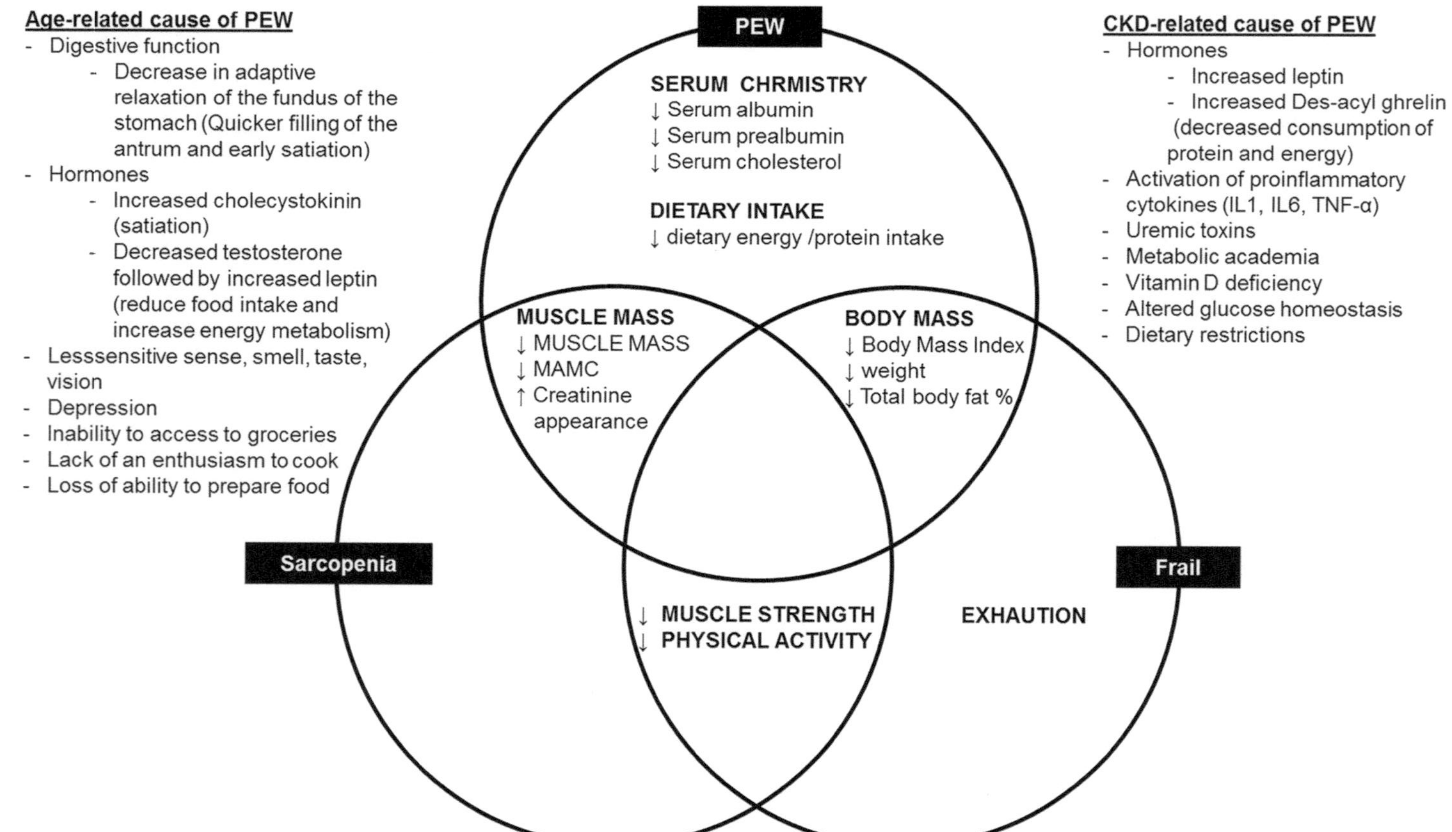

Fig. 16.1 Age- and chronic kidney disease-related causes of protein energy wasting (PEW), and the relationships between PEW, sarcopenia, and frailty

Table 16.1 Core nutritional targets and their purpose in elderly patients with chronic kidney disease

	Items	Target	Purpose
1	Energy	30–35 kcal/kg/day	Avoid risk of PEW
2	Protein		
	Low protein diet (LPD)	0.6–0.8 g/kg/day	Preserve kidney function (i.e., reduce nitrogen waste products, uremic symptoms, glomerular hyperfiltration, proteinuria, oxidative stress, metabolic acidosis; improve mineral metabolism, insulin resistance, blood pressure) and delay dialysis initiation
	KA/EAA supplemented very LPD (SVLPD)	0.3–0.4 g/kg/day, supplemented by KA/EAA	
	Low protein diet with plant-dominant (PLADO)	0.6–0.8 g/kg/day, >50% plant-based sources	Preserve kidney function, delay dialysis initiation, reduce inflammation, improve gut microbiome and GI motility
3	Sodium	<2300 mg/day	Correct elevated blood pressure and fluid retention

KA ketoacid, *EAA* essential amino acid, *PEW* protein-energy wasting, *GI* gastrointestinal

kidney health outcomes, which include amelioration of GFR decline, a reduction in proteinuria, mitigation of uremic toxin accumulation, and better control of hyperphosphatemia, hyperparathyroidism, and hyperkalemia; these effects of protein restriction may in turn preserve kidney function and avert or delay the onset of uremic symptoms in patients with advanced CKD [18–20].

There are limited randomized controlled studies that have examined the effects of dietary protein restriction on kidney outcomes specifically in older adults with CKD. However, low-protein diets may have kidney-protective effects in both older and younger patients based on inferences drawn from studies showing similar effect estimates for CKD outcomes among patients across a wide range of ages [21]. A recent study stratified 352 patients with stages 3–5 CKD by age (i.e., >65 vs. <65 years of age) showed that higher dietary protein intake was associated with a faster decline in eGFR in the overall cohort and in elderly patients after a median follow-up 4.2 years [22]. In an analysis of adults from the National Health and Nutrition Examination Survey (NHANES) who were stratified into 1994 participants with eGFR <60 mL/min/1.73 m^2 vs. 25,605 participants with eGFR ≥60 mL/min/1.73 m^2, respectively, there was effect modification of the association between the amount of dietary protein intake and mortality risk on the basis of age. Among participants who had preserved kidney function (i.e., eGFR ≥60 mL/min/1.73 m^2), high dietary protein intake scaled to absolute body weight (ABW) (i.e., ≥1.4 g/kg ABW/day) was associated with lower mortality risk in younger (<65 years old) but not in older (≥65 years old) adults after taking into account differences in sociodemographics, comorbidity status, and body mass index (BMI) [23].

It should be strongly emphasized that the underlying premise of dietary protein restriction in non-dialysis dependent (NDD) CKD is that patients maintain sufficient energy intake despite consuming a lower amount of protein. Maintaining adequate caloric intake helps patients avoid impaired nutritional status and the development of PEW [7]. In general, older adults have higher requirements for protein intake than that of younger persons due to age-related anabolism [24, 25], and patients with CKD tend to have reduced appetite and lower energy and protein consumption than older adults without CKD [26]. If overall energy intake is inadequate, dietary protein may be low which precludes the need for dietary protein restriction. Moreover, inappropriate or excessive restriction of dietary protein intake in older adults with CKD is a risk factor for worsening appetite and development of sarcopenia or PEW, which leads to loss of muscle and fat mass, cachexia, and heightened mortality risk [5]. Thus, it is important to prescribe dietary protein restriction carefully with the help of a dietitian using a tailored approach by first assessing a patient's overall health condition as well as their daily dietary intake appropriately (i.e., estimated dietary protein intake using 24-h urine collection).

Supplemented Protein Restriction and Plant-Dominant Low-Protein Diet (PLADO) in Elderly Patients with Chronic Kidney Disease

There are various options available for low-protein diets. For example, a supplemented very low protein diet (0.3–0.4 g/kg/day) accompanied by substitutes such as ketoacid analogs (KAs) or essential amino acids (EAAs) may enhance the salutary effects of dietary protein restriction by providing a sufficient balance of EAAs [27, 28]. The favorable effects of supplemented very low protein diets include improved serum albumin levels [29, 30], reductions in proteinuria [27, 28], decreased progression of CKD [30–32], and minimal to no changes in lean body and fat mass [33, 34]. In elderly patients with advanced NDD-CKD, a randomized controlled trial showed that a very low protein diet (defined as 0.3 g/kg/day of dietary protein intake) supplemented with KAs, EAAs, and vitamins delayed dialysis initiation by approximately 11 months as compared to the control group who did not undergo dietary protein restriction [35]. In this study, the mortality rates were similar between the two groups.

The plant-dominant low-protein diet (PLADO) is also a patient-centered low protein diet in which patients consume a dietary protein intake of 0.6–0.8 g/kg/day composed of >50% plant-based sources, administered by dietitians trained in NDD-CKD care [36]. It has been well established that not only the amount of dietary protein but also its type and source lead to different CKD outcomes. A longitudinal analysis of 1374 older female patients (mean age 75 years) including 367 participants with baseline eGFR levels <60 mL/min/1.73 m^2 showed that higher intake of plant protein was associated with slower decline in eGFR after 10 years of follow-up, and there was no difference in this association between the subgroup of patients without (eGFR $\geq$60 mL/min/1.73 m^2) or with CKD (eGFR <60 mL/min/1.73 m^2) [37]. Higher dietary intake of plant protein was also associated with lower mortality risk among adults aged $\geq$65 years old as well as in the overall group (median ages were 62 years old) in an age-stratified subgroup analysis (<60, 60–65, $\geq$65 years old) of a large prospective cohort of 237,036 male and 179,068 female patients without kidney failure who underwent 16 years of observation [38]. There are ongoing studies examining the efficacy of the PLADO diet in CKD patients examining whether a PLADO diet may confer a protective effect on kidney health outcomes and a favorable microbiome balance given its richness in minerals, vitamins, dietary fiber, antioxidants, and lesser generation of dietary acid loads and uremic toxins (i.e., trimethylamine n-oxide [TMAO], indoxyl sulfate, and p-cresyl sulfate).

Potassium Intake in Elderly Patients with Chronic Kidney Disease

Potassium is an essential nutrient needed for the maintenance of normal cellular function. Kidneys, as well as to a lesser degree, the colon play an important role in regulating potassium homeostasis and its excretion in response to changes in dietary potassium intake [39]. In contrast to healthy adults in whom relatively higher amounts of dietary potassium intake are recommended to prevent hypertension and cardiovascular disease [40], dietary potassium restriction has been the longstanding paradigm in treating and preventing hyperkalemia and its life-threatening complications (malignant arrhythmia, sudden cardiac death) in patients with advanced CKD [41]. Given the weak relationship between dietary potassium intake and serum potassium and the paucity of data examining the impact of dietary potassium restriction on outcomes in patients with kidney disease, there has been growing concern about the potential risks of this management strategy among patients with reduced GFR [42]. Limited studies have examined the association between dietary potassium intake and serum potassium levels and mortality among the elderly with kidney disease. A cross-sectional study among 95 NDD-CKD patients with a median age of 67 years showed no relationship between dietary potassium intake obtained by 3-day food records and serum potassium levels including hyperkalemia defined as a serum potassium level >5.0 mEq/L [43]. In regard to the association of dietary potassium intake on mortality, adults with lower dietary potassium intake scaled to total energy intake as well as those with low potassium intake largely from animal-based sources showed higher mortality risk independent of socio-demographics, comorbidities, socioeconomic status, lifestyle factors, and BMI, among adult participants from the National Health and Nutrition Examination (NHANES) study with eGFRs <60 mL/min/1.73 m^2 (mean age 73 years) [44]. Future studies are needed to elucidate the association between dietary potassium intake and outcomes, specifically in elderly patients with kidney disease.

Phosphorus Intake in Elderly Patients with Chronic Kidney Disease

Dietary phosphorus restriction is one of the cornerstones of the therapeutic treatment for hyperphosphatemia [45]. Since protein and phosphorus in food are closely correlated, in NDD-CKD dietary phosphate tends to be concomitantly reduced within the context of appropriate dietary protein restriction [46]. However, if patients have preferences for eating processed foods or have to rely on these food sources (i.e., due to socioeconomic status or inability to prepare meals), more attention to dietary phosphorus intake may be required even with appropriate dietary protein restriction to take into account the risk of greater intake of processed foods with high phosphorus bioavailability [47]. Dietary phosphate is found in two types of sources (i.e., organic vs. inorganic sources). Organic types include animal- and plant-derived phosphorus sources, and inorganic phosphorus sources include food additives found in processed foods. The degrees of phosphorus bioavailability vary depending on its source (i.e., 40–60% in animal-derived vs. 20–40% in plant-derived phosphorus, respectively) and type (i.e., approximately 100% in inorganic phosphorus). Plant-derived phosphate, which largely occurs in the form of phytates, has lower bioavailability because of the lack of the degrading enzyme phytase in humans [46].

Although traditional recommendations suggest maintaining dietary phosphorus intake between 800 and 1000 mg/day in patients with stages 3–5 CKD, the efficacy and safety of this recommendation have not yet been established [41]. There are a few studies that have examined the effects of dietary phosphorus restriction on CKD progression which have shown no association between dietary phosphorus intake and CKD progression in the younger CKD population [48, 49]. Studies of dietary phosphorus intake and kidney outcomes in the elderly CKD population have also been sparse with mixed findings. For example, in a small retrospective cohort study of 175 patients with stages 2–5 CKD (mean age of 65 years), higher phosphorus excretion per creatinine clearance (i.e., a surrogate measure for phosphorus intake) was associated with a higher risk of CKD progression [50]. In a prospective study of 1105 adults participants with eGFRs <60 mL/min/1.73 m^2 (mean ages were 71, 70, and 67 years old in lowest, middle, and highest phosphorus intake tertiles, respectively), high dietary phosphorus intake ascertained by 24-h dietary recall was associated with a very modest increase in serum phosphorus levels (a 100 mg/day increase in dietary phosphate ~0.009 mg/dL [0.006–0.011] increase in serum phosphorus) but was not associated with increased mortality over an average of 6.5 years of follow-up [51]. In a subgroup analysis from a retrospective study of 415 patients receiving maintenance hemodialysis, the lowest tertile of dietary phosphorus intake was associated with higher mortality risk in older (≥60 years old) but not in younger (<60 years old) adults [52]. Future studies are needed to elucidate the association between dietary phosphorus intake and outcomes in older patients with kidney disease.

Fiber Intake in Elderly Patients with Chronic Kidney Disease

There is increasing recognition of the health benefits of higher dietary fiber intake (i.e., improved blood pressure, glycemic control, dyslipidemia, gastrointestinal motility/constipation, and gut microbiota composition). Thus far, meta-analyses consisting of studies with relatively small sample sizes and inclusive of both younger and older patients with kidney disease have consistently shown the benefits of fiber supplementation on the reduction of uremic toxins including serum creatinine [53], p-cresyl sulfate [54, 55], and indoxyl sulfate [55]. Interestingly, a study conducted by Wu et al. revealed that the underlying age of patients (i.e., $\leq$60 or >60 years) was not an influential factor in these effects [54]. Furthermore, existing evidence including a study of 1105 participants with eGFRs <60 mL/min/1.73 m^2 (mean age $\geq$65 years old) [56] and a meta-analysis including studies in elderly patients with kidney disease [57] have shown the beneficial effects of higher dietary fiber intake on survival in patients with kidney disease. Further studies are warranted to evaluate the effects of dietary fiber intake and outcomes (i.e., constipation, all-cause and cardiovascular mortality) in this population.

Regarding dietary fiber intake, guidelines for people with kidney disease have been mixed, particularly due to concern that foods rich in fiber typically contain higher potassium content, which is traditionally restricted in people with kidney disease for the purposes of preventing and treating hyperkalemia [58]. However, greater consumption of plant-based fruits and vegetables which are rich sources of potassium, glucose, fructose, and fiber might provide salutary benefits in patients with kidney disease including with elderly based on the premise that (a) potassium intake concomitantly consumed with glucose/fructose reduces postprandial increases in serum potassium concentrations by facilitating intracellular potassium deposition [59], and (b) fermentable fiber increases the excretion of potassium into feces [60]. Based on these observations, a larger study of the impact of dietary fiber intake on CKD outcomes in the elderly population is needed.

Sodium Intake in Elderly Patients with Chronic Kidney Disease

Given that the role of sodium in the pathophysiology of hypertension has been recognized and that hypertension and CKD are closely related, a low sodium or low salt diet is widely considered a cornerstone in the treatment of hypertension in CKD patients as well as in the general population [61]. However, there is a paucity of studies examining the effects of sodium restriction in elderly patients with CKD. Age-related changes in sodium homeostasis (i.e., decreased total body sodium, with increased total body potassium), as well as changes in GFR, renal blood flow, and sodium-regulating hormonal systems (i.e., renin-angiotensin-aldosterone axis), may be responsible for the greater sodium sensitivity in older adults with CKD [62]. However, sodium restriction should be carefully implemented by regularly assessing patients' blood pressure and serum and blood sodium levels. Of note, dietary restriction including sodium restriction can cause the loss of appetite, insufficient dietary intake, sarcopenia and/or PEW, and hospitalization or other adverse clinical outcomes [63]. Thus, dietary restrictions, especially those implemented in older adults with CKD who have a higher risk of these complications, should be conducted within the context of individually tailored programs that are administered by specialty clinicians including dietitians with training and experience in NDD-CKD care.

Conclusion

Precision nutritional management that uses a tailored approach in prescribing the amount and sources of dietary protein as well as other nutrients is particularly needed in elderly patients with CKD in order to ameliorate GFR decline and risk of kidney failure. Given the heightened risk of developing PEW in older adults with CKD, close attention is needed to ensure adequate energy and nitrogen balance when administering a low-protein diet and other dietary interventions.Financial Support and SponsorshipThe authors are supported by research grants from the NIH/NIDDK: R01-DK122767 (CMR), R01-DK124138 (CMR, KKZ), K24-DK091419 (KKZ), R44-DK116383 (KKZ); and the Japan Society for the Promotion of Science Overseas Research Fellowship (YN).

Conflicts of Interest None of the authors have relevant disclosures to report.

References

1. Mallappallil M, Friedman EA, Delano BG, Mcfarlane SI, Salifu MO. Chronic kidney disease in the elderly: evaluation and management. Clin Pract (Lond). 2014;11:525–35.
2. Chao CT, Wang J, Huang JW, Chan DC, Chien KL. Frailty predicts an increased risk of end-stage renal disease with risk competition by mortality among 165,461 diabetic kidney disease patients. Aging Dis. 2019;10:1270–81.
3. Koppe L, Fouque D, Kalantar-Zadeh K. Kidney cachexia or protein-energy wasting in chronic kidney disease: facts and numbers. J Cachexia Sarcopenia Muscle. 2019;10:479–84.
4. Wu PY, Chao CT, Chan DC, Huang JW, Hung KY. Contributors, risk associates, and complications of frailty in patients with chronic kidney disease: a scoping review. Ther Adv Chronic Dis. 2019;10:2040622319880382.
5. Narasaki Y, Rhee CM, Kramer H, Kalantar-Zadeh K. Protein intake and renal function in older patients. Curr Opin Clin Nutr Metab Care. 2021;24:10–7.
6. Morley JE. Nutrition and the kidney in the elderly patient. In: American Society of Nephrology online geriatric nephrology curriculum. Washington, DC: American Society of Nephrology; 2009. p. 1–3.

7. Hanna RM, Ghobry L, Wassef O, Rhee CM, Kalantar-Zadeh K. A practical approach to nutrition, protein-energy wasting, sarcopenia, and cachexia in patients with chronic kidney disease. Blood Purif. 2020;49:202–11.
8. Kiebalo T, Holotka J, Habura I, Pawlaczyk K. Nutritional status in peritoneal dialysis: nutritional guidelines, adequacy and the management of malnutrition. Nutrients. 2020;12:1–14.
9. Oliveira EA, Zheng R, Carter CE, Mak RH. Cachexia/protein energy wasting syndrome in CKD: causation and treatment. Semin Dial. 2019;32:493–9.
10. Carré JE, Affourtit C. Mitochondrial activity and skeletal muscle insulin resistance in kidney disease. Int J Mol Sci. 2019;20:2751.
11. Inaguma D, Koide S, Ito E, Takahashi K, Hayashi H, Hasegawa M, Yuzawa Y. Ratio of blood urea nitrogen to serum creatinine at initiation of dialysis is associated with mortality: a multicenter prospective cohort study. Clin Exp Nephrol. 2018;22:353–64.
12. Seki M, Nakayama M, Sakoh T, Yoshitomi R, Fukui A, Katafuchi E, Tsuda S, Nakano T, Tsuruya K, Kitazono T. Blood urea nitrogen is independently associated with renal outcomes in Japanese patients with stage 3-5 chronic kidney disease: a prospective observational study. BMC Nephrol. 2019;20:115.
13. Baragetti I, De Simone I, Biazzi C, Buzzi L, Ferrario F, Luise MC, Santagostino G, Furiani S, Alberghini E, Capitanio C, Terraneo V, Milia V, Pozzi C. The low-protein diet for chronic kidney disease: 8 years of clinical experience in a nephrology ward. Clin Kidney J. 2020;13:253–60.
14. Giovannetti S, Maggiore Q. A low-nitrogen diet with proteins of high biological value for severe chronic uraemia. Lancet. 1964;1:1000–3.
15. Ko GJ, Kalantar-Zadeh K, Goldstein-Fuchs J, Rhee CM. Dietary approaches in the management of diabetic patients with kidney disease. Nutrients. 2017;9:824.
16. Klahr S, Levey AS, Beck GJ, Caggiula AW, Hunsicker L, Kusek JW, Striker G. The effects of dietary protein restriction and blood-pressure control on the progression of chronic renal disease. Modification of diet in Renal Disease Study Group. N Engl J Med. 1994;330:877–84.
17. Levey AS, Adler S, Caggiula AW, England BK, Greene T, Hunsicker LG, Kusek JW, Rogers NL, Teschan PE. Effects of dietary protein restriction on the progression of advanced renal disease in the modification of diet in renal disease study. Am J Kidney Dis. 1996;27:652–63.
18. Koppe L, Fouque D. The role for protein restriction in addition to renin-angiotensin-aldosterone system inhibitors in the management of CKD. Am J Kidney Dis. 2019;73:248–57.
19. Morris A, Krishnan N, Kimani PK, Lycett D. Effect of dietary potassium restriction on serum potassium, disease progression, and mortality in chronic kidney disease: a systematic review and meta-analysis. J Ren Nutr. 2020;30:276–85.
20. Yan B, Su X, Xu B, Qiao X, Wang L. Effect of diet protein restriction on progression of chronic kidney disease: a systematic review and meta-analysis. PLoS One. 2018;13:E0206134.
21. Levey AS, De Jong PE, Coresh J, Nahas MEL, Astor BC, Matsushita K, Gansevoort RT, Kasiske BL, Eckardt K-U. The definition, classification, and prognosis of chronic kidney disease: a KDIGO controversies conference report. Kidney Int. 2011;80:17–28.
22. Watanabe D, Machida S, Matsumoto N, Shibagaki Y, Sakurada T. Age modifies the association of dietary protein intake with all-cause mortality in patients with chronic kidney disease. Nutrients. 2018;10:1744.
23. Narasaki Y, Okuda Y, Moore LW, You AS, Tantisattamo E, Inrig JK, Miyagi T, Nakata T, Kovesdy CP, Nguyen DV, Kalantar-Zadeh K, Rhee CM. Dietary protein intake, kidney function, and survival in a nationally representative cohort. Am J Clin Nutr. 2021;114:303–13.
24. Krok-Schoen JL, Archdeacon Price A, Luo M, Kelly OJ, Taylor CA. Low dietary protein intakes and associated dietary patterns and functional limitations in an aging population: a NHANES analysis. J Nutr Health Aging. 2019;23:338–47.
25. Phillips SM, Paddon-Jones D, Layman DK. Optimizing adult protein intake during catabolic health conditions. Adv Nutr. 2020;11:S1058–69.
26. Lee SW, Kim YS, Kim YH, Chung W, Park SK, Choi KH, Ahn C, Oh KH. Dietary protein intake, protein energy wasting, and the progression of chronic kidney disease: analysis from the KNOW-CKD study. Nutrients. 2019;11:121.

27. Di Iorio BR, Marzocco S, Bellasi A, De Simone E, Dal Piaz F, Rocchetti MT, Cosola C, Di Micco L, Gesualdo L. Nutritional therapy reduces protein carbamylation through urea lowering in chronic kidney disease. Nephrol Dial Transplant. 2018;33:804–13.

28. Liu D, Wu M, Li L, Gao X, Yang B, Mei S, Fu L, Mei C. Low-protein diet supplemented with ketoacids delays the progression of diabetic nephropathy by inhibiting oxidative stress in the KKAy mice model. Br J Nutr. 2018;119:22–9.

29. Li A, Lee HY, Lin YC. The effect of ketoanalogues on chronic kidney disease deterioration: a meta-analysis. Nutrients. 2019;11:957.

30. Milovanova L, Fomin V, Moiseev S, Taranova M, Milovanov Y, Lysenko Kozlovskaya L, Kozlov V, Kozevnikova E, Milovanova S, Lebedeva M, Reshetnikov V. Effect of essential amino acid кetoanalogues and protein restriction diet on morphogenetic proteins (FGF-23 and Klotho) in 3b-4 stages chronic Kidney disease patients: a randomized pilot study. Clin Exp Nephrol. 2018;22:1351–9.

31. Satirapoj B, Vongwattana P, Supasyndh O. Very low protein diet plus ketoacid analogs of essential amino acids supplement to retard chronic kidney disease progression. Kidney Res Clin Pract. 2018;37:384–92.

32. Wang M, Xu H, Chong Lee Shin OL, Li L, Gao H, Zhao Z, Zhu F, Zhu H, Liang W, Qian K, Zhang C, Zeng R, Zhou H, Yao Y. Compound A-keto acid tablet supplementation alleviates chronic kidney disease progression via inhibition of the NF-kB and MAPK pathways. J Transl Med. 2019;17:122.

33. Bellizzi V, Calella P, Hernández JN, González VF, Lira SM, Torraca S, Arronte RU, Cirillo P, Minutolo R, Montúfar Cárdenas RA. Safety and effectiveness of low-protein diet supplemented with ketoacids in diabetic patients with chronic kidney disease. BMC Nephrol. 2018; 19:110.

34. Garibotto G, Sofia A, Parodi EL, Ansaldo F, Bonanni A, Picciotto D, Signori A, Vettore M, Tessari P, Verzola D. Effects of low-protein, and supplemented very low-protein diets, on muscle protein turnover in patients with CKD. Kidney Int Rep. 2018;3:701–10.

35. Brunori G, Viola BF, Parrinello G, De Biase V, Como G, Franco V, Garibotto G, Zubani R, Cancarini GC. Efficacy and safety of a very-low-protein diet when postponing dialysis in the elderly: a prospective randomized multicenter controlled study. Am J Kidney Dis. 2007;49:569–80.

36. Kalantar-Zadeh K, Joshi S, Schlueter R, Cooke J, Brown-Tortorici A, Donnelly M, Schulman S, Lau WL, Rhee CM, Streja E, Tantisattamo E, Ferrey AJ, Hanna R, Chen JLT, Malik S, Nguyen DV, Crowley ST, Kovesdy CP. Plant-dominant low-protein diet for conservative management of chronic kidney disease. Nutrients. 2020;12:1931.

37. Bernier-Jean A, Prince RL, Lewis JR, Craig JC, Hodgson JM, Lim WH, Teixeira-Pinto A, Wong G. Dietary plant and animal protein intake and decline in estimated glomerular filtration rate among elderly women: a 10-year longitudinal cohort study. Nephrol Dial Transplant. 2021;36:1640–7.

38. Huang J, Liao LM, Weinstein SJ, Sinha R, Graubard BI, Albanes D. Association between plant and animal protein intake and overall and cause-specific mortality. JAMA Intern Med. 2020;180:1173–84.

39. Kovesdy CP, Regidor DL, Mehrotra R, Jing J, Mcallister CJ, Greenland S, Kopple JD, Kalantar-Zadeh K. Serum and dialysate potassium concentrations and survival in hemodialysis patients. Clin J Am Soc Nephrol. 2007;2:999–1007.

40. US Department of Agriculture and US Department of Health and Human Services. Dietary Guidelines For Americans, 2020–2025. Washington, DC: US Government Publishing Office; 2020. Dietaryguidelines.gov. Accessed 7 Jan 2021.

41. Ikizler TA, Burrowes JD, Byham-Gray LD, Campbell KL, Carrero JJ, Chan W, Fouque D, Friedman AN, Ghaddar S, Goldstein-Fuchs DJ, Kaysen GA, Kopple JD, Teta D, Yee-Moon Wang A, Cuppari L. KDOQI clinical practice guideline for nutrition in CKD: 2020 update. Am J Kidney Dis. 2020;76:S1–S107.

42. Kovesdy CP. Metabolic acidosis and kidney disease: does bicarbonate therapy slow the progression of CKD? Nephrol Dial Transplant. 2012;27:3056–62.

43. Ramos CI, González-Ortiz A, Espinosa-Cuevas A, Avesani CM, Carrero JJ, Cuppari L. Does dietary potassium intake associate with hyperkalemia in patients with chronic kidney disease? Nephrol Dial Transplant. 2021;36:2049–57.
44. Narasaki Y, You AS, Malik S, Moore LW, Bross R, Cervantes MK, Daza A, Kovesdy CP, Nguyen DV, Kalantar-Zadeh K, Rhee CM. Dietary potassium intake, kidney function, and survival in a nationally representative cohort. Am J Clin Nutr. 2022;116:1123.
45. Narasaki Y, Rhee CM. Dietary therapy for managing hyperphosphatemia. Clin J Am Soc Nephrol. 2020;16:9–11.
46. Kalantar-Zadeh K, Gutekunst L, Mehrotra R, Kovesdy CP, Bross R, Shinaberger CS, Noori N, Hirschberg R, Benner D, Nissenson AR, Kopple JD. Understanding sources of dietary phosphorus in the treatment of patients with chronic kidney disease. Clin J Am Soc Nephrol. 2010;5:519–30.
47. Narasaki Y, Yamasaki M, Matsuura S, Morinishi M, Nakagawa T, Matsuno M, Katsumoto M, Nii S, Fushitani Y, Sugihara K, Noda T, Yoneda T, Masuda M, Yamanaka-Okumura H, Takeda E, Sakaue H, Yamamoto H, Taketani Y. Phosphatemic index is a novel evaluation tool for dietary phosphorus load: a whole-foods approach. J Ren Nutr. 2020;30:493–502.
48. Selamet U, Tighiouart H, Sarnak MJ, Beck G, Levey AS, Block G, Ix JH. Relationship of dietary phosphate intake with risk of end-stage renal disease and mortality in chronic kidney disease stages 3-5: the modification of diet in renal disease study. Kidney Int. 2016;89:176–84.
49. Williams PS, Stevens ME, Fass G, Irons L, Bone JM. Failure of dietary protein and phosphate restriction to retard the rate of progression of chronic renal failure: a prospective, randomized, controlled trial. Q J Med. 1991;81:837–55.
50. Kawasaki T, Maeda Y, Matsuki H, Matsumoto Y, Akazawa M, Kuyama T. Urinary phosphorus excretion per creatinine clearance as a prognostic marker for progression of chronic kidney disease: a retrospective cohort study. BMC Nephrol. 2015;16:116.
51. Murtaugh MA, Filipowicz R, Baird BC, Wei G, Greene T, Beddhu S. Dietary phosphorus intake and mortality in moderate chronic kidney disease: NHANES III. Nephrol Dial Transplant. 2012;27:990–6.
52. Brown-Tortorici AR, Narasaki Y, You AS, Norris KC, Streja E, Peralta RA, Guerrero Y, Daza A, Arora R, Lo R, Nakata T, Nguyen DV, Kalantar-Zadeh K, Rhee CM. The interplay between dietary phosphorous, protein intake, and mortality in a prospective hemodialysis cohort. Nutrients. 2022;14:3070.
53. Chiavaroli L, Mirrahimi A, Sievenpiper JL, Jenkins DJ, Darling PB. Dietary fiber effects in chronic kidney disease: a systematic review and meta-analysis of controlled feeding trials. Eur J Clin Nutr. 2015;69:761–8.
54. Wu M, Cai X, Lin J, Zhang X, Scott EM, Li X. Association between fibre intake and indoxyl sulphate/P-cresyl sulphate in patients with chronic kidney disease: meta-analysis and systematic review of experimental studies. Clin Nutr. 2019;38:2016–22.
55. Yang HL, Feng P, Xu Y, Hou YY, Ojo O, Wang XH. The role of dietary fiber supplementation in regulating uremic toxins in patients with chronic kidney disease: a meta-analysis of randomized controlled trials. J Ren Nutr. 2021;31:438–47.
56. Krishnamurthy VM, Wei G, Baird BC, Murtaugh M, Chonchol MB, Raphael KL, Greene T, Beddhu S. High dietary fiber intake is associated with decreased inflammation and all-cause mortality in patients with chronic kidney disease. Kidney Int. 2012;81:300–6.
57. Kelly JT, Palmer SC, Wai SN, Ruospo M, Carrero JJ, Campbell KL, Strippoli GF. Healthy dietary patterns and risk of mortality and ESRD in CKD: a meta-analysis of cohort studies. Clin J Am Soc Nephrol. 2017;12:272–9.
58. Su G, Qin X, Yang C, Sabatino A, Kelly JT, Avesani CM, Carrero JJ. Fiber intake and health in people with chronic kidney disease. Clin Kidney J. 2022;15:213–25.
59. Allon M, Dansby L, Shanklin N. Glucose modulation of the disposal of an acute potassium load in patients with end-stage renal disease. Am J Med. 1993;94:475–82.
60. Carlisle EJ, Donnelly SM, Ethier JH, Quaggin SE, Kaiser UB, Vasuvattakul S, Kamel KS, Halperin ML. Modulation of the secretion of potassium by accompanying anions in humans. Kidney Int. 1991;39:1206–12.

61. Borrelli S, Provenzano M, Gagliardi I, Michael A, Liberti ME, De Nicola L, Conte G, Garofalo C, Andreucci M. Sodium intake and chronic kidney disease. Int J Mol Sci. 2020;21:4744.
62. Luft FC, Weinberger MH, Fineberg NS, Miller JZ, Grim CE. Effects of age on renal sodium homeostasis and its relevance to sodium sensitivity. Am J Med. 1987;82:9–15.
63. Nagasawa Y. Positive and negative aspects of sodium intake in dialysis and non-dialysis CKD patients. Nutrients. 2021;13:951.

Chapter 17
Kidney Supportive Care

Tripta Kaur and Elizabeth Figuracion

Case Presentation

Henry is an 83-year-old man with progressive chronic kidney disease (CKD) in the setting of hypertension, diabetes, and peripheral vascular disease. He feels that he has a good relationship with his nephrologist who has followed him over the past 2 years. However, during this time his kidney function has incrementally declined and now his estimated glomerular filtration rate (eGFR) is 22 mL/min/1.73. He reports to his nephrologist that his main symptoms are fatigue ("I feel exhausted by the evening"), insomnia, and decreased appetite with 5-lb weight loss over the past 6 months. On exam, he is oriented, has mild temporal wasting, walks slowly down the hallway to the exam room, and has trace bilateral lower extremity edema. Henry has been widowed for the past 2 years but has good social support from his neighbors in his assisted living facility (ALF). He expresses that he can care for himself but needs help with groceries and cleaning. Due to his evident weight loss, a cystatin C is obtained and reveals that his true eGFR may be closer to 16 mL/min/1.73 m². After his nephrologist informs him about the changes in his kidney function, Henry becomes very quiet, however after a few moments he asks, "What does this mean for me?"

---

[1] Online calculator available.

T. Kaur (✉)
Nephrology and Palliative Care, Tufts Medical Center, Boston, MA, USA
e-mail: tkaur1@tuftsmedicalcenter.org

E. Figuracion
Palliative Care, Tufts Medical Center, Boston, MA, USA
e-mail: efiguracion@tuftsmedicalcenter.org

H. Kramer et al. (eds.), *Kidney Disease in the Elderly*,
https://doi.org/10.1007/978-3-031-68460-9_17

Introduction

The demographic of patients with kidney disease has evolved. Compared to 1972 when Medicare eligibility was expanded to include end-stage kidney disease (ESKD), adults with chronic kidney disease (CKD) are now older with more comorbidities [1, 2]. From 2015 to 2018, 36.8% of patients aged 65 years and older had CKD (defined as eGFR <60 mL/min/1.73 m^2 or urinary albumin creatinine ratio ≥30 mg/g). In 2019 the incidence and prevalence of ESKD was highest among individuals aged ≥75 years. Among these patients, 79% initiated in-center hemodialysis, 1.0% home hemodialysis, 7% peritoneal dialysis, and 12.9% received a kidney transplant [2]. In a cohort of patients with advanced kidney disease receiving care in the United States VA system, 53.3% of patients aged ≥85 years were treated with dialysis or were preparing to receive dialysis [3]. Elderly patients with kidney disease who undergo aggressive treatment options experience high symptom burden, negative impact on quality of life (QOL), and have increased risk for morbidity and mortality with low utilization of hospice services [3–5].

In studies that explore preferences in patients with advanced kidney disease, most patients expressed that improving QOL and addressing symptoms is very important (~60% to 80%) [6, 7]. In a Canadian cohort of patients with advanced CKD including kidney failure treated with dialysis or transplantation, only 17.8% reported prioritizing length of life and more than half (60.7%) of the patients on dialysis reported regret in starting dialysis [7]. Most patients preferred to die at home or in an inpatient hospice (65%) whereas 27.4% wanted to die in the hospital [7]. The active medical management of kidney disease without dialysis, also known as comprehensive conservative care (CCC), is an alternative to dialysis which focuses on preventative CKD management and optimizing QOL. The population-based incidence and prevalence of CCC in the US is unknown. In elderly patients with advanced CKD, the decision to pursue dialysis or CCC is complex and requires an integrated discussion of the patients' values and goals in the context of their prognosis with and without dialysis. Most patients with kidney disease have not had advanced care planning (ACP) discussions about treatment options and end-of-life care planning with their nephrologists and, only a minority have completed advanced directives [7–9]. Unfortunately, patients who were engaged in ACP discussions have reported a suboptimal experience [10]. Overall, older adults with advanced kidney disease will benefit from a comprehensive care model to address their dynamic needs from a patient-centered perspective. Currently, patients with kidney disease have lower utilization of palliative care and only ~20% enroll in hospice [1, 11]. In fact, most adults with CKD were unsure or had not heard about palliative care [7].

Palliative care is the active holistic care of individuals with a serious illness that aims to: (1) prevent, identify, and relieve physical, psychosocial, spiritual, and existential suffering; (2) improve the quality of lives of patients and their families, and (3) facilitate patient autonomy by aligning care with patients' values and priorities [12]. Palliative care can be incorporated at any stage of the patient's clinical course and can be provided alongside disease-directed therapies, such as dialysis and kidney transplantation. Palliative care does not hasten nor postpone death but rather works to positively influence a person's experience with illness and support patients and their families in the context of their cultural values and beliefs [12]. Palliative care has been shown to improve QOL and satisfaction with care and reduce hospitalizations and high intensity of care at the end of life. Hospice, which is a form of palliative medicine, is a philosophy and system of care designed to provide compassionate care at the end of life (prognosis of 6-months or less) when a patient's goals have shifted away from life-prolonging therapies and toward comfort and QOL [13].

In the United States, a limited number of physicians are formally trained to practice specialty palliative care. Therefore, it is imperative for all providers taking care of patients with kidney disease including nephrologists, advanced care providers, nurses, and social workers to have primary palliative care skills to implement kidney supportive care (Box 17.1).

Box 17.1 Essential Primary Palliative Care Skills [5]

• Education of overall medical condition
• Evaluation and communication of prognosis
• Basic advanced care planning discussions that elicit values and medical wishes to guide consistent treatment plans
• Assessment and management of physical and psychological symptoms
• Identification of clinical changes near the end of life

Kidney supportive care is the integration of palliative medicine into the care of all patients with kidney disease. Patients who would benefit from kidney supportive care include those with non-dialysis advanced and dialysis-dependent CKD, acute kidney injury (AKI), and kidney transplantation [1]. The goals of kidney supportive care are to optimize quality of life and prevent suffering through managing dynamic symptoms, helping patients and their families navigate complex treatment options, and supporting patients near the end of life.

In the following sections we will discuss the main domains of kidney supportive care which include (Fig. 17.1):

1. estimating prognosis to identify patients who would most benefit from kidney supportive care,
2. advanced care planning with shared decision-making (SDM) to promote goal-coordinate care,
3. the option of comprehensive conservative care (CCC),
4. transitions in dialysis to include a time-limited trial of dialysis, palliative dialysis, and withdrawal from dialysis,
5. symptom assessment and management, and
6. end of life care [1, 14].

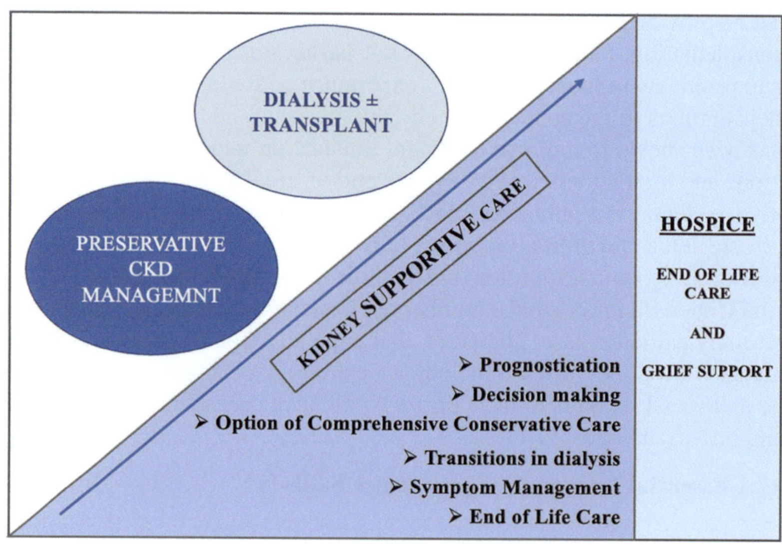

Fig. 17.1 Framework of kidney supportive care [1, 14]

Throughout the course of a patient's illness, the role of kidney supportive care can vary but generally increases with the progression of the patient's clinical trajectory and includes care at the end of life (Fig. 17.1). Specialty palliative care should be appropriately incorporated for further support in: (1) complex treatment-decision making and conflict resolution, (2) CCC, (3) refractory symptoms, and (4) end-of-life care [15].

Prognosis in Patients with Kidney Disease

Prognostication in patients with kidney disease is challenging. Predicting a patient's survival and quality of life with and without dialysis requires a full assessment of the patient's overall medical condition and prognostic factors. For patients who have multiple comorbidities, communicating with their relevant providers on their perspective of the patient's medical condition will help provide further insight into the patient's clinical trajectory [16]. General prognostic factors that help assess the risk of morbidity and mortality include age, comorbidities, and geriatric syndromes including functional and cognitive impairment, malnutrition, falls, and frailty (defined as increased vulnerability and decreased reserve to respond to health stressors) [17].

Prognosis with Dialysis

The adjusted mortality rate of Medicare beneficiaries aged 66–74 years receiving dialysis was approximately 10–15-fold higher compared to individuals not receiving dialysis [2]. Based on the United States Renal Data System (USRDS) the 1-year mortality rate after the initiation of dialysis for patients ≥65 years was ~30%. However, an analysis of Medicare beneficiaries showed a higher 1-year mortality rate after the initiation of dialysis of 54.5% in patients ≥65 years and ~68% in patients ≥85 years [2, 18]. Among patients >80 years old and patients >75 years old with comorbidities (cardiovascular disease, diabetes, dementia, cancer, and others), studies show that there is no survival benefit with dialysis as compared to non-dialysis care also known as CCC [2, 18–20]. In a single-center study of patients ≥70 years, the overall mean survival with dialysis (mean age 76) was 37.8 months vs. 13.9 months (≥1 year) with CCC (mean age 82). However, these patients who chose to initiate dialysis showed a significantly higher rate of hospital admissions, and approximately half of their survival time was spent in a hospital, traveling to and from dialysis and dialysis treatment, and recovering from dialysis with post-treatment fatigue. Patients aged ≥70 years receiving dialysis were also more likely to die in the hospital and experience a high intensity of care at the end-of-life compared to patients who chose CCC [21]. In a study of dialysis Medicare beneficiaries ≥65 years old, 76% were hospitalized, 48.9% had an intensive care unit admission, 29% had an intensive procedure, 20% were enrolled in hospice, and 44.8% died in the hospital in the final month of their life [22].

The impact of frailty and cognitive impairment in patients receiving dialysis further alters their clinical course. Frailty in a patient receiving dialysis is associated with a 2.68-fold higher risk of death and a 1.43-fold higher number of hospitalizations (independent of age, sex, comorbidity, and disability) [23]. Cognitive impairment and dementia in patients with advanced or dialysis-dependent CKD are associated with increased all-cause mortality. Patients with dementia have a 2.2-fold higher risk for death within 6 months of initiating dialysis compared to patients without cognitive impairment [24, 25].

Older adults who initiate dialysis have a high risk of functional loss and falls regardless of baseline functional status, and this decline in physical capability is associated with heightened mortality [26]. In a cohort of independent patients ≥80 years old, >30% required a private-caregiver or facility care 6-months after the initiation of dialysis [27], and furthermore, in a study of nursing home patients, 12-months after the initiation of dialysis 87% had died and only 13% maintained their pre-dialysis functional status [28].

Prior to initiation of dialysis, older adults with advanced CKD experience substantial declines in mental and physical health-related QOL. Based on current literature, there is high concern that QOL and symptom burden may be similar in elderly patients on dialysis as compared to comprehensive conservative care [29–32]. Interestingly, in a European cohort, De Rooij et al. demonstrated that initiating dialysis may help mitigate the decline but not improve QOL within the first year of dialysis initiation [33].

Prognosis Without Dialysis (or Comprehensive Conservative Care)

Current survival data in patients who elect CCC overall have been consistent. In a systemic review that analyzed prognosis with CCC the median survival (measured when the eGFR decreased to <15 mL/min/1.73 m^2) ranged between 6.3 and 23.4 months [34, 35]. As described above, in a single-center study of patients ≥70 years the average survival of patients on CCC was 13.9 months (≥1 year) [21]. Another study showed that patients with an average age of 82 years with a higher prevalence of dementia and comorbidities had a median survival of 16 months and 32% survived >12 months after the eGFR decreased below 10 mL/min/1.73 m^2 [32]. Dialysis as compared to CCC does not improve survival in patients >80 years old and patients >75 years old with comorbidities [2, 18–20]. Patients on CCC have lower rates of hospitalizations, tend to spend more time at home or in the community, and are more likely to die at home and elect hospice services [34].

Prognostication Tools

Prognostication is the culmination of the clinician's analytical assessment of the patient's overall health and clinical acumen. There are several validated renal prognostication tools available to help identify high-risk patients and support providers in evaluating which patients will most benefit from dialysis [35] (Box 17.2).

Box 17.2 Prognostication Tools in Kidney Disease
Prognostic tools to estimate mortality after the initiation of dialysis

- **Wick Score** (4): 6-month mortality

    - Age (≥80 2 pts), eGFR mL/min/1.73 m^2 (0–9.9 0 pt, 10–14.9 1 pt, ≥15 3 pts), atrial fibrillation (2 pts), chronic heart failure (2 pts), lymphoma (5 pts), metastatic cancer (3 pts), hospitalized in the last 6-months (2 pts).
    - Score range 0–19. Score <5 = <25% 6-month mortality and Score >12 = >50% mortality.

- **Thamer Score** (5): 3- and 6-months mortality

  - Age (<70 years 0 pts, 70–74 years 1 pt, 75–79 years 1 pt, 80–84 years 1 pt, 85–89 years 2 pts, ≥90 years 3 pt) and 1 pt each (albumin <3.5 g/dL, assistance with daily living, nursing home, cancer, heart failure, hospitalized more than once or >1 month in the last year).
  - Score range 0–9. Score of 4 = 17% mortality in 3-months/27% in 6-months and Score ≥8 = 39% mortality in 3-months/55% in 6-months.

- **Renal Epidemiology and Information Network (REIN) Score: Age ≥75** (7): 6-month mortality

  - Total dependence for transfers (3 pts), BMI <18.5 kg/m^2 (2 pts), peripheral vascular disease stage 3 or 4 (2 pts), chronic heart failure stage 3 or 4 (2 pts), severe behavioral disorder (2 pts), unplanned dialysis initiation (2 pts), active malignancy (1 pt), diabetes mellitus (1 pt), dysrhythmia (1 pt).
  - Score range 0–16. Score of 3–4 = 6-month mortality of 21–26% and Score ≥9 = 62–70% 6-month mortality.

- [1]**Integrated 6-month mortality tool** (3): 6-month mortality

  - Would I be surprised of this patient died in the next year?, serum albumin, age, dementia, peripheral vascular disease

- **Modified Charleston Comorbidity Index** (CCI) (6): 1-year mortality

  - Age (1 point for every 10 years older than 40) and Comorbidities (weighted score based on the type and number of comorbidities: 1 pt for each (coronary artery disease, congestive heart failure, peripheral vascular disease, cerebrovascular disease, dementia, chronic pulmonary disease, mild liver disease, diabetes), 2 pts for each (hemiplegia, moderate to severe renal disease, diabetes with end-organ damage, any tumor, leukemia, lymphoma), 3 pts for each (moderate or severe liver disease), 6 pts for (metastatic cancer or AIDS)
  - Score Range: 0–37. Score ≤3 = 3% 1-year mortality rate. Score ≥8 = 48% 1-year mortality rate.

Prognostication tool for the risk of progression to ESRD

- **See Footnote 1. The Kidney Failure Risk Equation:** 2- and 5-year probability (see Footnote 1)

  - Age, sex, estimated glomerular filtration rate (eGFR), and urinary albumin to creatinine ratio (ACR).

Adapted from Koncicki et al. [36]. Permission Requested. Additional Sources: [25, 37–45]

Estimation of Mortality After the Initiation of Dialysis

The *Wick Score, Thamer Score, REIN (Renal Epidemiology and Information Network) Score, Integrated 6-month mortality tool, Modified Charleston Comorbidity Index* and the *Surprise Question* are prognostic assessment tools designed to help estimate mortality after the initiation of dialysis and incorporate different combinations of the following prognostic factors: age, gender, eGFR mL/min/1.73 m^2, comorbidities, markers of nutrition, functional status, hospitalization events, and the surprise question [25, 37–45]. The *Surprise Question*, "Would I be surprised if this patient died in the next year?", is validated in patients with CKD and ESKD and helps capture the provider's global prognostic assessment and their clinical experience. Studies demonstrate that an answer of "no" to the *Surprise Question* has been associated with a 1-year mortality rate of 27% in patients with CKD Stage 4–5 and 29.4% in patients with ESKD which was 5 times and 3.5 times higher, respectively, when compared to answering "yes" [44, 45]. *The Fried Frailty Phenotype Criteria* helps identify frailty, a multifaceted overarching geriatric syndrome that encompasses a more comprehensive prognostic assessment than age and comorbidity alone. This physical frailty phenotype is defined as having at least 3 out of the 5 following criteria: unintentional weight loss >10 pounds in the past year, self-reported exhaustion, weakness (grip strength), slow walking speed, and low physical activity [46–48]. Lastly, the Karnofsky Performance Scale (KPS) is a functional assessment tool that ranges from 0 to 100 where 100 is normal, 70 is cares for self but is not able to perform normal activity, 40 is unable to live independently and requires special care, and 0 is dead [49–52].

The surprise question, KPS, The Fried Frailty Phenotype Criteria, and recognition of geriatric syndromes (to include dysphagia), worsening symptom burden, complications from dialysis, inability to tolerate dialysis, and multiple hospitalizations can help identify patients who are declining on dialysis [36].

Estimation of Progression to ESRD

The Kidney Failure Risk Equation tool helps estimate the 2- or 5-year risk of progression to kidney failure in patients with CKD Stage 3–5 using a 4-variable equation that includes age, sex, estimated glomerular filtration rate (eGFR), and urinary albumin to creatinine ratio (ACR) [53]. This tool, in combination with the clinician's observed trajectory of the patient's renal function, can help with prognostication without dialysis and provide a timeline to guide treatment options [54].

All these tools have several limitations which include generalizability and a focus on survival-based outcomes rather than patient-centered outcomes such as healthcare-related QOL. However, they can help mitigate prognostic uncertainty [40].

Decision Making in Advanced CKD

For elderly patients with advanced CKD, the decision to pursue versus forego dialysis and opt for CCC can be very challenging. Patients who proceed with dialysis (or a time-limited trial of dialysis) may hope for improved survival and maintain their independence. Based on their personal limitations, they may accept certain tradeoffs or burdens of dialysis. These tradeoffs can include time dedicated to dialysis and transportation, complications from dialysis and access failure, functional decline, and increased risk for hospitalizations due to acute illness and other comorbidities. Contrastingly, when a patient's goals are to focus on quality of life or preventing suffering rather than length of life, they may choose CCC. Studies show that most patients with kidney disease prefer a shared approach to decision making with their nephrologists [55] and want their nephrologists to discuss prognosis and end-of-life planning including withdrawal from dialysis [7, 55, 56]. Patients who discussed their overall medical condition and prognosis with their providers were less likely to report dialysis regret [57]. Advanced care planning (ACP) increases care consistent with patient goals and preferences.

ACP with shared decision making (SDM) is an ongoing process, in which competent patients, their family members/surrogate, and their health care providers develop a patient-centered preference-based care plan through interactive discussions to guide current and future medical care [dialysis ± kidney transplantation vs. CCC and end of life planning]. Essential components of ACP conversations include: (1) discussion of the patient's overall medical condition and prognosis and the risks/benefits of all treatment options, (2) clarification of prior discussions and medical documentation, and (3) reflection on the patient's goals/hopes, values/beliefs, fears and concerns. Making a recommendation based on expert opinion of the patient's prognosis and available treatment options and understanding of the patient's goals and values is an important component of SDM. In SDM the patient/surrogate guides the balance of partnership in decision making. Based on the patient/surrogate wishes, decisions may range from patient/surrogate-driven to physician-driven with varying degrees of partnership (shared decision-making continuum). A patient-centered recommendation not only helps support patients/surrogates who directly look to their providers for guidance but also promotes patient autonomy by fully informing the patient and allowing them to incorporate the provider's medical expertise into the decision process. Lastly, the patient's health care choices are accurately documented using advanced directives [58–60].

There are many different communication models that provide a framework to guide physicians in conducting ACP discussions. These SDM communication models include (1) Serious Illness Conversation Guide, (2) REMAP (Reframe, Emotion, MAP, Align, Propose a Plan), (3) SPIKES (Setting, Perception, Invitation,

Knowledge, Empathy, and Summary), and (4) SPIRES (Setup, Perceptions and perspectives, Invitation, Recommendation, Empathize, and Summarize) which is an adaptation of SPIKES created by Schell et al. for dialysis decision making [16, 61–63]. These models include similar communication themes. The following highlights the main communication principles from these standardized models and applies them to decision-making in patients with advanced CKD. This framework can be utilized for all types of ACP discussions including discussions about withdrawal from dialysis.

Set Up the Conversation

The first steps in preparing for an ACP discussion are to (1) introduce the purpose of the conversation, (2) highlight the importance of thinking about and preparing for the future, (3) ask permission to engage in discussion, and (4) decide together when and where the conversation should take place and which individuals should be present [54, 61]. For example, "Your kidney function is now at the point where it is very important for us to talk about how to best care for you going forward. Would it be okay if we plan a meeting to talk about this? Would you like to invite a family member or friend to support you during this discussion?" [16].

Assess Understanding

Before sharing information, it is important to elicit the patient's understanding of their kidney disease and overall medical condition, prognosis, and available treatment options (dialysis ± kidney transplantation vs. CCC). Understanding the patient's perspective of their medical condition shapes the subsequent discussion. It is helpful to first use broad open-ended questions followed by more directed questions as needed to elicit understanding. The following are communication examples [16, 54, 58]:

- *Medical Condition and Prognosis*: "What is your understanding of your overall health?" "Tell me how you feel about your medical problems?" "Tell me about your kidney disease." "How serious do you feel your kidney disease seems to be?" "How do you think your kidney disease will affect your life in the future?"
- *Treatment options*: "What have you been told about your treatment options for kidney disease?" "Have you heard of dialysis?" "What have you heard or been told about dialysis?" "Do you know anyone who has been on dialysis?" "What questions do you have about dialysis?" "What do you know about the different types of dialysis?" "What is your impression of dialysis as a possible treatment option?" "Have you heard about kidney transplantation? (If appropriate)" "Have you heard about a non-dialysis option called CCC?"

Ask About Information Preferences

An important part of the communication process is to determine how much and what information the patient wants to know about their overall medical condition and prognosis. Patients have a right to full disclosure to make informed decisions regarding their medical care, yet they may have different preferences about the types or extent of medical information they want to receive. The following are communication examples to elicit information preferences [36, 58, 64]:

- "Some people want to hear all the details about their kidney disease, others want to know the big picture, and sometimes people don't want to hear information directly and prefer to talk to a family member or friend. Which would you want?"
- "What kind of information do you want to know?"
- "How much information do you want to know about the future?" "How much do you want to know about the course of your kidney disease?" "How much and what kind of information do you want to know about prognosis?" "Do you want to know how people similar to you do on dialysis?"

If a patient states they do not want information about their medical condition and/or prognosis, it is important to understand why the patient does not want to know and acknowledge the patient's fear or concerns. Ask permission to rediscuss this topic later or, depending on the nature of the situation, talk to the person that the patient has designated to hear this information on their behalf. If the situation is urgent and the patient is unable to identify someone you can communicate with, share why you think it is very important to talk about this information today, express respect, and re-ask permission to proceed [64].

Share Information

Consider the patient's information preferences and discuss the patient's kidney disease in the context of their overall medical condition, review all treatment options (dialysis ± kidney transplantation vs. CCC), and communicate prognosis (or uncertainty in prognosis) with and without dialysis. Discuss prognosis not only in terms of time, but also in terms of effect on QOL such as functional trajectory (need for home caregiver or facility support), symptom burden and life impacts, and risk of developing medical complications, procedures, and hospitalizations [54]. Based on estimation of the patient's prognosis portray what life may be like with or without dialysis (CCC). The "Best Case/Worst Case" communication tool can be used to verbally and pictorially depict the best, most likely, and worst-case outcomes with dialysis vs. CCC. By visually mapping out the treatment options, it allows time for the patient to process the information and ask questions, and for the provider to elicit understanding. After completion of the diagram, ask "What are your thoughts and feelings about all of this?". This open-ended question can help initiate a discussion of the patient's goals and values in the context of these outcomes [65].

Provide Support

Strong emotions are commonly experienced during advanced care planning discussions. Acknowledging these emotions and providing empathy is important throughout these conversations. The mnemonic NURSE (Name: "I can see that this conversation is making you very nervous", Understand: "Talking about dialysis can be very scary." Respect: "You are asking all the right questions." Support: "I am here for you. We are going to work together to figure this out." Explore: "What concerns you the most about dialysis?" is one way to verbally address emotions. Another mnemonic to express empathy is SAVE (Support: "I am here to for you." Acknowledge: "Making this decision has been very hard on you." Validate: "Many people in this situation feel the way you do." Emotion naming: "You seem anxious.") At times emotions can become overwhelming and instead of outwardly expressing emotions (such as crying or anger) patients may become silent. A therapeutic silence, allowing for silence in the conversation, can allow the patient to process what has been said, experience their feelings, and formulate questions to continue talking [58].

Elicit Patient Goals and Values

By exploring a patient's hopes and expectations, concerns, worries, and sources of strength, and understanding their limitations/critical abilities, we can learn about the patient as a person and elicit their goals and values. Asking questions about hope provides insight into a patient's big-picture goals. Asking about patient's concerns, worries, and limitations (such as acceptable function) can highlight what burdens a patient is willing or not willing to tolerate to achieve their goals [16]. It is important to explore both health-related and personal aspects of their goals, concerns, and worries [54]. Also, understanding where the patient finds their inner strength (Family, Friendship, Religion/Spirituality) tells us more about their values, how patients cope with their illness, and sometimes how they approach decision-making [54, 58].

Koncicki et al. and Schell et al. developed communication examples to help elicit patients' hopes, concerns worries, and limitations in patients with kidney disease; the examples are as follows [14, 16, 58]:

Exploring Hopes and Expectations

- "What do you hope for in the future?" "What makes your life worth living?" "What is most important to you if your time is limited?" "What are you hoping to achieve with dialysis?" "What activities bring you pleasure and enjoyment?" "Is it important to you to live as long as possible, despite suffering, or to live without suffering for a shorter period of time?"

Exploring Concerns or Worries

- "What concerns you the most about dialysis?" "What worries you the most about your future?"

Exploring Limitations

- "Are their circumstances that would make your life not worth living?" "What level of function or independence is critical for you to have for an acceptable quality of life?" "In what situations do you think you would not want to continue dialysis?"

Some important communication strategies to encourage patients to share their goals and values include: (1) the use of open-ended questions, (2) minimal verbal (ex: "Hmm" or "Ah" or "Then?") and non-verbal (eye contact, nodding, and leaning forward) leads, (3) repetition (repeating key points so that the patient feels heard), (4) paraphrasing and reflecting (to ensure understanding of the patients' meaning), (5) clarifying responses (to help better understand the patients' feelings and allow the patient to reflect), and (6) lastly summarizing (to ensure that the patients' main message was appreciated) [58].

Make a Recommendation and Create a Care Plan

After evaluating and discussing the patient's overall medical condition, prognosis, and treatment options, and learning about what is most important to the patient, a recommendation can be formulated by translating the patient's priorities and estimated prognosis into a proposed treatment plan. Patients however may identify several priorities to which some may be contradictory. For example, an 87-year-old male with CKD, multiple comorbidities, and frailty may express that he hopes to spend as much time together with his wife and die peacefully in his home yet also wants to maintain his independence and live as long as he can with his wife. Explore these incongruent priories further to gain a better understanding of the patient's goals and focus on the priorities that are more attainable based on the patient's prognosis and treatment options. Therefore, in this patient with advanced CKD, as dialysis will likely not provide survival benefits over CCC, focus on the patient's priorities of time at home, maintaining the function, and a peaceful death to help formulate a treatment plan. Next, seek permission to make a recommendation by asking "Would it be helpful if I offered a recommendation?" Allow patients time to process the recommendation. Aligning the concept of making a recommendation with SDM, patients have the option to accept or decline a recommendation supporting their autonomy. If a patient/family does not accept the recommendation provide continued support by acknowledging the difficult situation, expressing commitment to working with the patent and family, and emphasizing the importance of continued open communication to develop a patient-centered care plan and arrange follow-up [59]. If the patient accepts the recommendation, re-review the discussion and recommendation, and outline a care plan together with the patient/family. Document the ACP discussion and notify relevant providers.

ACP discussions in patients with kidney disease should also include discussion of other life-sustaining treatment options such as cardiopulmonary resuscitation and intubation, artificial support, and end-of-life care planning. A health care proxy should be identified, and appropriate advanced directives should be completed to align with the patient's care plan.

Comprehensive Conservative Care

The goal of CCC is to optimize quality of life and live well without dialysis [66]. The Kidney Disease Improving Global Outcomes (KDIGO) conference on supportive care in 2013 and the Kidney Supportive Care Research Group (KSCRG: University of Alberta), have proposed clinical structures for CCC. The recommended process of CCC includes [1, 14, 66] the following:

- Continued shared decision-making as needed to support preference-based care.
- Clinical interventions that focus on patients' goals.

  - A tailored approach to CKD medical management to protect remaining kidney function, manage complications, and mitigate adverse events with the goal of enhancing quality of life.
  - Frequent symptom assessment with active management.

- Advanced care planning to identify the patient's wishes for (1) management of a crisis (an acute event or uncontrolled symptoms) and (2) end-of-life care, to include discussion of hospice.
- Consideration for referral (based on available resources) to specialty palliative care to incorporate an interdisciplinary team to help address complex symptom management and existential distress and provide psychosocial and spiritual support to patients and their families.

- Referral to case management to optimize services to help support patient's individual health care needs.
- Re-evaluation of the CCC plan based on patient's preferences as their clinical course advances.

The role and trajectory of CCC are highly variable and dependent upon the patient's kidney (eGFR 10–15 mL/min/1.73 m^2 vs. 5 mL/min/1.73 m^2) and overall medical condition and associated prognosis. Care may initially focus on preserving kidney function and managing complications of CKD alongside symptom management and later transition to symptom management and comfort closer to the end of life [14]. The frequency of clinical assessments and laboratory analysis will also change and initially may be ~ every 1–3 months and later become more infrequent with a need to transition to home-based care (to include hospice care) [1].

Given the paucity of data on CKD and symptom management in CCC, in 2015 a clinical working group led by the KSCRG and Alberta's Conservative Kidney Management Steering Committee comprising nephrologists, primary care providers, and palliative care and geriatric physicians, developed recommendations based on available evidence and expert opinion for (1) reducing the decline in kidney function and managing complications of advanced CKD in the context of addressing quality of life (see the following) and (2) symptom management [14, 66–68]. The recommendations are as follows:

Preservative CKD Management

- To help reduce decline in renal function, it is recommended to consider discontinuation of renin–angiotensin–aldosterone system (RAAS) inhibitors which can contribute to loss of glomerular filtration rate.
- Blood pressure targets can be relaxed and for most patients targeting a blood pressure less than 160/90 will be appropriate.
- Consider stopping statins as it may improve QOL and the side effects (myalgias) of statins have been shown to outweigh benefits in patients with life-limiting illness.
- Utilize diuretics and dietary sodium restriction as needed to optimize volume status in patients with dyspnea and bothersome lower extremity edema.
- To prevent fatigue and dyspnea, when indicated from an overall QOL standpoint, manage anemia using iron (oral ± IV based on tolerability and response with goal TSAT approximately >20%) and erythropoiesis-stimulating agents (ESAs) with goal Hg ~9 to 11 g/dL.
- Consider treatment of metabolic acidosis with prescription oral sodium bicarbonate or baking soda (sodium bicarbonate 650 mg tablet = ~1/8th teaspoon of baking soda) (goal CO_2 ~22 to 27 mmol/L) if fatigue, bone loss, muscle wasting, and malnutrition are affecting physical function and QOL and the patient is able to swallow and tolerate the medication burden.

- Regarding bone-mineral disease or calcium and phosphate metabolism, the recommendation is to stop monitoring the parathyroid hormone and re-educate patients and their families on liberalizing diet to optimize nutrition and QOL. Management of hyperphosphatemia with a moderate-phosphate-restricted diet ± phosphorous binders can be considered to treat restless leg syndrome and address myalgias, arthralgias, and pseudogout. Low-dose activated vitamin D (starting dose Calcitriol 0.25 mg PO three times per week) can also be used to prevent weakness, fatigue, and muscle loss.

Symptom Management

The above recommendations for CKD medical management in CCC should be applied based on the patient's overall condition and functional status. A web-site called Conservative Kidney Management (https://www.ckmcare.com/PractitionerPathway/AtAGlance) is a comprehensive resource to guide health care professionals in supporting patients on CCC and educating patients and their families about CCC [66].

Transitions in Dialysis

Time Limited Trial of Dialysis

In patients with advanced CKD and AKI when (1) the prognosis with dialysis is unclear or (2) there is a conflict between the nephrologist and patient/family or among providers about initiating dialysis, the use of a time-limited trial (TLT) of dialysis can promote preference-based care and increase informed-decision making to resolve conflicts, respectively [36, 69–71]. A time-limited trial (TLT) of dialysis is a goal-directed trial of dialysis over a defined period to determine if dialysis can help the patient achieve their specific goals without significant burden or suffering [36, 69–71]. This patient-centered process is guided by clinical markers of improvement or decline. Schell et al. coined the phrases (1) "patient-specific milestones", the goals that the patient hopes to attain with dialysis, to identify the parameters of dialysis success, and (2) "pause points", health conditions or situations that are unacceptable to the patient (critical limitations), to identify circumstances that the patient would not want to continue dialysis [36].

It is important to communicate with the patient and family that the hope is for the patient to benefit from dialysis based on their goals; however, if the patient's predetermined milestones are not achieved with dialysis or critical limitations develop, stopping dialysis and providing maximum comfort may best align with the patient's wishes [36]. A TLT of dialysis can also give patients and families time to process the patient's condition and prepare for the end of life [67]. The timeframe to evaluate the benefits and burdens of dialysis will vary based on the individual and whether the patient has AKI or progressive CKD. Generally, patients with AKI are critically ill in the hospital and therefore require reassessment on a scale of days to weeks. Whereas patients with kidney failure may require re-evaluation closer to weeks to months after the initiation of dialysis [36, 69]. During re-evaluation meetings it is important to consider that as patients' clinical courses unfold, they can experience different phases of their illness and their milestones and pause points may also change. The patient's care plan should be flexible and redirected based on their new outlook and goals [36].

The main purposed components for the framework of a TLT of dialysis include the following [36, 69–72].

- Involve the patient's support system to include their health care decision maker, family, and friends as desired in this process. Also include other relevant providers as needed and consider incorporating specialty palliative care for additional psychosocial and spiritual support and conflict resolution.
- Discuss the uncertainty in the patient's time- and function-based prognosis and the potential benefits and burdens of dialysis.
- Explore the patients' goals, values, and priorities.
- Introduce the purpose of a TLT of dialysis. If appropriate, based on the patients' specific goals, suggest a TLT of Dialysis.
- Elicit "patient-specific milestones" and "pause points".
- Discuss how the "patient-specific milestones" and "pause points" will help guide whether to continue or discontinue dialysis at the end of a time-limited trial of dialysis.
- Determine a medically appropriate time frame to evaluate the effect of dialysis.
- Summarize the proposed care plan and check for patient/family understanding.
- Document the conditions of the TLT of dialysis (who was present, what was discussed, the rationale for TLT, the identified milestones and pause points, the length of the trial, and potential actions at the end of the trial).
- At the purposed timeframe evaluate the patient's/family's perspective of the impact of dialysis on the individual [How do you think you are doing overall? Do you feel that dialysis is helping you meet your goals? Do you feel burdened by dialysis?]. Through this discussion, re-assess the "patient-specific milestones" and "pause points". If the decision is to continue with dialysis, negotiate another timeframe to reassess the effect of dialysis. If the patient/family wishes to stop dialysis, implement or create an end-of-life care plan.

Palliative Dialysis

As dialysis therapy itself can negatively affect a patient's healthcare experience, in addition to implementing primary palliative care skills to support dialysis patients, a palliative approach to dialysis therapy is also needed [71, 73]. Burdens related to dialysis therapy include (1) physical and psychological/emotional symptoms, (2) cognitive impairment and physical function decline, (3) dialysis treatment and transport time, (4) procedures for dialysis access, (5) complications of dialysis (infection, hypotension) which can result in hospitalizations, (6) dietary restrictions, (7) high pill burden, (8) social (loss of employment and change in social standing in the community and family) and (9) economic impacts.

Palliative dialysis, or a palliative approach to dialysis, is a patient-goal concordant approach to dialysis that focuses on improving QOL and reducing symptom burden and transitions away from conventional dialysis where the goal is to optimize rehabilitation and survival. There is no currently available data on outcomes with palliative dialysis, but the intent is to tailor dialysis based on the patient's personal goals to reduce suffering. For individuals who have a limited life expectancy (approximately <1 year) and dialysis is negatively impacting their QOL and interfering with their personal goals, in addition to the option of stopping dialysis, a palliative approach to dialysis could be considered. Palliative dialysis in some circumstances could represent a transition to withdrawal of dialysis by giving patients and their families more time together as well as time to process the patient's condition and prepare for the end of life [73].

Grubbs et al. proposed a palliative approach to dialysis that includes (1) the use of central venous catheters to reduce procedural burden, (2) acceptance of lower dialysis adequacy to reduce the burden of dialysis time, (3) allowance of hypertension to avoid symptoms, (4) liberalization of diet (more permissive hyperphosphatemia and hyperparathyroidism) to help support nutrition and QOL, (5) simplified medication regimens (stop statins), and (6) reduced laboratory monitoring. However, there are several providers (comfort with primary palliative care skills), economical, and infrastructural barriers (need for staff-assisted home dialysis and hospice support for patients actively on dialysis) to palliative dialysis. Economically, the current incentivized reimbursement model for dialysis patients is based on attaining performance metrics that were designed for conventional disease-directed dialysis and include measures of dialysis adequacy, hemoglobin, and phosphorous levels, and reducing central venous catheter use. These metrics do not align with a palliative approach to dialysis and this patient-centered care can financially impact dialysis providers. Policy and infrastructural changes are needed for the widespread clinical application of palliative dialysis [1, 71, 73].

Withdrawal from Dialysis

The second most common reason for death in dialysis patients is the elective withdrawal of dialysis. Rates of dialysis withdrawal in the US are variable and have been reported to be as low as ~10% and as high as ~50% [11, 74, 75]. In a single-center US study of maintenance hemodialysis patients, acute medical complications (51%), failure to thrive/frailty (22%), and chronic debility (18%) were the most common reasons for withdrawal [11]. Other factors associated with dialysis withdrawal include older age, Medicaid insurance (a marker for impoverishment), disability (OR 31.2), palliative care consult within 6 months, and hospitalizations within 30 days [11, 74, 75]. Comorbidity burden has not been found to be associated with dialysis withdrawal which supports studies that demonstrate perceived QOL in ESRD patients is not associated with comorbidities [74]. After withdrawal of dialysis, median survival is approximately 7 days but is variable and dependent upon the individuals' residual renal function and overall medical condition [11]. Hospice is utilized in only ~20% of dialysis patients and is more commonly provided to patients who electively withdrew from dialysis (37% vs. 7% non-withdrawals) [11].

It is important to identify patients receiving maintenance dialysis who are declining and approaching the end of life. Re-addressing their "patient-specific milestones" and "pause points" will highlight the benefits and burdens of dialysis and determine if dialysis is helping the patient attain their goals or is rather prolonging their suffering. These discussions can help the patient and their family process and prepare for the end of life and may result in the consideration of palliative dialysis or withdrawal from dialysis. Other patients may independently voice their desire to stop dialysis, prompting the need for goals of care discussion.

The following outlines a process to approach all patients who are contemplating withdrawal from dialysis [36, 71]:

1. Assess the patient's decision-making capacity and overall understanding of dialysis and what will happen if the patient stops dialysis. If the patient does not have decision-making capability, involve the patient's health care decision-maker.
2. Holistically explore from a physical, psychosocial, and spiritual perspective the underlying reasons why the patient/surrogate is considering withdrawing from dialysis.
3. Identify and address potential modifiable factors:

    (a) Physical:

       - Underlying medical diseases.
       - Challenges with dialysis treatment to include dialysis modality and time, and the location of the dialysis center (distance from home).
       - Uncontrolled symptoms.

    (b) Psychological: Depression or anxiety.
    (c) Social: Feelings of being a burden to one's family. Other personal conflicts.
    (d) Economical: Burden of the cost of continued treatment, medications, diet restrictions, and transportation.
    (e) Existential and spiritual distress.

4. After identifying and attempting to modify these factors, if the patient/surrogate continues to express that they want to stop dialysis their wishes should be respected.
5. Counsel the patient/surrogate on survival after stopping dialysis and create an end-of-life care plan with a recommendation for hospice care and completion of the POLST (Physician Orders for Lift Sustaining Treatment) form [71].

Table 17.1 Domains of signs/symptoms and life impacts in patients with CKD and ESKD [4]

Signs and symptoms (prevalence (%))	Life impacts (prevalence (%))
Pain/discomfort (57%): bodily pain/discomfort, muscle pain/cramps, muscle soreness, feeling unwell, dizziness	Psychological/emotional strain (49%): anxiety, depression, mood changes/disorders/irritability, impact on self-image
Energy/fatigue (42%): fatigue, lack of energy, lethargy, tiredness, shortness of breath, weakness	Cognitive impairment (27%): memory, attention, concentration, confusion
Sleep-related (28%): poor sleep quality, difficulty sleeping, daytime sleepiness, short sleep duration, restless legs syndrome, drowsiness	Dietary habit disruption (23%): avoid specific foods, control the amount of food, restrict the volume of liquid intake, difficulty knowing foods permitted
GI-related: (18% anorexia, 18% nausea): general GI symptoms, nausea, appetite loss/anorexia, constipation, diarrhea	Physical function decrement (43%): inability to work or difficulties working, unable to practice self-care (dressing, transferring), physical limitations, limited activity performance, mobility limitation
Urinary-related: frequent urination, restricted ability to urinate, nocturia, urinary tract infections	Interference with social relationships (34%): negative impact on sexual life. General social impact, negative impact on families, marriages, and social circles, and decreased social interactions had a prevalence of <50%, however are common in clinical practice
Skin, hair, nails related (25%): itching/pruritus, dry skin, skin infections, hypothermia, nail deterioration	Other: poor general health perception
Other: taste alteration, thirst, macrovascular/microvascular diabetic complications, pallor	

Symptom Assessment and Management

Patients with CKD and ESKD experience significant symptom burden and impact on health-related quality of life. Symptom etiology is multifactorial and is a result of the progression of kidney disease, comorbid conditions, and the treatment of kidney disease, such as dialysis. The burden of these symptoms and their impact on quality of life can increase as the patient's kidney disease and overall medical condition progress [4]. Understanding the patient's experience of kidney disease helps identify symptoms to develop management strategies and guides informed treatment decisions [2, 4].

Flythe et al. conducted an extensive literature review of signs/symptoms and the impact on QOL reported by patients with CKD and ESKD and developed a comprehensive categorization. Seven domains of signs and symptoms and six domains of life impacts were identified [4] (Table 17.1).

Studies suggest that the nephrology community is not adept at recognizing and treating symptoms of kidney disease. However, this is an essential component in the supportive care of kidney patients and should be conducted across all care settings, to include clinics, hospitals, and dialysis centers [1]. Unless patients are directly asked, many will not express their symptoms to their providers. Thus, symptom assessment tools can be utilized to assist providers in identifying symptoms by promoting patient communication and monitoring a patient's symptoms over time. The following are current validated tools for symptom assessment [1]:

- Integrated Palliative Care Outcome Scale Renal (IPOS-Renal).
- Edmonton Symptom Assessment Revised: Renal (ESAS-Renal).
- Dialysis Symptom Index (DSI).
- Pain assessment: Brief Pain Inventory.

The management of symptoms not only includes pharmacologic and nonpharmacologic approaches to address symptoms directly, but also requires (1) evaluation of reversible underlying conditions that could be contributing to the symptoms and (2) understanding the nature (physical, psychological, social, and spiritual) and extent of the patient's symptoms to guide appropriate therapies (Table 17.2). Pharmacological treatments have some limitations, and it is important to help manage patient's expectations. Incorporating an interdisciplinary team composed of social workers, chaplains, counselors, and specialty palliative care can help address the multifaceted nature of symptoms also known as total symptoms [1].

End of Life Care

Due to current national policy, hospice care in kidney disease is limited to patients with kidney failure who forgo dialysis and opt for CCC and patients who electively withdraw from dialysis. Patients receiving maintenance dialysis can qualify for hospice if the patient has an estimated prognosis of 6 months and a poor prognosis is associated with a diagnosis other than kidney failure (e.g., malignancy, dementia, etc.). Therefore, patients receiving maintenance dialysis with a prognosis of <6 months without such conditions are not eligible for hospice care until they choose to withdraw from dialysis. Patients who elected CCC also have barriers to hospice care. Medications routinely used to manage complications of advanced CKD such as ESAs for anemia-related symptoms and newer-generation potassium binders (patiromer and sodium zirconium cyclosilicate) are generally not included in hospice formularies [82]. Specialty palliative care can be incorporated in patients of all ages at any stage of kidney disease and should be utilized to fill the current gaps in hospice care in the US [15].

Table 17.2 General approach to symptom management for patients with CKD and ESRD [1, 67, 76–81]

Symptom	Causes: address possible reversible factors	Pharmacological treatment (Dose adjustment based on eGFR and dialysis status)	Nonpharmacological treatment
Pain	– Metabolic derangements leading to bone disease – Peripheral neuropathy – Musculoskeletal: osteoarthritis	– Utilize the WHO analgesic ladder – Avoid morphine, codeine, hydrocodone, tapentadol, meperidine, and extended-release tramadol – Safer opioids: oxycodone, tramadol, fentanyl, dilaudid, and methadone – Neuropathy: gabapentin/pregabalin, duloxetine (avoid in dialysis)/venlafaxine, tramadol, amitriptyline, methadone, or topical lidocaine and capsaicin	– PT, OT, heat/cold therapies – Cognitive behavioral therapy, relaxation therapies/guided imagery, other forms of psychotherapy – Spine or joint injections, neurolytic blocks, spinal analgesics – Complementary: acupuncture, massage, music, and art therapy
Fatigue	– Dialysis-related hypotension – Rapid osmotic shifts during dialysis – Mood and sleep disorders – Malnutrition – Anemia – Medication side effects – Metabolic acidosis – Hypo-/hyperthyroidism, adrenal insufficiency – Vitamin D deficiency	– Erythropoietin (EPO) and iron (IV/PO) for treatment of anemia – Evaluate and treat underlying conditions	– Exercise and PT if tolerated – Sleep hygiene – Nutrition optimization – Energy conservation strategies – Complementary treatments
Sleep disturbance	– May be related to pain or other symptoms – Primary sleep disorders – Sleep apnea – Restless legs syndrome (RLS)	– Sleep aid medication if other disorders are excluded: eszopiclone/zolpidem/zaleplon, trazodone, mirtazapine, doxepin, melatonin – RLS: gabapentin, pramipexole/ropinirole/rotigotine	– Sleep hygiene techniques – Exercise if tolerated

(continued)

Table 17.2 (continued)

Symptom	Causes: address possible reversible factors	Pharmacological treatment (Dose adjustment based on eGFR and dialysis status)	Nonpharmacological treatment
Pruritus	– Uremic: complex mechanisms; secondary hyperparathyroidism, hyperphosphatemia, calcium phosphate deposition in the skin – Xerosis – Anemia – Primary dermatological conditions – Other systemic condition	– Gabapentin, pregabalin – Difelikefalin (dialysis patients) – Phosphate binders, 1,25 di-OH vitamin D – EPO and iron (IV/PO)	– Dietary phosphate restriction – Emollient therapy for dry skin – Avoidance of extreme temperatures – Can consider: UVB therapy, acupuncture
Anorexia	– Uremia – GI: dysgeusia, gastroparesis, mechanical – Nausea and vomiting – Dry mouth (medication induced)	– Antiemetics (see below) – If no response, trial of appetite stimulants: dronabinol, mirtazapine, olanzapine – Dry mouth: saliva substitute, lip balm, stimulation of saliva with sour foods/candies	– Liberalize dietary restrictions
Depression	– Multifaceted syndrome: metabolic, psychosocial, spiritual, and existential	– First line: selective serotonin reuptake such as sertraline	– Exercise – Cognitive behavioral therapy
Nausea/vomiting	– Uremia – Medications – GI: constipation, delayed gastric emptying	– Ondansetron, metoclopramide, olanzapine or haloperidol	– Small, regular meals – Avoid strong smells and alcohol – Manage constipation – Oral hygiene – Relaxation therapies, acupuncture
Dyspnea	– Pulmonary edema or infection – Anxiety – Anemia	– Treat underlying conditions: diuretics, antibiotics, EPO + iron (IV/PO) – Consider low-dose opioids near the end of life	– Fans – Careful positioning – Relaxation techniques

eGFR estimated glomerular filtration rate, *GI* gastrointestinal, *OT* occupational therapy, *PT* physical therapy, *UVB* ultraviolet B

Case Presentation Continued

The nephrologist communicates the importance of talking more about his kidney condition and about the next steps. He asks Henry a series of questions about his information preferences, and Henry replies "Don't hold anything back doctor. I want to know everything. I want to know how much time I have left and what my life might look like." Together they decide to have a meeting in 2-weeks and Henry would like to have the support of his stepdaughter and friend. The nephrologist elicits that his stepdaughter is his health care proxy.

In the interim, his nephrologist reviews Henry's medical record and communicates with his primary care provider to gain a better picture of his medical condition. Henry is of advanced age (83 years old), has multiple comorbidities, is displaying physical frailty but no recent falls, has a Karnofsky Performance Scale (KPS) of 70, does not have evidence of cognitive impairment on Montreal Cognitive Assessment, and his albumin level has decreased to 3.4 correlating with his recent weight loss. Based on the Kidney Failure Risk Assessment tool his risk of needing dialysis is ~24% in 2 years and 58% in 5 years. Based on the integrated 6-month mortality tool, his mortality rate 6 months after the initiation of dialysis is 35%. His nephrologist and primary care provider feel that they would not be surprised if the patient died in the next year. His nephrologist is very concerned that dialysis may not provide a survival benefit over CCC and given the patient's frailty, he will be at higher risk for further functional decline, development of cognitive impairment, falls, and morbidity, and inpatient mortality.

Two-weeks later, Henry, his stepdaughter Sarah, and his friend Diane meet with the nephrologist in the office. After introductions, the nephrologist asks Henry "What is your understanding of your kidney condition?" Henry explains that he has had problems with his kidneys for a very long time but more recently his kidneys have gotten much worse. He also expresses that he does not know much about dialysis. The nephrologist elicits Sarah and Diane's understanding as well. He then asks permission to share more information about Henry's overall medical condition, treatment options (dialysis and CCC), and prognosis. To communicate prognosis, his nephrologist draws a diagram explaining the best, most likely, and worse-case scenarios of dialysis vs. CCC based on the patient's prognosis. Through this discussion, Henry, Sarah, and Diane were able to clarify questions regarding dialysis, CCC, symptom burden, and what life may look like on dialysis. Henry also started to voice concerns about each pathway and his nephrologist prompted Henry to tell him more about these concerns and fears and asked about his hopes and expectations for the future. Henry expressed that his main goals are to maintain his independence and continue to live in the independent section of his ALF. He also hopes to improve his appetite so he can eat the food he loves and have more energy to socialize with his neighbors. He expresses a desire that he never wants to live in a nursing home and stated, "I rather die than be in a nursing home" and he does not want to die in the hospital. He is very concerned about dialysis and feels uneasy with the idea of needing procedures and possibly even having to go to the hospital because of a problem. Henry becomes visibly overwhelmed with this decision process. His nephrologist asked Henry if it would be helpful if he made a recommendation and Henry expressed that he would like to hear his opinion. His nephrologist states, "It sounds like most of your goals are about trying to feel better, maintaining your independence, and spending time with your family and friends. I can hear that living in a nursing home is unacceptable to you and you are very concerned about dialysis and its complications. Based on this, I recommend CCC." Henry exhales a sigh of relief and states "I agree. At this time, I just want to enjoy the time I have left with Sarah and Diane and when my time comes let me go." Sarah and Diane support Henry's decision. Henry and his nephrologist establish a CCC plan and Henry also elects to be DNR/DNI. He is started on mirtazapine to help with sleep, appetite, and depression which was later identified by his nephrologist.

Eight months later Henry's priorities shift, and he now expresses that his most important goal is to be alive to meet his first great-grandchild who will be born in 2-months. His eGFR is now 5 mL/min/1.73 m^2, and he has intermittent hyperkalemia despite high dose patiromer, and shows diuretic resistance with lower extremity edema and dyspnea on exertion. His nephrologist organizes another goals of care discussion with Henry and Sarah, and based on his new priorities, together they decide to conduct a trial of dialysis. Henry's "milestones" with dialysis are to (1) live long enough to meet his great-grandchild and (2) improve his symptoms of shortness of breath and lower extremity edema which are now affecting his mobility. He explicitly states his "pause points" and expresses that he would want to stop dialysis if he could no longer care for himself and needed to go to a nursing home. They decide that they will re-evaluate how he is doing 1-month after he initiates dialysis.

A tunneled dialysis catheter is placed successfully, and Henry is started on dialysis. At the 1-month re-assessment, Henry reports that he is feeling much better regarding his leg swelling and breathing and continues to live in his ALF. However, he is very tired all the time, feels that dialysis days are very long, and his appetite remains poor. Henry is motivated by his goals to continue with dialysis and 1 month later he meets his new great-granddaughter. Shortly thereafter Henry starts to become weaker and has a prolonged complicated hospitalization resulting in him no longer being able to care for himself in his home environment. His nephrologist meets him in the hospital and after a long conversation with Henry, Sarah, and Diane, Henry makes the decision to stop dialysis. As per Henry's wishes, home hospice is arranged in Sarah's home, and Henry dies 10 days later surrounded by his family and friends.

Conclusion

Kidney supportive care is a comprehensive care model that focuses on improving the lives of patients with kidney disease. Patient-centered communication to guide preference-based care, symptom recognition and management, and end-of-life care

are essential components to support elderly patients with kidney disease. There are many barriers to translating this care model into a system-wide clinical practice, including education, the development of an infrastructure, and current medical policies. The intent of this chapter is to educate and empower all providers taking care of patients with kidney disease to practice kidney palliative care skills to optimize the care of this unique patient population.

References

1. Gelfand SL, Scherer JS, Koncicki HM. Kidney supportive care: core curriculum 2020. Am J Kidney Dis. 2020;75(5):793–806.
2. United States Renal Data System. 2021 USRDS annual data report: epidemiology of kidney disease in the United States. Bethesda, MD: National Institutes of Health, National Institute of Diabetes and Digestive and Kidney Diseases; 2021.
3. Wong SPY, Hebert PL, Laundry RJ, Hammond KW, Liu C-F, Burrows NR, et al. Decisions about renal replacement therapy in patients with advanced kidney disease in the US Department of Veterans Affairs, 2000–2011. Clin J Am Soc Nephrol. 2016;11(10):1825–33.
4. Flythe JE, Karlsson N, Sundgren A, Cordero P, Grandinetti A, Cremisi H, et al. Development of a preliminary conceptual model of the patient experience of chronic kidney disease: a targeted literature review and analysis. BMC Nephrol. 2021;22(1):233.
5. Kaur T, Koncicki H. Education in palliative care during nephrology fellowship: where are we?. Kidney News Online. 2021. https://www.kidneynews.org/.
6. Saeed F, Sardar MA, Davison SN, Murad H, Duberstein PR, Quill TE. Patients' perspectives on dialysis decision-making and end-of-life care. Clin Nephrol. 2019;91(5):294–300.
7. Davison SN. End-of-life care preferences and needs: perceptions of patients with chronic kidney disease. Clin J Am Soc Nephrol. 2010;5(2):195–204.
8. Oskoui T, Pandya R, Weiner DE, Wong JB, Koch-Weser S, Ladin K. Advance care planning among older adults with advanced non-dialysis-dependent CKD and their care partners: perceptions versus reality? Kidney Med. 2020;2(2):116–24.
9. Ramer SJ, Koncicki HM. To dialysis and beyond: the nephrologist's responsibility for advance care planning. Kidney Med. 2020;2(2):102–4.
10. Frazier R, Levine S, Porteny T, Tighiouart H, Wong JB, Isakova T, et al. Shared decision making among older adults with advanced CKD. Am J Kidney Dis. 2022;80:599.
11. Chen JC-Y, Thorsteinsdottir B, Vaughan LE, Feely MA, Albright RC, Onuigbo M, et al. End of life, withdrawal, and palliative care utilization among patients receiving maintenance hemodialysis therapy. Clin J Am Soc Nephrol. 2018;13(8):1172–9.
12. Radbruch L, De Lima L, Knaul F, Wenk R, Ali Z, Bhatnaghar S, et al. Redefining palliative care—a new consensus-based definition. J Pain Symptom Manag. 2020;60(4):754–64.
13. Tatum PE, Mills SS. Hospice and palliative care. Med Clin North Am. 2020;104(3):359–73.
14. Davison SN, Levin A, Moss AH, Jha V, Brown EA, Brennan F, et al. Executive summary of the KDIGO controversies conference on supportive care in chronic kidney disease: developing a roadmap to improving quality care. Kidney Int. 2015;88(3):447–59.
15. Gelfand SL, Schell J, Eneanya ND. Palliative care in nephrology: the work and the workforce. Adv Chronic Kidney Dis. 2020;27(4):350.
16. Schell JO, Cohen RA. A communication framework for dialysis decision-making for frail elderly patients. Clin J Am Soc Nephrol. 2014;9(11):2014–21.
17. Carlson C, Merel SE, Yukawa M. Geriatric syndromes and geriatric assessment for the generalist. Med Clin North Am. 2015;99(2):263–79.

18. Wachterman MW, O'Hare AM, Rahman O-K, Lorenz KA, Marcantonio ER, Alicante GK, et al. One-year mortality after dialysis initiation among older adults. JAMA Intern Med. 2019;179(7):987.

19. Verberne WR, Geers ABMT, Jellema WT, Vincent HH, van Delden JJM, Bos WJ. Comparative survival among older adults with advanced kidney disease managed conservatively versus with dialysis. Clin J Am Soc Nephrol. 2016;11(4):633–40.

20. Misra M, Oreopoulos D, Vonesh E. Dialysis or not? A comparative survival study of patients over 75 years of age with chronic kidney disease stage 5. Nephrol Dial Transplant. 2008;23(5):1768–9.

21. Carson RC, Juszczak M, Davenport A, Burns A. Is maximum conservative management an equivalent treatment option to dialysis for elderly patients with significant comorbid disease? Clin J Am Soc Nephrol. 2009;4(10):1611–9.

22. Kreuter W. Treatment intensity at the end of life in older adults receiving long-term dialysis. Arch Intern Med. 2012;172(8):661.

23. McAdams-DeMarco MA, Law A, Salter ML, Boyarsky B, Gimenez L, Jaar BG, et al. Frailty as a novel predictor of mortality and hospitalization in individuals of all ages undergoing hemodialysis. J Am Geriatr Soc. 2013;61(6):896–901.

24. Cheung KL, LaMantia MA. Cognitive impairment and mortality in patients receiving hemodialysis: implications and future research avenues. Am J Kidney Dis. 2019;74(4):435–7.

25. Cohen LM, Ruthazer R, Moss AH, Germain MJ. Predicting six-month mortality for patients who are on maintenance hemodialysis. Clin J Am Soc Nephrol. 2009;5(1):72–9.

26. Li M, Tomlinson G, Naglie G, Cook WL, Jassal SV. Geriatric comorbidities, such as falls, confer an independent mortality risk to elderly dialysis patients. Nephrol Dial Transplant. 2007;23(4):1396–400.

27. Jassal SV, Chiu E, Hladunewich M. Loss of independence in patients starting dialysis at 80 years of age or older. N Engl J Med. 2009;361(16):1612–3.

28. Kurella Tamura M, Covinsky KE, Chertow GM, Yaffe K, Landefeld CS, McCulloch CE. Functional status of elderly adults before and after initiation of dialysis. N Engl J Med. 2009;361(16):1539–47.

29. van Loon IN, Goto NA, Boereboom FT, Verhaar MC, Bots ML, Hamaker ME. Quality of life after the initiation of dialysis or maximal conservative management in elderly patients: a longitudinal analysis of the geriatric assessment in older patients starting dialysis (GOLD) study. BMC Nephrol. 2019;20(1):108.

30. Engelbrecht BL, Kristian MJ, Inge E, Elizabeth K, Guldager LT, Helbo TL, et al. Does conservative kidney management offer a quantity or quality of life benefit compared to dialysis? A systematic review. BMC Nephrol. 2021;22(1):307.

31. Da Silva-Gane M, Wellsted D, Greenshields H, Norton S, Chandna SM, Farrington K. Quality of life and survival in patients with advanced kidney failure managed conservatively or by dialysis. Clin J Am Soc Nephrol. 2012;7(12):2002–9.

32. Brown MA, Collett GK, Josland EA, Foote C, Li Q, Brennan FP. CKD in elderly patients managed without dialysis: survival, symptoms, and quality of life. Clin J Am Soc Nephrol. 2015;10(2):260–8.

33. de Rooij ENM, Meuleman Y, de Fijter JW, Le Cessie S, Jager KJ, Chesnaye NC, et al. Quality of life before and after the start of dialysis in older patients. Clin J Am Soc Nephrol. 2022;17(8):1159–67.

34. O'Connor NR, Kumar P. Conservative management of end-stage renal disease without dialysis: a systematic review. J Palliat Med. 2012;15(2):228–35.

35. Couchoud C, Hemmelgarn B, Kotanko P, Germain MJ, Moranne O, Davison SN. Supportive care: time to change our prognostic tools and their use in CKD. Clin J Am Soc Nephrol. 2016;11(10):1892–901.

36. Koncicki HM, Schell JO. Communication skills and decision making for elderly patients with advanced kidney disease: a guide for nephrologists. Am J Kidney Dis. 2016;67(4):688–95.

37. Thorsteinsdottir B, Hickson LTJ, Giblon R, Pajouhi A, Connell N, Branda M, et al. Validation of prognostic indices for short term mortality in an incident dialysis population of older adults >75. PLoS One. 2021;16(1):e0244081.

38. Wick JP, Turin TC, Faris PD, MacRae JM, Weaver RG, Tonelli M, et al. A clinical risk prediction tool for 6-month mortality after dialysis initiation among older adults. Am J Kidney Dis. 2017;69(5):568–75.

39. Thamer M, Kaufman JS, Zhang Y, Zhang Q, Cotter DJ, Bang H. Predicting early death among elderly dialysis patients: development and validation of a risk score to assist shared decision making for dialysis initiation. Am J Kidney Dis. 2015;66(6):1024–32.

40. Couchoud C, Labeeuw M, Moranne O, Allot V, Esnault V, Frimat L, et al. A clinical score to predict 6-month prognosis in elderly patients starting dialysis for end-stage renal disease. Nephrol Dial Transplant. 2008;24(5):1553–61.

41. Beddhu S, Bruns FJ, Saul M, Seddon P, Zeidel ML. A simple comorbidity scale predicts clinical outcomes and costs in dialysis patients. Am J Med. 2000;108(8):609–13.

42. Rattanasompattikul M, Feroze U, Molnar MZ, Dukkipati R, Kovesdy CP, Nissenson AR, et al. Charlson comorbidity score is a strong predictor of mortality in hemodialysis patients. Int Urol Nephrol. 2011;44(6):1813–23.

43. Hemmelgarn BR, Manns BJ, Quan H, Ghali WA. Adapting the Charlson comorbidity index for use in patients with ESRD. Am J Kidney Dis. 2003;42(1):125–32.

44. Javier AD, Figueroa R, Siew ED, Salat H, Morse J, Stewart TG, et al. Reliability and utility of the surprise question in CKD stages 4 to 5. Am J Kidney Dis. 2017;70(1):93–101.

45. Moss AH, Ganjoo J, Sharma S, Gansor J, Senft S, Weaner B, et al. Utility of the "surprise" question to identify dialysis patients with high mortality. Clin J Am Soc Nephrol. 2008;3(5):1379–84.

46. Fried LP, Tangen CM, Walston J, Newman AB, Hirsch C, Gottdiener J, et al. Frailty in older adults: evidence for a phenotype. J Gerontol Ser A Biol Med Sci. 2001;56(3):M146.

47. Sy J, Johansen KL. The impact of frailty on outcomes in dialysis. Curr Opin Nephrol Hypertens. 2017;26(6):537–42.

48. Worthen G, Tennankore K. Frailty screening in chronic kidney disease: current perspectives. Int J Nephrol Renov Dis. 2019;12:229–39.

49. Karnofsky DA, Burchenal JH. The clinical evaluation of chemotherapeutic agents in cancer. In: MacLeod CM, editor. Evaluation of chemotherapeutic agents. New York: Columbia University Press; 1949. p. 196.

50. McClellan WM, Anson C, Birkeli K, Tuttle E. Functional status and quality of life: predictors of early mortality among patients entering treatment for end stage renal disease. J Clin Epidemiol. 1991;44(1):83–9.

51. Ifudu O, Paul HR, Homel P, Friedman EA. Predictive value of functional status for mortality in patients on maintenance hemodialysis. Am J Nephrol. 1998;18(2):109–16.

52. Ritchie JP, Alderson H, Green D, Chiu D, Sinha S, Middleton R, et al. Functional status and mortality in chronic kidney disease: results from a prospective observational study. Nephron Clin Pract. 2014;128(1–2):22–8.

53. Tangri N, Grams ME, Levey AS, Coresh J, Appel LJ, Astor BC, et al. Multinational assessment of accuracy of equations for predicting risk of kidney failure. JAMA. 2016;315(2):164.

54. Mandel EI, Bernacki RE, Block SD. Serious illness conversations in ESRD. Clin J Am Soc Nephrol. 2016;12(5):854–63.

55. Barrett TM, Green JA, Greer RC, Ephraim PL, Peskoe S, Pendergast JF, et al. Preferences for and experiences of shared and informed decision making among patients choosing kidney replacement therapies in nephrology care. Kidney Med. 2021;3(6):905.

56. Couchoud CG, Beuscart J-BR, Aldigier J-C, Brunet PJ, Moranne OP. Development of a risk stratification algorithm to improve patient-centered care and decision making for incident elderly patients with end-stage renal disease. Kidney Int. 2015;88(5):1178–86.

57. Saeed F, Ladwig SA, Epstein RM, Monk RD, Duberstein PR. Dialysis regret. Clin J Am Soc Nephrol. 2020;15(7):957–63.

58. Shega JW, Paniagua MA. Communication and teamwork. In: Essential practices in hospice and palliative medicine. Chicago, IL: AAHPM; 2017.
59. Jacobsen J, Blinderman C, Alexander Cole C, Jackson V. "I'd recommend …" how to incorporate your recommendation into shared decision making for patients with serious illness. J Pain Symptom Manag. 2018;55(4):1224–30.
60. Kon AA. The shared decision-making continuum. JAMA. 2010;304(8):903.
61. Serious illness conversation guide—ariadne labs. Serious illness conversation guide. Ariadne Labs: A Joint Center for Health Systems Innovation (www.ariadnelabs.org) and Dana-Farber Cancer Institute. Revised April 2017. Licensed under the Creative Commons Attribution-Non Commercial-Share Alike 4.0 International License, http://creativecommons.org/licenses/by-nc-sa/4.0/. Serious illness conversation guide CONVERSATION FLOW PATIENT-TESTED LANGUAGE SI-CG 2017-04-18; 2015 [cited 2022 Aug 16]. https://www.ariadnelabs.org/wp-content/uploads/2017/05/SI-CG-2017-04-21_FINAL.pdf.
62. Childers JW, Back AL, Tulsky JA, Arnold RM. REMAP: a framework for goals of care conversations. J Oncol Pract. 2017;13(10):e844.
63. Baile WF, Buckman R, Lenzi R, Glober G, Beale EA, Kudelka AP. Spikes—a six-step protocol for delivering bad news: application to the patient with cancer. Oncologist. 2000;5(4):302–11.
64. Back A, Arnold RM, Tulsky JA, Fryer-Edwards K, Baile WF. Mastering communication with seriously ill patients: balancing honesty with empathy and hope. New York, NY: Cambridge University Press; 2010.
65. Grubbs V. Time to recast our approach for older patients with ESRD: the best, the worst, and the most likely. Am J Kidney Dis. 2018;71(5):605–7.
66. Conservative Kidney Management. [cited 2022 Aug 2023]. https://www.ckmcare.com/PractitionerPathway/AtAGlance.
67. Davison SN, Tupala B, Wasylynuk BA, Siu V, Sinnarajah A, Triscott J. Recommendations for the care of patients receiving conservative kidney management. Clin J Am Soc Nephrol. 2019;14(4):626–34.
68. Schell JO, Arnold RM, Davison SN. Components of CKM. UpToDate. 2021 [cited 2022 Aug 23]. https://www.uptodate.com/contents/kidney-palliative-care-conservative-kidney-management#.
69. Scherer JS, Holley JL. The role of time-limited trials in dialysis decision making in critically ill patients. Clin J Am Soc Nephrol. 2015;11(2):344–53.
70. Siropaides CH, Arnold R. Time-limited trials for serious illness. Palliative Care Network of Wisconsin. 2020 [cited 2022 Aug 27]. https://www.mypcnow.org/fast-facts/.
71. Moss AH. Integrating supportive care principles into dialysis decision making: a primer for palliative medicine providers. J Pain Symptom Manag. 2017;53(3):656.
72. Moss AH, Singer D, Rettig R, Price CA, Newmann JM, Kitsen J, et al. Shared decision-making in the appropriate initiation of and withdrawal from dialysis. Rockville: Renal Physicians Associations; 2010. [cited 2022 Aug 27].
73. Grubbs V, Moss AH, Cohen LM, Fischer MJ, Germain MJ, Jassal SV, et al. A palliative approach to dialysis care: a patient-centered transition to the end of life. Clin J Am Soc Nephrol. 2014;9(12):2203–9.
74. Ko GJ, Obi Y, Chang TI, Soohoo M, Eriguchi R, Choi SJ, et al. Factors associated with withdrawal from dialysis therapy in incident hemodialysis patients aged 80 years or older. J Am Med Dir Assoc. 2019;20(6):743.
75. Wetmore JB, Yan H, Gilbertson DT, Liu J. Factors associated with elective withdrawal of maintenance hemodialysis: a case-control analysis. Am J Nephrol. 2020;51(3):227–36.
76. Raghavan D, Holley JL. Conservative care of the elderly CKD patient: a practical guide. Adv Chronic Kidney Dis. 2016;23(1):51–6.
77. Portnoy RK. Treatment of cancer pain. Lancet. 2011;377(9784):2236–47.
78. Koncicki HM, Unruh M, Schell JO. Pain management in CKD: a guide for nephrology providers. Am J Kidney Dis. 2017;69(3):451–60.

79. Scherer JS, Combs SA, Brennan F. Sleep disorders, restless legs syndrome, and uremic pruritus: diagnosis and treatment of common symptoms in dialysis patients. Am J Kidney Dis. 2017;69(1):117–28.
80. Lu E, Schell JO, Koncicki HM. Opioid management in CKD. Am J Kidney Dis. 2021;77(5):786–95.
81. Verduzco HA, Shirazian S. CKD-associated pruritus: new insights into diagnosis, pathogenesis, and management. Kidney Int Rep. 2020;5(9):1387–402.
82. Grubbs V. ESRD and hospice care in the United States: are dialysis patients welcome? Am J Kidney Dis. 2018;72(3):429–32.

Index

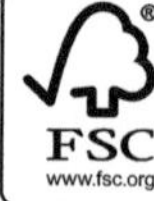

MIX
Papier aus verantwortungsvollen Quellen
Paper from responsible sources
FSC® C105338

If you have any concerns about our products,
you can contact us on
ProductSafety@springernature.com

In case Publisher is established outside the EU,
the EU authorized representative is:
Springer Nature Customer Service Center GmbH
Europaplatz 3, 69115 Heidelberg, Germany

Printed by Libri Plureos GmbH
in Hamburg, Germany